THYROID HORMONES

Biosynthesis, Physiological Effects, and Mechanisms of Action

STUDIES IN SOVIET SCIENCE

LIFE SCIENCES

1973

MOTILE MUSCLE AND CELL MODELS
N. I. Arronet
PATHOLOGICAL EFFECTS OF RADIO WAVES
M. S. Tolgskaya and Z. V. Gordon
CENTRAL REGULATION OF THE PITUITARY-ADRENAL COMPLEX
E. V. Naumenko

1974

SULFHYDRYL AND DISULFIDE GROUPS OF PROTEINS
Yu. M. Torchinskii
MECHANISMS OF GENETIC RECOMBINATION
V. V. Kushev

1975

THYROID HORMONES: Biosynthesis, Physiological Effects, and Mechanisms of Action
Ya. Kh. Turakulov, A. I. Gagel'gans, N. S. Salakhova, A. K. Mirakhmedov, L. M. Gol'ber, V. I. Kandror, and G. A. Gaidina

STUDIES IN SOVIET SCIENCE

THYROID HORMONES

Biosynthesis, Physiological Effects, and Mechanisms of Action

Ya. Kh. Turakulov, A. I. Gagel'gans, N. S. Salakhova, and A. K. Mirakhmedov

Institute of Biochemistry
Academy of Sciences of the Uzbek SSR, Tashkent

and

L. M. Gol'ber, V. I. Kandror, and G. A. Gaidina

Institute of Experimental Endocrinology and Hormone Chemistry
Academy of Medical Sciences of the USSR, Moscow

Edited by
Ya. Kh. Turakulov

Translated from Russian by
Basil Haigh

Translation Editor
Donald H. Ford
State University of New York
Downstate Medical Center
Brooklyn, New York

Springer Science+Business Media, LLC

Library of Congress Cataloging in Publication Data

Main entry under title:

Thyroid hormones.

(Studies in Soviet science)
Translation of Tireoidnye gormony.
Includes bibliographies.
1. Thyroid hormones. I. Turakulov, I͡Alkin Khalmatovich. II. Series. [DNLM: 1. Thyroid hormones—Biosynthesis. 2. Thyroid hormones—Physiology. WK202 T596]
QP572.T5T5713 612'.44 75-28119
ISBN 978-1-4899-2707-1

The original Russian text, published by Fan in Tashkent in 1972, has been corrected by the authors for the present edition. This translation is published under an agreement with the Copyright Agency of the USSR (VAAP).

ТИРЕОИДНЫЕ ГОРМОНЫ
А. И. Гагельганс, Г. А. Гайдина, Л. М. Гольбер, В. И. Кандрор,
А. К. Мирахмедов, Н. С. Салахова, Я. Х. Туракулов

TIREOIDNYE GORMONY
A. I. Gagel'gans, G. A. Gaidina, L. M. Gol'ber, V. I. Kandror,
A. K. Mirakhmedov, N. S. Salakhova, Ya. Kh. Turakulov

ISBN 978-1-4899-2707-1 ISBN 978-1-4899-2705-7 (eBook)
DOI 10.1007/978-1-4899-2705-7

Originally published by Consultants Bureau, New York in 1975
Softcover reprint of the hardcover 1st edition 1975

Foreword

Western knowledge of progress in biomedical research in Russia is severely limited by the scarcity of Russian journals available to us as well as the fact that few of us can read Russian. Therefore, it is of special significance that this recent contribution to the Russian scientific literature has been translated into English.

This publication, *Thyroid Hormones,* brings to us a detailed analysis of recent work in Russia, and in particular in the Laboratory of Hormone Biochemistry, Institute of Biochemistry, Academy of Science of the Uzbek SSR and the Laboratory of Pathological Physiology, Institute of Experimental Endocrinology and Hormone Chemistry, Academy of Medical Science of the USSR. The review illustrates the parallel pathways of investigation taken by investigators in Russia and in the West, indicating where the results have complemented each other or stimulated new questions and approaches. Consequently, the book provides an excellent review of the contributions made by Russian scientists in thyroid research and couples it with Western thought on these subjects to produce a complete review of the thyroid hormones.

The large amount of data provided and the inclusion of multiple viewpoints toward specific problems provides an excellent survey of the mechanisms of biosynthesis and control of hormone formation, physiological effects of the hormones, and the molecular mechanisms involved in thyroid hormone action.

It is evident from the book that despite tremendous advances during the last two decades, the final chapters on our understanding of the thyroid gland have yet to be written. Many questions still remain to be answered concerning biosynthesis and peripheral metabolism of the hormones.

Further, the mechanisms of action are still only partially elucidated. Thus, while Turakulov and his colleagues have created an admirable survey of what we know and understand, they have also indicated where our knowledge is weak, inconsistent, or not available. They have, in a sense, indicated the directions our investigations might logically take in order to eventually enable us to attain a complete understanding of the thyroid gland and its functions.

Donald H. Ford

Preface to the English-Language Edition

The thyroid hormones, their biosynthesis, physiological effects, and molecular mechanism of action still engage the attention of biochemists, physiologists, and endocrinologists.

Despite the tremendous advances made in the last two decades in the study of this problem, many details of the biosynthesis, peripheral metabolism, and, in particular, the mechanism of action of the thyroid hormones still remain unexplained.

The great interest shown in the study of the thyroid gland is explained, first, by the powerful action of thyroid hormones on many physiological processes in the body and on cell metabolism and, second, by the important place of thyroid pathology in the general structure of endocrine diseases. Although the foci of endemic goiter have now been largely eradicated, thyrotoxicosis is still widespread and in some countries endemic goiter is still a problem.

In the last decade much progress in the study of the biochemistry of thyroid hormones has been made through research into the mechanisms of biosynthesis of the thyronine structure and of thyroglobulin and in the regulation of these processes and the molecular mechanism of action of thyroid hormones. Research on some aspects of this problem has been undertaken in the Soviet Union also.

In B. V. Aleshin's laboratory in Khar'kov, morphological, physiological, and biochemical evidence of the existence of parahypophyseal effects on the thyroid gland from the nervous system have been obtained. Recent investigations have confirmed that after division of the sympathetic nerves running from the cervical sympathetic ganglia to the thyroid gland not only is the absorption of iodide by the thyroid reduced, but the composition of the iodine-containing components is altered [14].

New facts on the iodoproteins of the thyroid gland, on changes in the physicochemical properties and fluorescence spectra of the iodoamino acids, and the conformation of the thyroglobulin molecule in various forms of thyroid pathology have been obtained at the Institute of Biochemistry.

To study the action of thyroid hormones on the mechanism of energy conversion in the mitochondria, experiments are being carried out at the present time to determine the permeability of the mitochondrial membrane to H^+ and K^+ ions and to various anions (predominantly of oxidation substrates) under normal conditions and in thyrotoxicosis.

As a result of these experiments it is becoming clear how the thyroid hormones affect the pathways of utilization of the H^+ gradient in the mitochondria under physiological conditions and whether their uncoupling effect is linked with the induction of proton conductance, as is postulated by Mitchell's chemo-osmotic theory with respect to classical uncouplers.

Finally, the recognition that the mitochondria are the primary "target" of the thyroid hormones brings with it the need to seek for specific components with high affinity for thyroxine and triiodothyronine.

Endocrine correlations between the mother and fetus are being studied in many laboratories. At the Institute of Biochemistry, Academy of Sciences of the Uzbek SSR in Tashkent, and at the Institute of Biology of Development, Academy of Sciences of the USSR in Moscow, M. S. Mitskevich has obtained new data concerning the formation of the fetal thyroid gland in the prenatal period of development, the permeability of the placenta, and the rate of deiodization in the fetus depending on the level of function of the maternal thyroid gland and hypothalamohypophyseal system. The authors hope that publication of this monograph in English will help to inform readers in the West of research on thyroid hormones in progress in the Soviet Union.

Preface

In the last decade the biochemistry of hormones and hormonal regulation has remained in the forefront of attention of biochemists, physiologists, endocrinologists, specialists in the field of bio-organic chemistry, and biologists and physicians in many different fields. As in the past, attention has been focused on the chemical structure, biosynthesis, and mechanism of action of hormones. Much progress has been made in the investigation of protein-peptide pituitary hormones, the releasing factors of the hypothalamic centers, and the new thyroid hormone thyrocalcitonin. As a result of rapid progress in the methods of protein chemistry, within a short time nearly all the hormones of protein-polypeptide nature have been obtained in a pure form, the primary structure of many of them has been established, and some have been synthesized in the laboratory. A problem on the current agenda is the synthesis of insulin on a commercial scale. Problems concerned with the biosynthesis and metabolism of the protein and other groups of hormones are being successfully studied.

New ideas have been expressed on the mechanism of action of hormones at the cellular and molecular levels. To explain the hormonal regulation of cellular activity, the view that hormones act on the genetic apparatus of the cell and thereby regulate specific protein synthesis has received the greatest support. This idea, first expressed in 1961 by Clever on the basis of his observation on the action of ecdysone on puffs (swellings on chromosomes) of insects, and subsequently developed into an orderly theory of the regulation of the genetic activity of the cell by hormones by Karlson, has received wide support from many research workers studying the mechanism of action of other hormones. Abundant experimental evidence on the precise localization of the primary action of hormones and on the molecular interaction between hormones and the specific receptor structures controlling the protein-synthesizing system of the cell has now been gathered.

Research into the biochemistry of thyroid hormones in recent years has developed chiefly in the direction of the study of the structure and biosynthesis of thyroglobulin and the mechanism of action of thyroxine on intracellular processes. The stages of biosynthesis of thyroglobulin and the exact localization of these processes in the follicles have been established, the function of the ribosomes and polysomes of the thyroid gland in the synthesis of the peptide chain forming the basis of the thyroglobulin molecule has been explained, and the presence of other proteins than thyroglobulin in the thyroid gland has been demonstrated. The action of thyroxine on oxidative phosphorylation, on ionic transport, and on the functioning of the genetic system of the cell has been thoroughly investigated.

Our knowledge of the physiological effects and action of the thyroid hormones on the general course of metabolism in the body, and of the principal stages in the intrathyroid metabolism and the transport of iodine, about which there was already considerable information in the literature, has been supplemented during this period by new facts. Our knowledge of the regulation of thyroid function has increased in extent, expecially in connection with the productive theory of Sutherland et al. [485] of the role of cyclic 3′,5′-adenosine monophosphate (c-AMP) in the production of the hormonal effect and also with the progress made in the study of the nervous regulation and action of hypothalamic thyrotropin-releasing factor.

Most attention is paid in this monograph to the present state of our knowledge of the biosynthesis and mechanism of action of thyroid hormones and to certain other aspects of the biochemistry and physiology of the thyroid gland which have recently been the subject of intensive research.

The monograph is a collective work of authors from two laboratories — the Laboratory of Hormone Biochemistry, Institute of Biochemistry, Academy of Sciences of the Uzbek SSR and the Laboratory of Pathological Physiology, Institute of Experimental Endocrinology and Hormone Chemistry, Academy of Medical Sciences of the USSR — and it surveys their main achievements in the field of study of the biosynthesis, physiological effects, and mechanism of action of the thyroid hormones.

Contents

Introduction

The thyroid gland is a major component of the endocrine system. It occupies an important place in the general hormonal balance of the body and exerts a powerful regulatory influence over body functions: its growth, development, and metabolism.

All the biological functions of the body are under the general control of the higher levels of the nervous system, and the endocrine glands are major intermediaries through which this nervous control is effected at the cellular and intracellular level by the secretion of chemical agents known as hormones.

The activity of the thyroid gland is itself under the direct control of a hormone of the anterior lobe of the pituitary gland, which controls other endocrine glands also. The anterior pituitary influences the whole course of metabolism by liberating trophic hormones into the circulation which regulate the functions of the endocrine glands and by the direct action of a special hormone — growth hormone — on the other organs and tissues. To use a familiar metaphor, if the pituitary is the conductor of the endocrine orchestra, the thyroid gland plays the part of the first violin. As the chief organ of iodine metabolism the thyroid gland appears at a certain stage of evolution of the animal kingdom. It is found in all vertebrates and in certain of the Chordata. Concentration of iodine may also be observed in an extremely primitive form in the Ascidiacea and Amphioxidae.

Although no rudimentary, biochemically differentiated thyroid function evidently occurs in the invertebrates, all the tissues of these animals, nevertheless, do contain iodine. Some of them may accumulate it in considerable amounts. The biosynthesis of iodized tyrosines as components of the scleroproteins does take place, but it has no importance as a hormonal function. There is firm evidence that iodoproteins of the thyroglobulin type appear in the higher vertebrates for the first time in the Protochordata. The biochemical mechanism of their formation is identical in all the Chordata and is definitively fixed in the time of its appearance.

The location of the thyroid gland varies in different animals. In man it is classically described as a flattened bilobar pink structure weighing 25–30 g, situated at the level of the thyroid cartilage on either side of the larynx. The macroscopic appearance and microscopic picture of the gland vary considerably with age.

The thyroid gland has several functions in connection with the iodine metabolism of the body: (1) It actively concentrates iodide from the circulating blood and converts it into organically bound iodine and physiologically active specific hormones; (2) it acts as a reservoir of thyroid hormones, which it fixes as thyroglobulin and stores in its follicles; (3) it regulates the liberation of this stored hormone under the constant and restraining control of the thyroid-stimulating hormone of the pituitary; (4) it is a very efficient assimilator of iodine liberated during metabolism of the thyroid hormones, which it stores should an exogenous supply of iodine be deficient.

The hormone is stored in the gland itself chiefly as thyroglobulin in the bound state, which is its reserve form, and is liberated by the thyrotropic hormone of the anterior pituitary, which controls proteolysis. The transport forms of the thyroid hormones, consisting of thyroxine and a small quantity of 3,5,3′-triiodothyronine, circulate in the blood stream, mainly bound to the plasma proteins. The very small proportion of the hormone in the free state is the active part. The protein-bound hormone (measured as protein-bound iodine, or PBI) is not physiologically active. In the generally accepted view, free thyroxine and triiodothyronine are the substances which actually penetrate through the cell membrane and evidently interact with the receptor surfaces of the cell structures.

Until the last decade it was popularly held that a particularly active form of the thyroid hormones exists at the cellular level, and many workers attempted to explain the period elapsing between the time of administration of thyroxine and the manifestation of its physiological effect on the body by the need for the thyroxine molecule to be modified into the active form of the hormone.

However, this view has not been confirmed experimentally. The hypothetical active form of the hormone (tetraiodothyroacetic acid) — widely distributed in the tissues after administration of thyroxine — has been shown to have only 10–40% of the activity of the hormone. Tetraiodothyroacetic acid and the other analogs formed from thyroxine by oxidative deamination are now no longer regarded as active forms of the hormone. However, this does not dispose of the problem of "activation" of the thyroxine molecule, but, as Barker [38] suggests, the activation may take place by deiodination at the cellular level during realization of the hormonal effect.

Two major discoveries made at about the same time at the end of the 1930s and beginning of the 1940s were important events in the study of the physiology and biochemistry of the thyroid hormones. These were the introduction of thyrostatic agents and the use of radioactive iodine in clinical practice and experimental research. Success achieved in the elucidation of the precise mechanisms of hormone formation in the thyroid gland, of metabolism of thyroid hormones in the body, and of the effect of various intrinsic and extrinsic factors on many aspects of thyroid function are unquestionably the result of the use of radioactive iodine ^{131}I. This technique has been particularly useful in conjunction with the other modern techniques of paper chromatography and electrophoresis. These methods have yielded new facts which could not have been obtained by the methods of classical chemical analysis. As a result of progress in the investigation of iodine metabolism, detailed information about the principal pathways of thyroid hormone formation in the gland and of the degradation and distribution of the hormones at the peripheral tissue level is available.

A new chapter in the physiology and biochemistry of thyroid hormones began in 1952 when the important iodinated compound 3,5,3′-triiodothyronine was first discovered simultaneously by two groups of workers, Gross and Pitt-Rivers [188] in England and Roche, Michel, and Lissitzky [424] in France. It was soon shown that this compound is the second thyroid hormone, with greater physiological activity than thyroxine.

This discovery stimulated the development of further research into all aspects of the biochemistry of the thyroid hormones and led to an increase in the breadth and depth of our knowledge, especially in regard to transport, tissue metabolism, and the mechanism of action of these substances.

The extensive use of ^{131}I-labeled thyroxine and triiodotyrosine, in conjunction with radiochromatography and histoautoradiography, opened new paths for the study of the tissue metabolism of thyroid hormones.

The use of these methods provided more accurate and detailed information about such processes as the transport of the hormones in the blood, their penetration through the cell membrane and binding in the intracellular space, and the metabolism of thyroxine in connection with the mechanism of its hormonal effect. Important advances in this field include the decisive proof of the role of free thyroxine in the blood and the peripheral effect and the rate of metabolism and action of the hormone on the anterior pituitary. Mention must also be made of detailed investigations of the principles governing the binding of thyroxine by serum protein and the discovery of disturbances of the transport of the hormone caused by genetic changes in the concentration of serum thyroxine-binding proteins.

The opinion widely held by workers attempting to explain the long latent period before manifestation of the physiological effect of thyroxine by the binding of the hormone with blood proteins, which could delay changes in the level of the circulating free hormone, merits attention. These proteins, acting as a buffer for thyroxine, prevent an untoward increase in free blood concentration after the administration of large doses of the hormone.

Investigations into the fate of thyroxine once it has penetrated into the cell have shown the existence of intracellular thyroxine-binding and triiodothyronine-binding proteins that differ from the serum thyroxine-binding protein. Although the data on the function of these proteins in intracellular thyroxine metabolism are by no means exhaustive, they can be presumed to be concerned with regulating the supply of free thyroxine for metablism. The action of the hormone is considered to be accompanied by transformation in its molecule. Although neither the importance of the changes taking place in the structure of thyroxine for the manifestation of its activity nor the precise localization of those changes has yet been finally settled, most investigators associate transformations in the molecule with the process of deiodination.

However, before we can fully understand the link between conversions in the thyroxine molecule and the production of its hormonal effect, we need much more information about the intimate details of the mechanism of its action.

On the basis of the extensive research conducted in recent years, chiefly by Tata's group, it is now clearly recognized that the mechanism of action of physiological doses of thyroid hormones *in vivo* and *in vitro* is connected with stimulation of the biosynthesis of specific proteins. However, the manifestation of this action requires a certain latent period after introduction of the hormone into the body or its addition to the system *in vitro*. Meanwhile, the effects of thyroxine on the structure and function of mitochondria are well known; these effects can be observed under certain conditions within a few minutes, i.e., virtually without a latent period, as Hoch [219] has shown recently. There are now two hypotheses to explain the mechanism of action of thyroid hormones on protein biosynthesis. The first is based on a cytoplasmic mechanism of action of the hormone, namely the mitochondrially dependent stimulation of translation activity, independent of the synthesis of new RNA molecules; the other is based on a nuclear effect of the hormone, leading to activation of the gene and of the translation process, and to an increase in ribosomal synthesis on the template of newly formed mRNAs. It is possible that these two mechanisms whereby thyroxine stimulates protein synthesis represent two phases of the realization of the intracellular effect of the hormone. The initial phase depends on mitochondrial activity while the subsequent phase depends on an increase in protein synthesis through the nuclear apparatus of the cell.

An exhaustive study of the primary reactions of these two stages in the action of thyroid hormones and of the mechanism linking them together is an essential condition for a general theory of the place of hormonal stimulation in the regulation of the principal manifestations of cell activity: protein biosynthesis, oxidative phosphorylation, and ion transport. The action of thyroid hormones on these fundamental processes lies at the basis of all its diverse physiological effects.

PART I

Hormones of the Thyroid Gland

The basic function of the thyroid gland is to produce and secrete thyroxine into the blood. This is the principal hormone of the thyroid gland and has the distinctive property of containing iodine in its molecule. The formation of thyroxine, like that of its less iodinated analog, triiodothyronine (which is hormonally more active but is present in the body in much smaller quantities), and also of the other iodinated amino acids, takes place within the framework of the specific protein of the thyroid gland—thyroglobulin. The globulin itself contains large quantities of organically bound iodine. Thus, thyroid hormone formation is based on two continuous and closely interconnected fundamental processes: the circulation of iodine inside the thyroid gland and the biosynthesis of thyroglobulin. These processes are strikingly precise in the way they ensure production of the required amounts of thyroid hormones for the physiological needs of the organism. They require a constant inflow of structural materials and energy, and the whole course of metabolism of the gland, with its rich blood supply and its fine regulatory mechanism, is designed to this end.

The circulation of iodine in the thyroid gland includes the following successive stages: fixation of the blood iodide by the thyroid gland, its oxidation into elementary iodine, the biosynthesis of the thyroid hormones and their accumulation as thyroglobulin, the enzymic hydrolysis of the protein and liberation of iodinated amino acids from the thyroglobulin molecule, and, finally, the secretion of the finished hormone into the circulation. These successive stages in hormone biosynthesis are clearly reflected in the morphology of the follicle—the functional unit of the thyroid gland (Figures 1 and 2).

The follicles are cavities surrounded by epithelial cells with a secretory function. These cavities are filled with a liquid protein-mucopolysaccharide mass known as colloid, into which the microvilli on the apical surface of the

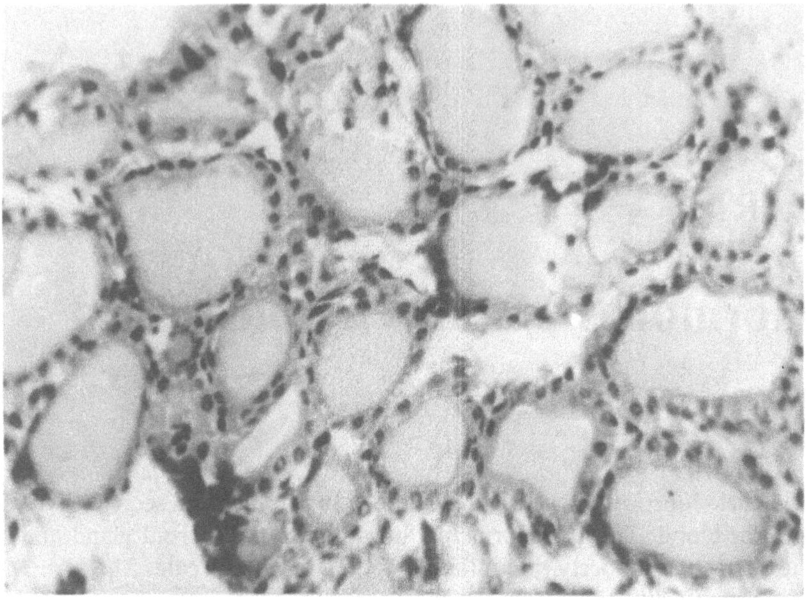

Fig. 1. Histological structure of the thyroid gland of the normal rat, 270X.

epithelial cells project. The colloid consists chiefly of a specifically iodine-containing protein, thyroglobulin. The role of the colloid and epithelial cells in the function of the follicles is inseparably connected with the whole course of iodine metabolism in the thyroid gland and with thyroglobulin synthesis. Another characteristic feature of follicle architecture is the close connection between the outer surface of the follicle and the rich network of blood vessels.

The performance of the unique endocrine function by the thyroid gland is a process which requires the combined participation of all elements of the follicles, all the intracellular structures, and all the chemical components of the epithelial cells either as substrates, as enzymes, or as energy-yielding material.

Chemical Components of the Thyroid Gland

Like any other organ the thyroid gland contains proteins, nucleic acids, lipids, carbohydrates, vitamins, and minerals. The principal chemical components determining the hormonal secretion of the gland are iodine-containing compounds — thyroglobulin and iodinated amino acid, which

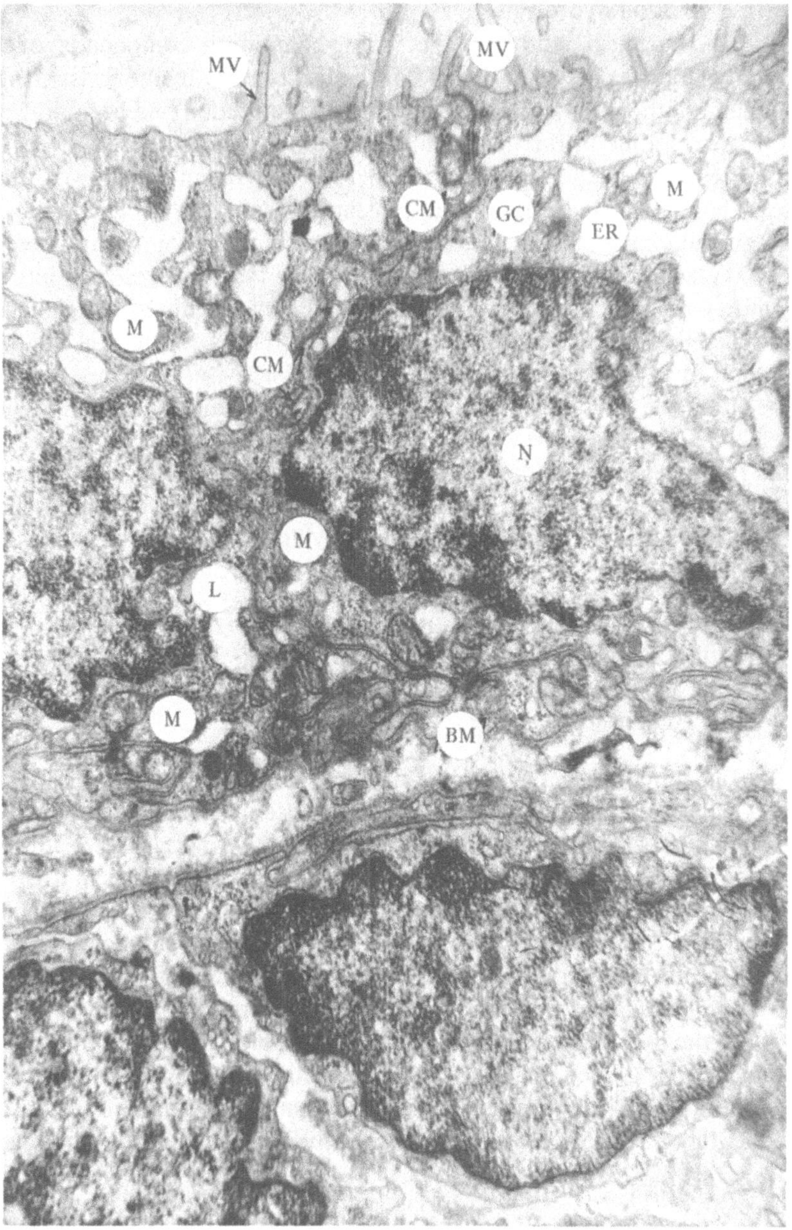

Fig. 2. Ultrastructure of thyroid gland cells of a normal rat, 21,500X. M–mitochondria, GC–Golgi complex, CM–cytoplasmic membrane, MV–microvilli, ER–endoplasmic reticulum, BM–basement membrane, N–nucleus, L–lipid.

occur mainly in the bound form in the protein molecule and are liberated in the free form on hydrolysis.

The chemical study of the iodine-containing compounds of the thyroid gland was begun at the end of the last century by the Swiss chemist Baumann, although as long ago as in the 1850s attention had been drawn to the role of iodine in the development of goiter. During a search for the active principle of the thyroid gland in 1895–96, Baumann showed that a firmly bound iodine compound is constantly present in it. This discovery was an important step in the study of the chemical composition of the thyroid gland and its endocrine function. Since that time research into the chemistry and biochemistry of the iodinated components of the gland has continued intensively and without interruption. This work quickly led to the isolation of iodinated proteins with hormonal activity, and these proteins were found to contain an iodinated amino acid, diiodotyrosine. A little later, the active hormone of the gland, thyroxine, was discovered and isolated from these protein preparations as an individual chemical compound. In the middle of the present century, with the introduction of new methods of chemical analysis (paper chromatography and the use of the radioactive isotopes of iodine) several other iodinated amino acids were discovered in digests of the thyroid gland and in the blood and other less intensively iodinated proteins, differing from thyroglobulin.

Iodinated Amino Acids

The composition of the iodinated compounds formed in the thyroid gland and secreted into the blood stream has been adequately studied. The first iodinated compound to be identified in the thyroid gland was diiodotyrosine; this iodinated derivative of tyrosine was discovered in 1896 by Drechsel (cited in [422]) almost at the same time as Baumann investigated the chemical composition of the gland. The presence of large quantities of diiodotyrosine in the thyroid gland was confirmed in 1931 by Harrington and Randall [203]. However, this compound has no hormonal activity.

By the hydrolysis of iodothyroglobulin several active substances were obtained, all of which proved to be imperfectly purified breakdown products of the iodine-containing protein. Much patient research has led to the production of a pure preparation with the biological action of thyroid gland

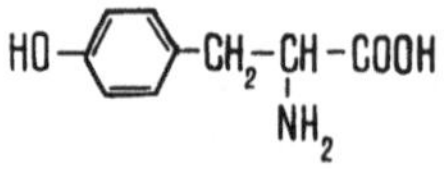

Tyrosine

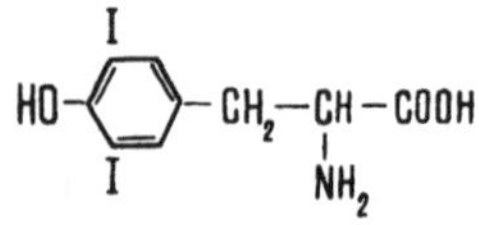

3,5-Diiodotyrosine

tissue. This goal was reached by Kendall, who in 1915 isolated crystalline thyroxine from a digest of thyroglobulin. The next stage in the study of thyroid hormones was the establishment of the formula of thyroxine by Harrington in 1926 and its synthesis by Harrington and Barger in 1927 (cited by Trendelenburg [522]). Methods for the biological assay of the hormonal activity of thyroid preparations based on elevation of the basal metabolism in rodents or the acceleration of metamorphosis in tadpoles were then developed.

In the 1940s iodinated proteins with thyroid activity were obtained from casein and other proteins. Although reports of the preparation of such proteins actually began to appear in the early 1930s, the problem was not finally solved until 1939, when Ludwig and von Mutzenbecher [292] succeeded in isolating crystalline thyroxine from iodinated casein and other proteins. This was confirmed a little later by Harrington and Pitt-Rivers [201]. Pure thyroglobulin was isolated at the same time. An important discovery in thyroid hormone chemistry was the synthesis of thyroxine from diiodotyrosine, described in 1939 by von Mutzenbecher.

In the thyroid gland itself thyroxine accounts for about three-quarters of the total content of thyroid hormones. It has been isolated in the pure form after enzymic or barium hydrolysis of the gland, and it also contains the greater part of the hormonal iodine in the plasma.

Until 1948 three iodine-containing substances were thus known to be present in the thyroid gland: diiodotyrosine, thyroxine, and thyroglobulin. With the introduction of radiochromatographic techniques, rapid advances were made in the study of the composition of iodine-containing components of thyroid gland digests. After hydrolysis of the thyroid gland, Fink and Fink [142] in 1948 demonstrated the presence of another iodinated tyrosine derivative, 3-monoiodotyrosine, and in 1952 Roche, Michel, and Lissitzky discovered iodinated histidine in the hydrolysis products. At the same time a very important iodinated compound of the thyroid gland — 3,5,3′-triiodothyronine — was discovered almost simultaneously by two groups of workers: by Gross and Pitt-Rivers in England and by Roche, Michel, and Lissitzky in France (cited in [422]).

Reports were soon published of the discovery of two other iodinated components: 3,3′,5′-triiodothyronine and L-3,3′-diiodothyronine, by

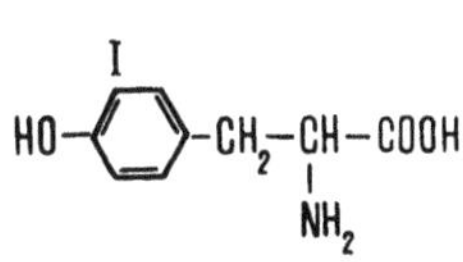

3-Monoiodotyrosine

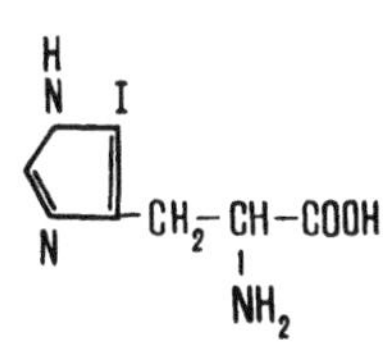

Monoiodohistidine

Roche and Michel and their group [425, 428]. The first of these compounds, an isomer of the L-3,5,3′-triiodothyronine, was found to be almost inactive against goiter, whereas the other, with two atoms of iodine in the two phenol rings of the thyronine (L-3,3′-diiodothyronine), has about 80% of the activity of thyroxine. The identification of these iodinated amino acids was confirmed by comparing their properties with those of synthetic iodothyronines. The presence of 3,3′-diiodothyronine and 3,3′,5′-triiodothyronine as components of thyroglobulin was disputed for some time because many workers were unable to reproduce the results obtained by Roche and Michel and their group. The opinion was held that these compounds are breakdown products of iodothyronines resulting from irradiation by the large doses of radiactive iodine used in the experiments. By a series of later investigations, however, Roche et al. [426] conclusively proved that these two new iodothyronines are in fact components of thyroglobulin.

The composition of iodinated components of the thyroid gland has not been finally settled by these discoveries. In the last few years several new iodine-containing components have been discovered in thyroid digests. In 1958 Hillmann et al. [217] reported finding thyroxamine, the structural formula of which is given below, in thyroid digests and in the plasma. This observation was not confirmed by other workers [392]. Later, however, Hillmann et al. [218] obtained further evidence in support of their claim: after injecting ^{131}I into rats they confirmed the presence of thyroxamine by radiochromatography and isolated it from digests of the gland by co-crystallization. Hillmann and Taslimi consider that thyroxamine is formed in the thyroid gland by the decarboxylation of thyroxine, although some of it may be peripheral in origin.

This component, incidentally, was studied intensively by Thibault and Lachaze [512] as long ago as 1951 in experiments in which thyroxine was incubated with segments of small intestine. However, no further evidence has subsequently been obtained to suggest that thyroxamine is a product of biological metabolism of thyroxine. It is also remarkable that thyroxamine is only sparingly soluble under the conditions usually used in biological research. This must be taken into account when the possible biological role of this substance is interpreted, despite its considerable thyroxine-like activity.

An event of much greater significance for understanding the biosynthesis of thyroid hormones is the identification of 4-hydroxy-3,5-diiodophenylpyruvic acid (DIPPA) in the thyroid gland [483]. The importance of

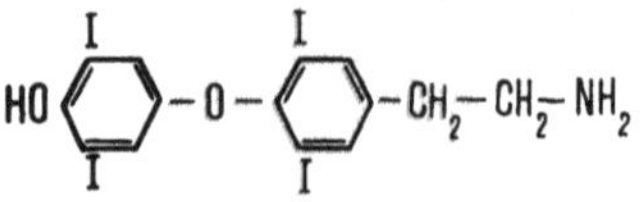

Thyroxamine

DIPPA as a normal component of thyroid tissue is that in earlier experiments *in vitro* it was shown that thyroxine can be formed by the condensation of DIPPA with diiodothyronine (DIT), which exists in both the free and the bound state in the thyroglobulin molecule.

Other new iodinated products are 2,4-diiodohistidine, which was discovered in the thyroid gland by Block et al. [55], and 2,6-diiodohydroquinone, recently found by Ljungren [286]. Whereas the physiological role of the first component is unknown, the second may play the role of an intermediate product in the synthesis of thyroid hormones, according to the workers who discovered it.

The following iodinated derivatives of tyrosine are thus known in the thyroid gland: 3-monoiodotyrosine, 3,5-diiodotyrosine, minimal quantities of 2- or 4-monoiodohistidine, none of which possess hormonal activity. The thyroid hormones include four iodinated components, all derivatives of the same structure, i.e., L-thyronine or β-4-(4-hydroxyphenoxyphenyl)-L-aminopropionic acid.

The iodinated derivatives of thyronine correspond to the formulas for 3,3′-diiodothyronine [429], 3,5,3′-triiodothyronine [188], 3,3′,5′-triiodothyronine, and thyroxine or 3,5,3′,5′-tetraiodothyronine. These thyronine derivatives are the hormonal products of the thyroid gland, which it secretes into the blood stream.

All the natural iodinated amino acids isolated from the thyroid gland are derivatives of L-isomers of tyrosine and thyronine with the L-configuration, and they possess optical activity. The hormonal activity of the D-isomers of thyroxine and triiodothyronine, as I shall show later, is incomparably less than the activity of their natural opposite numbers.

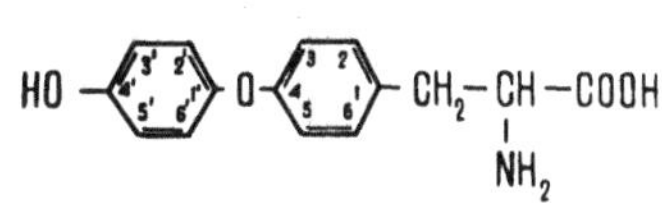

Thyronine (T)

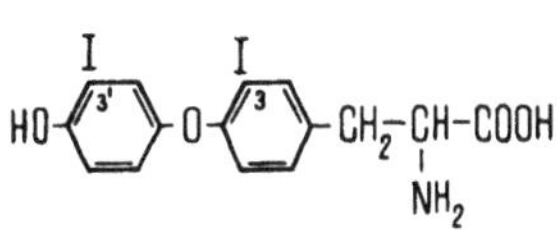

3,3′-Diiodothyronine (T_2).

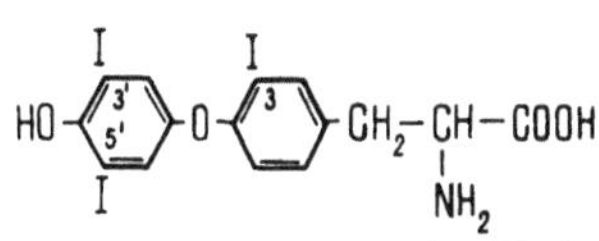

3,3′,5′-Triiodothyronine (T_3′)

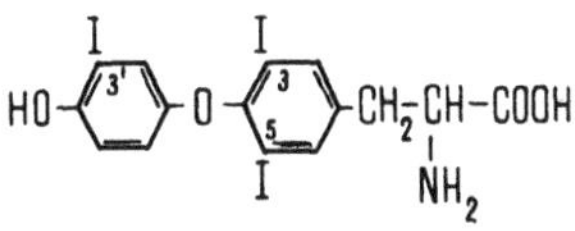

3,5,3′-Triiodothyronine (T_3)

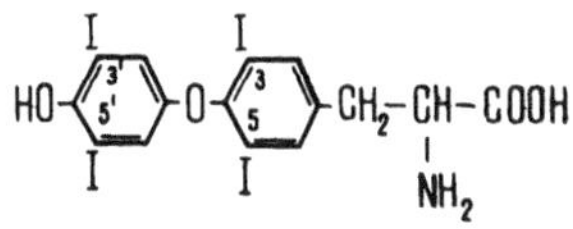

3,5,3′,5′-Tetraiodothyronine (T_4)

Harrington et al. [202] proposed the following abbreviations for the iodinated amino acids and their derivatives from the thyroid gland, which have been generally accepted and will be used in this book: (T) thyronine, (T_1) monoiodothyronine, (T_2) diiodothyronine, (T_3) triiodothyronine, (T_4) thyroxine, (MIT) monoiodotyrosine, and (DIT) diiodotyrosine. The position of the iodine atom in the first and second benzene rings is shown by numbers: For example, T_3 represents the 3,5,3′-form and $T_{3'}$ the 3,3′,5′-form of triiodothyronine.

The quantitative ratio between the various iodinated components in thyroglobulin varies considerably, but its content of iodinated tyrosines is particularly high; data obtained by different workers attribute 50–70% of the total iodine content of the gland to these compounds. The iodinated thyronines account for only 25–30% of the total iodine [157, 526]. Frey and Flock [157] give the following quantitative proportions of the individual iodine-containing components after hydrolysis of thyroglobulin in a neutral medium: MIT 28%, DIT 40%, T_4 20%, T_3 3%, and iodide 7%. These figures reflect the distribution of iodine among the individual iodinated compounds composing thyroglobulin, and they are evidently more accurate than the values obtained by Taurog [505] after alkaline hydrolysis of the protein: MIT 22%, DIT 24%, T_4 22%, and iodide 14%. Pitt-Rivers and Rall [390] investigated the relative percentages of iodine-containing compounds in the thyroid gland when equilibrium was established between the blood and the gland after injection of ^{131}I and found that I, MIT, DIT, T_4, and T_3 accounted for 13, 20, 16, 18, and 3%, respectively, of the total activity in the thyroid gland.

The MIT/DIT and iodotyrosines/iodothyronines ratios are often looked upon as indicators of the intensity of hormone formation. Under normal conditions the first ratio is usually close to 0.5 and the second to 2.5–3.0, but their values depend to a great degree on the time elapsing after the injection of ^{131}I, the amount of iodine in the diet, and the functional state of the gland. In experiments with radioactive iodine, Bois and Larsson [57] showed that DIT formation is inhibited in the thyroid gland of rats on an iodine-deficient diet or when receiving added propylthiouracil and thyrotropic hormone and that virtually all the iodine exists as MIT.

Proteins of the Thyroid Gland

The term proteins of the thyroid gland is usually applied to the iodinated proteins constituting the specific components of the gland and not to the structural proteins of the follicular epithelial cells or cell organelles.

The main component of the thyroid follicles is the glycoprotein thyroglobulin, which accounts for 70% or more of the dry weight of the gland. It is not only a reserve form of the thyroid hormones, preserving the finished structures of the thyroid hormones in a bound state in its molecule, but it is also the template on which all stages in the biosynthesis of thyroxine and triiodothyronine are enacted. As a reserve hormone thyroglobulin is chiefly stored inside the thyroid follicles as colloid. Finished molecules of thyroglobulin and its subunits or immature forms are also found in both a free and a bound form in the epithelial cells, where they may be in a state of continuous migration, in the process of synthesis or completion of the molecule, or undergoing iodination on the way into the interior of the follicles or migrating from the follicles to the basal end of the cells.

Besides thyroglobulin, other proteins have been found in the thyroid gland. With the ultracentrifuge no fewer than five protein components have been isolated from thyroid tissue treated with an isotonic solution. Thyroglobulin accounts for 80% of the total [430]. The other soluble proteins, distinguished by their sedimentation properties in the ultracentrifuge, are formed at least partially by dissociation of thyroglobulin into subunits containing different amounts of iodine, etc.

However, besides these fractions, differing only in their sedimentation coefficient, two other types of proteins, differing in their physicochemical properties, their degree of iodination, and the composition of their iodized components from thyroglobulin, have also been found in normal thyroid tissue. One of them closely resembles serum albumin and is called thyroalbumin; the other type of these proteins is insoluble and is bound with the cell particles, hence the name particulate protein. Their content in the normal thyroid gland is small, and it varies considerably in certain pathological states of the gland.

Thyroglobulin

Thyroglobulin is a complex protein containing iodine and carbohydrates, with a sedimentation coefficient of 19 S and molecular weight of 660,000; it is the principal protein synthesized in the thyroid gland. Most of the iodine of the gland is found in its molecule, linked by covalent bonds. The halogen is incorporated into the protein in the form of iodinated amino acids, and the iodine content in the thyroglobulin determines its content in the colloid and in the gland as a whole.

Our knowledge of the structure and properties of thyroglobulin has been greatly augmented in recent years with new facts obtained by modern methods of protein analysis. However, before these methods could be used, it was first necessary to develop a technique for preparing thyroglobulin in a pure form.

In their efforts to develop methods of isolating iodinated proteins from the thyroid, investigators aimed at obtaining homogeneous products which could be looked upon as pure, at determining whether the thyroid contains a mixture of iodoproteins corresponding to different levels of halogenation, and if so, how to separate them.

In order to obtain pure undenatured proteins, extraction at 0°C with isotonic sodium chloride solution of frozen sections of the organ and precipitation of the iodoproteins with ammonium sulfate between 35 and 45% saturation were suggested. The homogeneity of the specimens thus obtained could be verified by their sedimentation rate in the ultracentrifuge and by electrophoretic fractionation [207]. It has not yet been established whether one or more thyroglobulins are present in the thyroid gland.

These problems were later reexamined by Derrien et al. [109], Stanley [478], and Eastey et al. [126], using a new method of isolation of thyroglobulin developed by Derrien et al. [109]. This method, which yields thyroglobulin in the undenatured form, is based on the principle of fractional precipitation of proteins from thyroid gland extracts by saturation to certain concentrations with potassium sulfate or with a mixture of equal quantities of mono- and dipotassium sulfate. Three fractions of thyroglobulin were isolated from thyroid extracts by this method. Their solubility remained constant in the presence of certain neutral salts and under appropriate conditions of pH and temperature, and they were electrophoretically and immunologically homogeneous. The solubility of the pure, undenatured preparations of thyroglobulin was independent of the content of iodine and iodinated amino acids. In addition, under certain conditions, this protein was identical in its composition in all fractions isolated by successive precipitation in increasing concentrations of neutral salts. Hence it follows that the iodine content in thyroglobulin is highly variable and cannot be used as a criterion of the purity of the preparation.

However, the study of heterogeneity of thyroglobulin called for the development of finer methods of preparative fractionation. Column chromatography with DEAE-cellulose after preliminary fractionation with ammonium sulfate was suggested in 1959. The protein isolated by this method was electrophoretically homogeneous and of uniform amino acid composition, but its rate of elution varied [59, 416]. The rate of elution was found to depend on the iodine content: Molecules of thyroglobulin with a lower iodine content were eluted faster.

A method of isolation of thyroglobulin by gel filtration through Sephadex G-200 without preliminary salt extraction was published in 1963; the semipurified extract was applied directly to the column [378]. This method, like that of filtration through a column with 8% agarose, as suggested by Van Zyl and Edelhoch [540], gives effective separation of thyroglobulin from absorbed molecules of proteins, macroglobulins, and serum proteins.

To investigate some aspects of thyroglobulin structure, Pyzhova and Ioffe (working in the laboratory of hormone biochemistry of the Institute of

Biochemistry in Tashkent) tested several methods of preparing thyroglobulin in the pure form. They developed their own modification, consisting of the following stages: extraction of slices of the gland with three volumes of 0.9 N NaCl for 24 h at 4°C, centrifugation and filtration to remove particles of lipids, ultrafiltration to concentrate the extract, and chromatography through Sephadex G-200 and an ion-exchange column. The protein thus obtained gave one spot during electrophoresis on paper and agar gel, while on ultracentrifugation it gave three peaks corresponding to three thyroglobulin fractions, of which the principal peak was a protein with a sedimentation coefficient of 19 S.

Investigations of the physicochemical properties, studies by ultracentrifugation on a sucrose density gradient, and the study of the individual stages of biosynthesis and the immunochemical properties of thyroglobulin [453] have recently confirmed the earlier observations on the heterogeneity of its molecule. Protein fractions with sedimentation coefficients of 3–8 S, 12 S, 14–16 S, 17–19 S, 27 S, and 32–35 S have been isolated.

Following electrophoresis in 3 M urea at pH 6.5 on starch gel, thyroglobulin separates into two zones as a result of the partial dissociation of the original molecule into two subunits [295]. Dissociation of 19 S thyroglobulin into two subunits with a sedimentation coefficient of about 9.5 S is also observed at a neutral pH, after removal of the salts, or in the presence of the anionic detergent sodium dodecyl sulfate [476].

On electrophoresis of thyroglobulin preparations on polyacrylamide gel, two components are found, more of one than of the other.

If the monomer is regarded as the smallest unit which can be obtained without cleavage of the covalent bond, the thyroglobulin monomer is the 12 S subunit, the 18 S subunit is a dimer, 27 S a tetramer, and 35 S a hexamer.

Lissitzky et al. [283] determined the minimal molecular weight of the polypeptide chains of sheep thyroglobulin by ultracentrifugation and by gel filtration of the S-carboxymethylated derivative of thyroglobulin on Sephadex G-200. They concluded from the values of the molecular weight obtained that sheep 19 S thyroglobulin consists of 8 polypeptide chains, each with a molecular weight of 80,000, and that the 12 S subunit of the thyroglobulin molecule contains two different polypeptide chains, each with a molecular weight of 80,000.

Other evidence of the heterogeneity of the 12 S subunit of thyroglobulin has been reported. Salvatore et al. [448], for instance, showed that native 12 S thyroglobulin isolated from the guinea pig thyroid contains only one-tenth of the iodine of the 19 S thyroglobulin obtained from the same preparation. It was shown that this naturally occurring thyroid protein did not arise from 19 S thyroglobulin and did not dimerize into 19 S thyroglobulin. Although it does not interact with undissociated 19 S thyroglobulin, it combines with the 12 S subunit arising from the 19 S subunit with the formation of a hybrid thyroglobulin molecule. This shows that thyroglobulin consists of two different 12 S subunits, one of which is equivalent to the natural 12 S molecule.

Investigations with bovine 19 S thyroglobulin revealed differences between the thyroglobulin molecules to correspond with their ability to dissociate into 12 S subunits under the influence of guanidine or urea, compounds acting on noncovalent bonds. Two types of thyroglobulin molecules were discovered: one capable of dissociating, in which the two 12 S subunits are held together by noncovalent interactions and which dissociate readily in 6 M guanidine, and one which does not dissociate, consisting of two 12 S subunits held together by one or more S–S bonds. In turn, the 12 S subunit contains two chains with a molecular weight of 165,000 that form dimers with disulfide cross-linkages.

The question of the number of polypeptide chains in the thyroglobulin molecule likewise has not been finally settled. Its determination is difficult because of the virtual impossibility, with present methods, of separating the single chains formed after reduction and alkylation of thyroglobulin.

There is some evidence to show that thyroglobulin consists of four peptide chains [476]. According to these observations, the N-terminal amino acids of human thyroglobulin are two aspartic acid residues, one serine residue, and one glycine residue. Different results were obtained on determination of the N-terminal amino acids of pig thyroglobulin by the phenylisothiocyanate method [113], by which they were identified as aspartic acid, asparagine, and glycine. Other experiments have shown that the N-end of the pig thyroglobulin molecule contains tyrosine, 3,5-diiodotyrosine, and thyroxine. Experiments conducted jointly with Pyzhova and Ioffe [402, 403] demonstrated the presence of two peptide chains and showed that the two terminal amino acids are glycine and alanine. It is difficult to explain the difference between these results.

Investigations have shown that thyroglobulin contains 202 hemicystine residues per molecule, all in the oxidized form [349]; it therefore contains 101 disulfide groups. Complete reduction of these bonds leads to the formation of polypeptide chains with an approximate molecular weight of 165,000.

Thyroglobulin contains several amino acids capable of binding iodine; the degree of their iodination varies, however, with the physiological conditions. During alkaline or enzymic hydrolysis of thyroglobulin, iodinated derivatives of tyrosine and thyronine, together with the principal amino acids characteristic of the specific protein of the thyroid gland, are liberated.

Many determinations of the amino acid composition of thyroglobulin have been made. Although the results are similar, they are not completely identical. The figures obtained by Lipman et al. [278] for the number of amino acid residues of thyroglobulin (calculated as having a molecular weight of 650,000, made up of protein 578,000, carbohydrates 65,000, and iodinated amino acids 7000) differ considerably from those obtained by Pierce et al. [385] and those given by Berzin in his book *The Biochemistry of Hormones* [53].

Pierce et al. [385] determined the amino acid composition of thyroglobulin from normal and goitrous thyroid glands. No difference was found in the composition of the amino acids, in the total carbohydrate content per protein molecule, or in the type of the sugar residues.

The amino acid composition of the thyroglobulin of the normal human thyroid gland as reflected in results obtained by three groups of workers is given in Table I. The possible causes of differences in the amino acid composition of thyroglobulin as shown by results obtained in different laboratories will not be discussed, more especially because differences have been found when preparations of thyroglobulin from the thyroid gland of some species of animals have been investigated. They can evidently be explained by differences in the methods used to obtain, purify, and analyze the preparations. Determination of the primary structure of the protein molecule will provide a sound basis for the discussion of these results, but by that time the results of new tests ought to be available.

Thyroglobulin is sparingly soluble in water and acids but readily soluble in solutions of alkalies and neutral salts. It is precipitated from alkaline solutions by acids. Thyroglobulin has a characteristic ultraviolet absorption spectrum with two maxima: one at 2800 Å, dependent on the presence of aromatic amino acids and tryptophan in the molecule, and another at 3200–3300 Å. The latter is dependent on the presence of the chromophore groups of thyroxine and diiodotyrosine and is consequently more specific for thyroglobulin.

Much of the thyroglobulin molecule consists of arginine, leucine, and serine, and altogether there are about 140 tyrosyl + iodotyrosyl + iodothyronine residues. The ratio between them varies depending on the degree of iodination, but even if the iodine concentration is 1% (highly iodinated thyroglobulin) only 50 of the 280 potential sites of iodination are occupied. After iodination under rigorous conditions *in vitro* many tyrosyl residues remain uniodinated.

The degree of iodination of the thyroglobulin molecule has an effect on the number and type of iodinated amino acids, the protein structure, and the density [93]. The secondary and tertiary structure of thyroglobulin and, in particular, the surroundings of the tyrosyl residues, determining the ef-

TABLE I. Amino Acid Composition of Human Thyroglobulin

	After Pierce et al. [385]		After Lipman et al. [278]	After Berzin [53]
	g amino acid residues/100 g protein	moles amino acid residues/mole protein (mol. wt. 660,000)	moles amino acid residues/mole protein (mol. wt. 650,000)	g amino acid residues/100 g protein
Aspartic acid	5.9	339	387	8.4
Glutamic acid	12.4	634	708	15.3
Threonine	3.8	248	235	5.3
Serine	5.3	402	498	10.8
Proline	4.4	299	368	7.0
Glycine	3.2	367	427	3.7
Alanine	3.8	349	437	7.4
Valine	4.6	303	318	1.45
Isoleucine	2.4	140	133	2.4
Leucine	7.5	437	490	12.8
Hemicystine	2.9	187	153	3.6
Methionine	1.3	65	66	1.3
Lysine	3.4	175	124	3.4
Histidine	1.4	68	63	2.2
Arginine	5.9	250	359	12.7
Amino nitrogen	0.9	408	357	2.3
Tyrosine	3.2	129	129	3.2
Phenylalanine	5.3	238	268	6.7
Tryptophan	–	–	69	2.1
Thyroxine	–	–	–	0.21
Triiodothyronine	–	–	–	0.05
Diiodotyrosine	–	–	–	0.5
Monoiodotyrosine	–	–	–	0.6
Monoiodohistidine	–	–	–	0.02
Hexosamine	–	–	–	1.8

fectiveness of condensation of the iodinated tyrosines and the formation of hormonally active structures, depends chiefly on the number and type of the iodoamino acids. If thyroglobulin preparations obtained from iodine-deprived glands are iodinated *in vitro* up to a normal iodine content, the number of and ratio between the iodinated amino acids change to those characteristic of normal thyroglobulin.

The values obtained by Crombrughe et al. [92] for the content of iodinated amino acids in thyroglobulin are compared in Table II with the degree of iodination of normal human thyroglobulin and thyroglobulin isolated from a goiter, and in Table III with thyroglobulin from a goiter iodinated *in vitro*. The results obtained by Saatov in experiments conducted in the author's laboratory to determine the composition of the iodinated

TABLE II. Content of Iodinated Amino Acids in Thyroglobulin Compared with Degree of Iodination (Data of Crombrughe et al. [92])

Total iodine, %	Tyrosine	MIT	DIT	T_4	Number of iodine atoms
		For normal human thyroglobulin			
0.36	125.8	6.9	3.3	2.4	21 (0.4%)
0.50	126.9	6.8	4.4	2.7	27 (0.52%)
0.80	111.4	9.8	10.8	3.9	48 (0.92%)
1.12	89.1	10.5	14.9	6.9	68 (1.3%)
		For thyroglobulin isolated from goiter			
0.05	124.5	5.2	1.3	0	7 (0.13%)
0.04	126.6	4.6	1.0	0	7 (0.13%)
0.14	121.9	4.8	2.1	0.6	9 (0.17%)
0.10	132.3	6.6	2.0	0	15 (0.3%)
0.02	115.8	4.9	0	0	5 (0.1%)

amino acids in thyroglobulin depending on the degree of iodination are given in Table IV.

However, differences are found in the distribution of iodinated amino acids in the thyroglobulin iodinated *in vivo* and *in vitro*. Ogawara et al. [361] recently showed that during iodination of thyroglobulin from a human goiter *in vitro*, followed by digestion with pronase, the content of $3,5,3'T_3$ and T_4 hormones is significantly lower. However, the content of biologically inactive iodothyronines $3,3',5'T_3$ and $3',5'T_2$ as well as of monoiodohistidine is much greater. According to these workers these differences are mainly due to the nonidentity of the mechanisms of the two types of iodination.

The low iodine content of iodoamino acids in thyroglobulin obtained from thyrotoxic patients after prolonged treatment with antithyroid prepa-

TABLE III. Content of Iodinated Amino Acids in Thyroglobulin from Goiter Iodinated *in Vitro*

Iodine added, moles/mole protein	MIT	DIT	T_4	Iodine content by chemical analysis, %	Iodine content, spectrophotometrically, %
0	4.6	1.0	0	0.05	0.13
15	9.8	3.4	0.5	0.18	0.35
45	10.1	9.1	0.8	0.83	0.90
95	9.8	13.5	3.5	0.95	0.97
195	11.7	23.3	6.0	1.0	1.56

TABLE IV. Content of Iodinated Amino Acids in Normal Thyroglobulin and in Thyroglobulin from Nodular Goiter (Data of Saatov [444])

Material tested	Total iodine, %	Moles/mole protein				Number of iodine atoms
		Tyrosine	MIT	DIT	T_4	
Normal thyroglobulin (bovine)	0.78		11.7	8.3	3.6	44 (0.84%)
Ditto	0.58	100	5.4	9.4	2.0	32 (0.61%)
Nodular goiter (euthyroid)	0.36	86.3	5.6	1.8	1.3	18 (0.34%)
Ditto	0.42	86.3	8.1	4.8	2.0	26 (0.5%)
Ditto	0.47	98	8.1	8.1	2.3	32 (0.6%)
Ditto		90	4.7	4.0	2.3	21 (0.4%)

rations may be increased by *in vitro* iodination up to the level of the thyroglobulin of normal human glands. This makes thyroxine synthesis by the intramolecular interaction between bound DIT and smaller molecules such as diiodophenylpyruvic acid appear perfectly feasible.

The carbohydrate components of thyroglobulin account for 8.5–10.6% of the molecule and consist of 23 heteropolysaccharide units of two types, differing in molecular weight and structure. The work of Cheftel et al. [80] and Spiro and Spiro [474] has shown that the small unit of the carbohydrate chain contains mannose and N-acetylglucosamine only, in the ratio of 5:1, while the large unit consists of five types of monosaccharides in a certain order: mannose, galactose, N-acetylglucosamine, sialic acid, and fucose. Each molecule of human thyroglobulin contains approximately 359 carbohydrate residues. Sialic acid or fucose are removed more easily and may perhaps occupy the terminal position of the carbohydrate unit and thus be linked with galactose.

The presence of two types of carbohydrate units presupposes the existence of two different polypeptide chains.

Mature 19 S thyroglobulin, for instance, is a polymer with a virtually constant structure consisting of subunits; these are 12 S half-molecules joined together by a noncovalent bond: The two half-molecules are complementary rather than completely identical. The basis of the molecule consists of 6 S subunits joined by disulfide bonds. The 19 S molecule arises through further iodination of thyroglobulin with a sedimentation coefficient of 17–18 S. By polymerization of the 19 S thyroglobulin larger analogs are obtained: a tetramer and hexamer with sedimentation coefficients of 27 S and 35 S, respectively.

The different fractions of thyroglobulin both in thyroid gland extracts and in purified preparations contain different quantities of iodine, which can be taken as an index of the degree of maturity of the molecule.

The question of possible changes in the properties of thyroglobulin under normal and pathological conditions of the thyroid gland has been the subject of several investigations. However, the data so far published do not justify the conclusion that differences exist in the amino acid composition of preparations of iodinated protein obtained from the normal thyroid gland or from the gland affected by adenoma or exophthalmic goiter. Differences are observed only in the total content and relative proportions of the iodinated amino acids.

Determination of the purity of thyroglobulin isolated from the same patient, but from normal and carcinomatous thyroid gland tissue, by electrophoresis and by immunological tests showed that the protein fractions in the two cases moved as single components but differed in mobility. In each case three or four antigenic components were found in the thyroglobulin.

Derrien et al. [109] also investigated the thyroglobulin of four species of mammals (ox, horse, dog, and pig) to see if they exhibit species-specific differences as has been shown, for example, in relation to insulin, hemoglobin, somatotropin, etc. These investigations revealed no differences between the thyroglobulins of the animals studied.

Other Thyroid Gland Proteins

A protein with properties similar to serum albumin has been particularly carefully studied. The view is still expressed that this protein is indistinguishable in its physicochemical properties and immunological characteristics from serum albumin [377]. In a recent paper on thyroid albumin Jonckheer and Karcher [233] gave a detailed account of the method of isolation of thyroid albumin from normal human thyroid gland and of its electrophoretic and immunological properties. Four fractions of this protein were obtained, two with the characteristics of serum albumin. Iodination affected the chromatographic behavior of the protein and its electrophoretic mobility. The main mass of thyroid albumin is iodinated. It contains 2.62 times more glycine than human serum albumin but less methionine. It can be concluded from these results that by far the greater part, if not all, of the thyroid albumin is an iodinated protein that differs from serum albumin.

Similar results have been obtained in the writer's laboratory by Saatov [444] and Dzhalilova and Saatov [124].

According to their observations, thyroalbumin in normal thyroid gland tissue accounts for 5–10% of the total protein content. In goiter and, in particular, in carcinoma of the thyroid gland the content was sharply increased at the expense of thyroglobulin which, in some cases of cancer and congenital goiter, was almost completely absent from a saline extract of the gland.

Investigation of the composition of the iodized components after acid hydrolysis of thyroalbumin showed that the digest contained the iodinated tyrosines MIT and DIT but not iodinated thyronines. Hormonally active structures are evidently not associated with the thyroalbumin molecule.

Besides soluble iodinated proteins, which include thyroglobulin and thyroalbumin, insoluble proteins have been found in the thyroid gland where they are connected with the nucleus or associated with particles (particulate protein). In the normal thyroid gland the insoluble protein contains 6–10% of the total iodine.

These proteins include two types of iodoproteins isolated by Robins et al. [418] from normal and abnormal human thyroid tissue and from normal sheep thyroid glands. One of these proteins, a particulate iodoprotein, was not extracted from tissue homogenates with 0.14 M NaCl, while the second, known as *S-1-iodoprotein*, although soluble in NaCl, differed from thyroglobulin in its other physicochemical properties.

In the course of an investigation of thyroglobulin biosynthesis, Spiro and Spiro [474] isolated an insoluble protein bound with subcellular particles. The protein, associated with light fractions, was isolated by treatment of the particles with 1% digitonin. The isolated protein resembled thyroglobulin in its immunochemical properties, electrophoretic mobility, and carbohydrate composition. The view of these authors that this protein is evidently a precursor of soluble thyroglobulin might be acceptable, but the considerable level of iodination makes this conclusion doubtful for we know that most iodination in the thyroid gland takes place in the colloid.

Proteins different from thyroglobulin, known as pathological thyroglobulins, have been described in various types of congenital thyroid disease with goiter in man and animals; these abnormal thyroglobulins have a low iodine content, mainly in the form of iodinated tyrosines. One such abnormal thyroglobulin component was isolated and studied by Roche et al. [427] from the thyroid of three patients with familial goiter. Earlier De Groot et al. [103] had reported the discovery of an unusual protein, containing iodotyrosines and iodothyronines linked together in peptides, in the blood of patients with congenital goiter. This protein is evidently a product of incomplete synthesis or irregular fragmentation of thyroglobulin. In other cases the appearance of abnormal iodoproteins in the circulation may be the result of incomplete proteolysis of thyroglobulin.

Metabolism in the Thyroid Gland

The whole course of metabolism in the thyroid gland tissue is directed toward the performance of its endocrine function, namely, the production of thyroid hormones. This process is closely linked with the circulation of iodine in the gland and with thyroglobulin biosynthesis, processes requiring a constant supply of structural materials and energy. Thyroglobulin biosynthesis unquestionably takes place on an RNA template, and the formation of the peptide chain of this complex protein is controlled by the course of nucleic acid metabolism.

The composition of nucleic acids in the normal thyroid gland and their modification in disease have been the subject of detailed investigations, particularly in the last five to ten years.

Research in the writer's laboratory [529, 535] has revealed considerable fluctuations in the nucleic acid content in the normal thyroid gland around mean levels of 17.53 ± 3.43 mg/100 ml for DNA and 11.29 ± 1.23 mg/100 ml for RNA.

The observations of Kasavina et al. [246] and of Atakhanova [30] show a statistically significant increase in the RNA content both in human euthyroid nodules and in goitrous glands of experimental animals. Changes in the DNA content are not statistically significant.

Investigations of the nucleotide composition of total and ribosomal RNA of the normal human thyroid and of the goitrous gland have not revealed any differences [30], but qualitative differences between some transfer RNAs have been found in the goitrous thyroid gland [32]. For example, fractionation of ^{14}C-thyronyl tRNA in normal thyroid gland on methylated albumin revealed two components, while in the tissue of a nodular euthyroid goiter a third isoacceptor component was found. No tRNAs for iodinated tyrosines [75] or iodinated thyronine [21] have been found in the thyroid gland. Meanwhile purified sheep tRNA was found to be active relative to uniodinated amino acids. This fact has a bearing on the hypotheses put forward to explain biosynthesis of the thyroid hormones, and it is indirect evidence that iodination of tyrosines with the formation of MIT and DIT and the formation of thyronine are secondary reactions and take place in the interior of the thyroglobulin molecule after incorporation of amino acids into the peptide chains. However, these findings do not rule out the possibility that a molecule of iodinated tyrosine or its modified analog is attached to the mono- or diiodotyrosine existing in a bound form in the peptide chain of thyroglobulin.

Determinations of the rate of RNA and DNA biosynthesis in the normal and goitrous thyroid gland from ^{14}C-uridine or 2-^{14}C-thymidine and on the synthesis of mononucleotides from their precursors have been published. The work of Khalikov and Seitmuratova [529] in the writer's laboratory showed that the intensity of incorporation of ^{14}C-uridine into newly synthesized RNA is 2.6 times higher, while the incorporation of ^{14}C-thymidine into DNA is 1.5 times higher in goitrous gland tissue than in the normal tissue surrounding the nodule. These results confirm the view that the acceleration of protein biosynthesis in goiter is due to increased synthesis of nucleic acids and, in particular, of RNA.

Khalikov [249], in the writer's laboratory, used 2-^{14}C-formic acid and ^{14}C-L-glycine as ribonucleoprotein precursors and also demonstrated the acceleration of mononucleotide synthesis in goitrous thyroid tissue. Injections of thyroxine were found to lower the RNA content in the thyroid gland considerably [310] while injection of methylthiouracil causes a marked increase in the RNA content in the thyroid gland accounted for by the morphological activity of the epithelial cells. Lindsey and Cohen [277] discovered a parallel increase in the weight of the thyroid gland and an increase in the content of acid-soluble nucleotides and RNA, which are influenced by antithyroid agents and iodine deficiency. The activity of enzymes concerned with RNA synthesis (uridine phosphorylase and uridine kinase) was more than doubled, and the incorporation of pyrimidine nucleotides into RNA was considerably intensified.

The experiments of Atakhanova [31] also showed a considerable increase in the RNA content per unit weight of the thyroid gland in rats after prolonged administration of the antithyroid agent 6-methylthiouracil.

Thyroid hormone formation is also inseparably linked with the conversion of carbohydrates and lipids with aerobic oxidation supplying energy for the various reactions in the production and secretion of the thyroid hormones. The important role of carbohydrate metabolism by direct oxidation and also of phospholipid metabolism in hormone formation is clearly revealed by the effects of thyroid-stimulating hormone on the gland. Morton and Schwartz [332], for instance, described the selective absorption of ^{32}P by thyroid phospholipids in cows under the influence of thyrotropic hormone. Freinkel and Ingbar [155] investigated the synthesis of thyroid hormone in slices of thyroid gland and found that the first stage of synthesis, the accumulation of iodine by the gland, depends on energy supplied by oxidative phosphorylation. The uptake of ^{32}P by individual phospholipid fractions varied and also depended on the metabolic state of the thyroid gland. Consequently, phospholipids in the gland can be subdivided into several fractions, each with its own metabolic characteristics. Kögl and Deenen [257], working with thyroid slices and homogenates, showed that the incorporation of phosphorus from $Na_2H^{32}PO_4$ into phospholipids is doubled on the addition of thyroid stimulating hormone (TSH).

Studies of glucose assimilation and metabolism and of the utilization and incorporation of inositol into lipids by thyroid gland slices have shown that all these processes are modified by TSH. Thyrotropin increases the assimilation of glucose and accelerates lipogenesis from it. The increase in CO_2 formation and in its incorporation into lipids is regarded as the result of activation of oxidative decarboxylation by phosphogluconate oxidation in the thyroid gland.

Dumont [118] found an increase in the rate of oxidation of glucose by the hexose monophosphate pathway by the action of TSH on the thyroid gland. Working with tissue slices, he found a much greater acceleration of $^{12}CO_2$ formation from glucose-1-^{14}C than from glucose-6-^{14}C.

It is not yet possible to judge how metabolic phenomena modify iodine metabolism in the thyroid gland, but from the experimental evidence so far obtained it can be stated that the initial stages of intrathyroid changes are connected with an increase in the uptake of extrathyroid glucose. The increase in glucose absorption makes the cofactors and substrates accessible for anabolic processes by activating the phosphogluconate pathway, including the provision of $NADPH_2$ for fatty acid synthesis.

In general it must be admitted that the data on chemical anatomy and metabolism of the thyroid gland are inadequate. Further research in this direction, particularly into the intimate connections between the metabolism of the gland and its hormone-forming function, could prove very fruitful.

The Biosynthesis of Thyroid Hormones

Thyroid hormone formation takes place in several successive but independent stages, involving the participation of different structural components of the follicles: the transfer of iodine from the blood into the gland, protein synthesis and iodination, the formation of the thyroid hormones, and their secretion. These stages are integrated into a unified and coordinated endocrine process in the general cell metabolism of the follicular epithelium of the thyroid gland.

Fixation of the Blood Iodides by the Thyroid Gland

The first and essential condition for the beginning of the intrathyroid metabolism of iodine is the uptake of iodides by the thyroid gland from the circulating blood. The ability to concentrate iodides from the blood is in fact the most important distinguishing feature of the thyroid gland.

Iodine ions are present in the blood plasma in very low concentrations (0.1–0.5 μg/100 ml), and to enable such a negligible quantity of iodine to participate in the metabolic cycle, a highly efficient mechanism of concentration is required to provide a continuous accumulation of iodides in the cells. Such a mechanism functions in the thyroid gland. The fixation of the blood iodides by the thyroid gland has two consecutive aspects: the accumulation of iodide and its oxidation into elementary iodine (I_2).

Iodine can react with thyroglobulin so as to enter into organic combination only in the elementary form. However, in the absence of organic iodine fixation, the thyroid gland can accumulate iodine on the same scale as the salivary glands or the gastric juice, i.e., up to a level 40–50 times higher than the plasma iodine concentration. This stage of iodine fixation must be distinguished from the next stage, when the iodide is oxidized to elementary iodine and rapidly incorporated into the protein molecule.

Free iodine is in equilibrium with the iodine of the circulating blood and also with the bound iodine which is in unstable combination with the colloidal system and can pass through membranes.

The autonomy of this first phase of intrathyroid iodine metabolism has been clearly revealed by research in which oxidation of iodides into I_2 in the gland was blocked by means of sulfonamides and thiourea derivatives. Such investigations were first carried out by Chaikoff's group [153] and by other workers who observed that, although in the presence of sulfonamides and thiouracil thyroid gland slices fix less iodine in the organic form, they nevertheless maintain their iodine-concentrating ability. The same result is found after administration of propylthiouracil to animals.

The thyroid gland, when blocked by thiouracil, can thus take up iodine and fix it in a concentration several hundred times greater than the plasma iodine concentration. Under these conditions iodine accumulates in the gland as salts of thyroglobulin, instead of being incorporated into iodinated amino acids. These salts constitute the *weakly combined iodine* (Figure 3). If the block is complete, the iodine in the thyroid gland is in re-

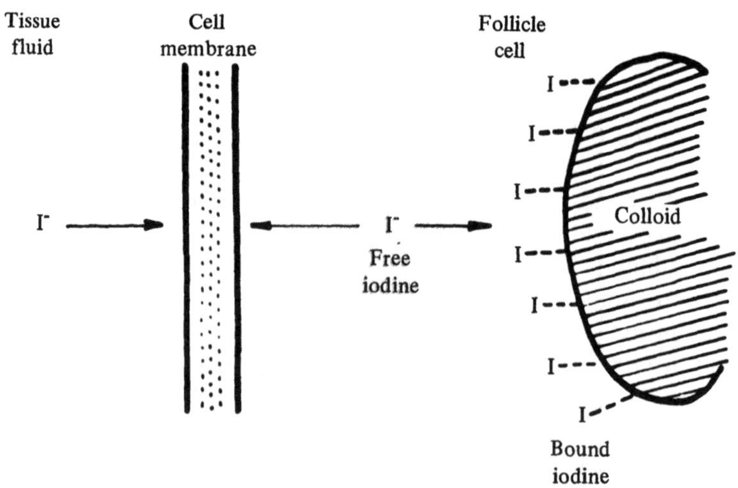

Fig. 3. Scheme showing the state of iodine in the thyroid gland.

versible equilibrium with the plasma iodide and, by contrast with iodine accumulating and bound in the organic form in the unblocked gland, it can easily be displaced by thiocyanate, perchlorate, and certain other anions [538].

Physiologically speaking, iodine is integrated into organic compounds immediately after its entry into the gland. Accordingly only a very small quantity of iodine, not more than 2% of the total content in the thyroid gland, exists as iodides and can return to the plasma. This agrees with observations showing that after only 1–2 min the ^{131}I accumulated by the unblocked thyroid gland cannot be displaced by thiocyanate. Some of the iodides in the gland are formed by dehalogenation of iodotyrosines liberated from the thyroglobulin during proteolysis. The mechanism of uptake of plasma iodine by the thyroid gland has not yet been fully explained despite much research.

In the modern view the thyroid uptake of iodine is regarded as *active transport*, a process linked with the simultaneous expenditure of energy provided by aerobic cell metabolism, for which triphosphopyridine nucleotide and oxygen must be present [47, 155].

Results obtained by Freinkel and Ingbar [155] show that an active metabolically linked process of oxidation is an essential condition for the transport of inorganic iodine into the thyroid gland against the concentration gradient. The transport of iodine is blocked by the addition of inhibitors of aerobic respiration (cyanide, azide, sulfide, arsenite, phloridzin, fluoroacetate, etc.) and also of many other compounds reacting with sulfhydryl groups (Hg, Zb, Cu, iodoacetate, bromoacetate, quinone, *p*-chloromercuribenzoate, 2,3-dimercaptoimidazole) but which do not necessarily influence tissue respiration, to the incubation medium.

The absorption of iodine is also reduced by the action of sulfonamides, inhibitors of oxidative phosphorylation (2,4-dinitrophenol, 2,4,6-trinitrophenol, etc.) and by high concentrations of iodide, thiocyanate, perchlorate, etc., and it is increased by the action of TSH [159]. The iodination of thyroglobulin is a reaction sensitive to thyroid-stimulating hormone. Antithyroid and other agents modify the effect of TSH in various ways. Iodide, in physiological concentrations, potentiates its action on the formation of bound iodine.

During incorporation of atoms of elementary iodine into the thyroglobulin molecule in the first period, iodotyrosines are synthesized in the gland; after 15 sec these can also be found in the form of free amino acids. Nevertheless, it is difficult to determine the origin of these free iodotyrosines: whether they appear as the result of iodination of tyrosine molecules or secondarily, in the course of the enzymic breakdown of iodinated thyroglobulin. As regards both the composition of the thyroglobulin and the form of the three amino acids, the iodotyrosines formed are subsequently used for the synthesis of iodinated thyronines.

In the modern view the synthesis of thyroid hormones embraces at least two processes: first, the synthesis of iodotyrosines, accompanied by the incidental iodination of histidine, and second, the condensation of two molecules of iodotyrosines with the formation of thyroxine and triiodothyronines. The deiodination of monoiodotyrosine and diiodotyrosine, evidently formed in excess and not utilized at that particular moment for the synthesis of iodinated thyronines, also takes place in the thyroid gland.

If iodine molecules are present, solutions of tyrosine and histidine can be iodinated very quickly by substitution of one hydrogen atom in the ring by one iodine atom.

The process of formation of iodotyrosines, given adequate amounts of iodine, takes place in the following order: Monoiodotyrosine is synthesized first and diiodotyrosine later [423].

During hydrolysis of thyroglobulin by a proteolytic enzyme, large quantities of mono- and diiodotyrosine are liberated as well as hormonally active iodothyronines. In the generally accepted view these iodotyrosines are not utilized for the synthesis of thyroxine and triiodothyronines, but the iodine is quickly removed from their molecule by enzyme action. The iodine liberated reenters the metabolic cycle and is utilized by the gland for hormone formation.

The enzyme participating in the mechanism of iodine conservation by the thyroid gland by recirculation of iodide from iodotyrosines after disintegration of thyroglobulin has now been sufficiently well studied. Attention was first drawn by Roche and co-workers to the presence of dehalogenases, capable of removing iodine from molecules of iodotyrosines, but not from iodothyronines, in the thyroid gland, liver, and kidneys. In 1957 Stanbury and Morris [477] located this enzyme in the microsomes and showed that it requires NADP as coenzyme. Iodotyrosine deiodinase differs from the deiodinases found in many tissues which deiodinate iodothyronines. This enzyme, investigated by Tata, is found in the soluble fraction of the cytoplasm and requires flavin mononucleotide and iron ions as coenzymes. Iodotyrosine deiodinase is found in the active form in several other tissues also (liver, kidneys, salivary glands). The system of deiodination acts by hydrogenation and is active only against derivatives of the L-form (DIT + 2H → MIT + 1H; MIT + 2H → tyrosine + 1H). It is generally accepted that its absence or slowing of the mechanism of iodotyrosine deiodination is the cause of certain forms of congenital disease in man leading invariably to hypothyroidism [47].

The iodide produced from the iodotyrosines as a result of deiodination in the thyroid gland has the same fate as iodide newly arriving from the circulation. Both are incorporated equally rapidly into the thyroglobulin molecule, and the relations between iodine arising from iodotyrosines and the iodide newly introduced into MIT and DIT molecules and into T_4 and T_3 are the same.

Roche and co-workers [424] made a full examination of the conditions of action of the deiodinating enzyme in animals, but there is no information in the literature on the volume of this reaction compared with the quantity of MIT and DIT formed. Is this activity sufficient for the rapid destruction of all iodinated tyrosines, so that these components do not enter the blood stream?

According to the opinion expressed in the literature concerning the participation of at least some free modified iodotyrosine molecules in the synthesis of thyronine structures, the deiodination process in the thyroid gland does not lead to total destruction of all iodinated tyrosines formed by proteolysis of thyroglobulin, to prevent them from appearing in the blood stream. Some of them can evidently be utilized after "activation" for synthesis of the iodothyronine structure without deiodination.

Formation of L-*Thyroxine and* L-*Triiodothyronine*

Since the time of the first synthesis of thyroxine by Harrington and Barger, L-3,5-diiodotyrosine has been regarded as its precursor in the thyroid gland. If the existing view on the formation of thyroxine within the thyroglobulin molecule is accepted, this process in the course of iodination of the protein can be explained in two ways: (1) by iodination of tyrosine residues and partial conversion of diiodotyrosine molecules into thyroxine; and (2) by the presence of thyronine in the ready-made form in the protein and its iodination with the direct formation of thyroxine.

The first explanation seems more probable, for the presence of thyronine in the protein has not yet been demonstrated, although on the other hand it is doubtful whether condensation of iodinated tyrosine residues contained in the protein molecule in a bound state is possible.

The general scheme of condensation of two diiodotyrosine molecules can be represented as follows:

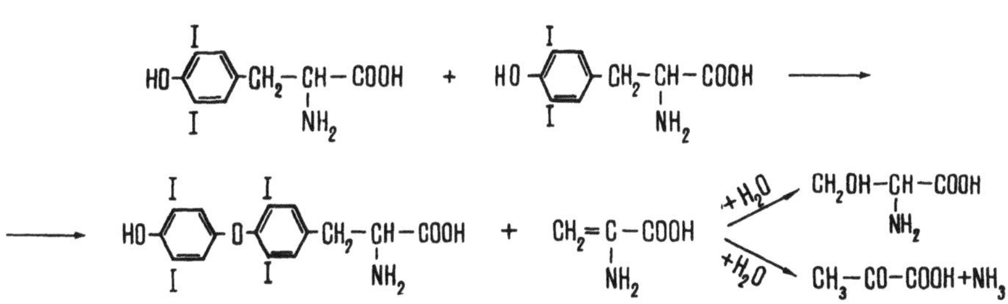

The alanine chain in this reaction is separated as dehydroalanine $CH_2{=}C(NH_2){-}COOH$ which is then hydrated into serine or pyruvic acid and ammonia. In this mechanism the diiodotyrosine molecules in the protein must be arranged stereochemically so that they can react with each other. In fact, however, not all tyrosine residues in the protein molecule are so arranged, and there is therefore less thyroxine in thyroglobulin than would be expected from a calculation based on the number of thyronine residues. The role of thyroglobulin in thyroxine synthesis cannot thus be regarded as fully understood. Although other proteins can also iodinate tyrosine with the formation of MIT and DIT, thyroglobulin is the only known protein capable of forming thyroxine *in vivo*. By iodination *in vitro* thyroglobulin can form more thyroxine, but not more diiodothyronine, than other proteins investigated, and the formation of T_4 is not changed in the presence of 8 M urea [127].

An important role in the formation of the thyronine structure is evidently played by the quaternary structure of thyroglobulin, as is shown by the fact that iodination takes place chiefly after the formation of 17–18 M thyroglobulin by noncovalent association of its subunits. However, comprehensive studies of the pattern of the increase in T_4 in the thyroglobulin molecule during iodination *in vitro*, and also of the reactivity of tyrosine residues, undertaken by Edelhoch and his group [128], show that the decisive role is played by the primary structure of the protein molecule. This is perfectly natural for, as has been conclusively proved, all higher forms of organization of the protein molecule are ultimately determined by its amino acid sequence. Recent data on the amino acid neighbors of T_4 in thyroglobulin have demonstrated the important role both of the degree of iodination and of the amino acid sequence in the molecule for thyroxine synthesis.

Of about 120 tyrosine residues in the thyroglobulin molecule, under normal conditions from 10 to 25 are iodinated and from 1 to 5 are in the form of thyroxine [408].

Investigations by Van Zyl and Edelhoch [540] have shown that when thyroglobulin is iodinated *in vitro* there is an increase in the DIT peaks and a decrease in the tyrosine residues. The environment of the tyrosyl groups determines the relative amounts of MIT and DIT synthesized. In another investigation Edelhoch and Perlman [130] studied the reactivity of monoiodotyrosyl and diiodotyrosyl residues in the thyroglobulin molecule in the reaction with N-acylimidazole and concluded that DIT residues are much more reactive than MIT. An increase in the ratio of T_4 and T_3 in thyroglobulin with an increase in the iodine content is explained by the rapid rise in DIT/MIT.

Attempts to investigate the link between thyroxine synthesis and the primary structure of thyroglobulin have frequently been undertaken. The terminal amino acids of the thyroglobulin molecule [113, 476] and the composition and structure of the peptides obtained by controlled enzymic hydrolysis of thyroglobulin with the production of a mixture of peptides of stable composition [22] have been studied. In a recently published paper, Dunn [119] took another step toward the discovery of the amino acid sequence of thyroglobulin. He describes the isolation and composition of fractions of thyroxine-containing peptides obtained after digestion of thyroglobulin by pronase and showed that only a few specific amino acids are constantly found next to T_4.

Pronase digestion was carried out under conditions where most MIT and DIT was liberated from ^{125}I-labeled rabbit thyroglobulin in the free form and T_4 and T_3 were linked in a peptide bond. The fraction of this hydrolysis product containing most of the iodine in the form of iodotyrosines was fractionated by gel diffusion into seven iodopeptides, in which T_4, glutamic acid, serine, aspartic acid, and alanine were the most frequent. Two-thirds of the total thyroxine of the thyroglobulin was found in the peptide fractions studied. By comparing the amino acid composition of all the thyroxine-containing peptides, Dunn concluded that the Ala-Ser-T_4-Glu-Asp sequence was the only combination not ruled out by the solution to the problem whether T_4 is bounded by a unique amino acid sequence. These four amino acids were also found to be in association with T_4 in human thyroglobulin [498]. This suggests that some particular environment of tyrosine residue is an essential condition for thyroxine biosynthesis.

Since Ludwig and Von Mutzenbecher [292] found that thyroxine can be formed from DIT during prolonged incubation, many investigations have been carried out to study the mechanism of this reaction with a change in the conditions under which it takes place and with the use of various DIT analogs and iodotyrosine peptides [392]; the important role of the conditions of oxidation was thereby established.

Edelhoch [128] wrote that T_4 is synthesized in many proteins, just as it is in thyroglobulin, by the reaction with iodine and including iodination and condensation. It is important to know the environment of the tyrosyl residues in the thyroglobulin molecule and also to determine whether tyrosine residues in the thyroglobulin molecule possess activity comparable with that found in models with low molecule weight. As was stated above, the necessary information has been obtained on these matters, but the mechanism of formation of the thyronine structure still remains unknown.

Two concepts with respect to this mechanism are at present being discussed. According to one of them, two DIT molecules in the composition of thyroglobulin react with each other to form T_4 with the elimination of serine or of a dehydroalanine residue. Early nonenzymic models were based on this concept [224, 392]. Acceptance of this scheme with interaction between two diiodotyrosines in the interior of the thyroglobulin molecule meets with

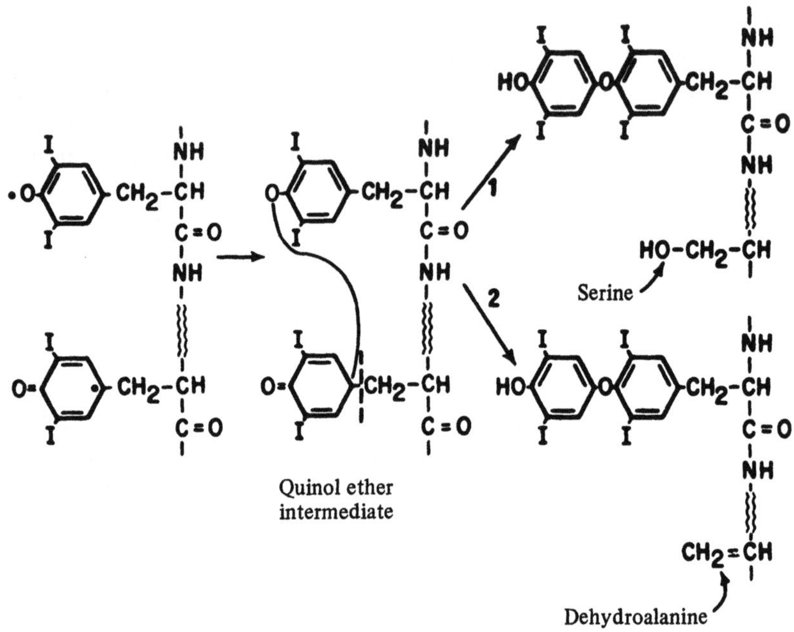

many difficulties because of stereochemical relations. Further, as was stated above, it requires proof of the conversion of one diiodotyrosine molecule in the peptide chain into a molecule of serine or alanine. A possible mechanism of condensation, put forward by Cahnmann on the basis of a similar mechanism suggested in 1942 by Johnson, Tewksbury, and Harrington (cited in [224]), is illustrated above.

Direct experimental proof of such a reaction has not yet been obtained. Other nonenzymic reaction models designed to explain the mechanism by which DIT is converted into T_4 in the thyroid gland suggest the participation of free iodotyrosines or their analogs. Proof of nonenzymic synthesis of thyroxine from DIT in a medium containing H_2O_2 and horseradish peroxidase was obtained previouly [259]. Lissitzky and Krotemberg [281] and Pavlovic-Hournac et al. [374] described the formation of T_4 from DIT during incubation of labeled DIT with orthodiiodohydroquinone, although no thyroxine was synthesized under these conditions from DIT alone.

Another hypothesis put forward first by Hillmann [216] assumes the formation of T_4 by condensation of residues of the DIT molecule in the composition of thyroglobulin with the keto analog of DIT. Many nonenzymic model reactions studied in recent decades have been based on this hypothesis. In the general form it postulates the synthesis of thyroxine in the thyroglobulin molecule by condensation of one free, so-called activated, molecule of iodotyrosine with the iodotyrosyl residue of the polypeptide chain of thyroglobulin [72, 312, 464] or with a free DIT molecule [317].

These investigations showed that diiodophenylpyruvic acid (DIPPA) is able to react *in vitro* not only with free DIT, but also with DIT residues in the thyroglobulin molecule. It was shown quite recently that the synthesis of T_4 from DIT and DIPPA takes place through a series of reactions [54, 354]. DIPPA is first converted into its enol tautomer. The enol tautomer of DIPPA is then oxidized through the formation of an intermediate free phenoxy radical into a hydroperoxide derivative, which finally condenses with DIT to form T_4. Surks et al. [483], after injecting radioactive iodine into a rat, found labeled DIPPA in the thyroid gland. This discovery was regarded as the only evidence of the biological role of DIPPA in T_4 formation by condensation with DIT. However, Blasi et al. [54] showed that the thyroid glands of several animals contain an enzyme system with ability: (1) to form DIPPA from DIT and (2) to convert the keto form of DIPPA into the enol tautomer. Indirect evidence was obtained that thyroid peroxidase can oxidize the enol form of DIPPA into its hydroperoxide derivative. According to these observations T_4 synthesis requires the presence of pyridoxal phosphate, *a*-ketoglutarate, a system generating hydrogen peroxide, and a thyroid postmitochondrial supernatant. The first stage of T_4 synthesis *in vitro* consists of transamination of DIT into DIPPA, which is evidently catalyzed by tyrosine transaminase present in the thyroid gland. The second state, tautomerization of DIPPA into the enol form, is brought about by the tautomerase present in the soluble fraction of the thyroid homogenate. The third stage, oxidation of diiodohydroxyphenolpyruvic acid into the hydroperoxide derivative, is catalyzed by a model peroxidase, similar to horseradish peroxidase, in the presence of a system generating hydrogen peroxide. It can be concluded from this indirect evidence that thyroid peroxidase can also catalyze this reaction. The course of biosynthesis, in accordance with the experimental data, can be represented as follows:

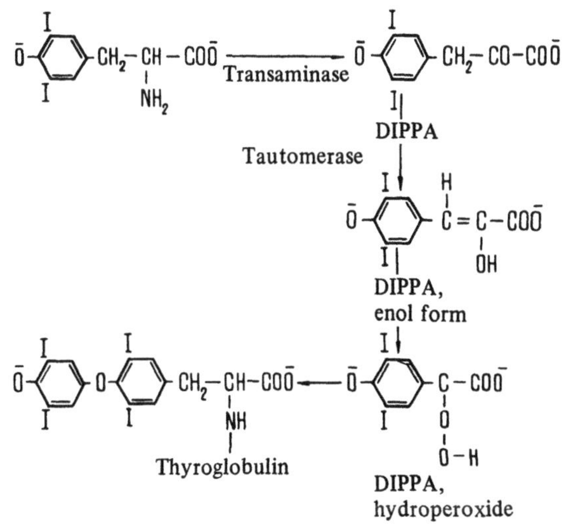

Cahnmann and Funakoshi [72] described a model system for the formation of 3,5,3′-triiodothyronine from 3-iodophenylpyruvic acid, DIT, and oxygen.

The evidence regarding the character of the side chain removed from the iodotyrosine during its condensation with the second iodotyrosine molecule is contradictory.

Meltzer and Stanaback [317] also showed that DIT reacts at room temperature and at neutral pH with DIPPA in the presence of oxygen with the formation of T_4 in a high yield. Shiba et al. [464] showed that DIPPA does not act as a catalyst in this reaction but forms the phenol moiety of T_4. Rattlesnake venom, used as a source of L-aminooxidases, converts DIT into T_4 in the presence of oxygen. DIPPA is first formed in this reaction by oxidative deamination. If the reaction between DIT and DIPPA is in fact a correct model of T_4 formation in the thyroid gland, the question of how DIPPA appears *in vivo* must be answered. It seems more likely that DIPPA is formed from DIT by transamination than by oxidative deamination. In a paper published recently Shiba et al. [465] described a nonenzymic model of thyroxine biosynthesis from DIT after the addition of glyoxalate to the medium. Under these circumstances the reaction proceeds through transamination by chelation of the metal with the Schiff's base of DIT and glyoxalic acid, followed by condensation of the 4-hydroxy-3,5-diiodophenylpyruvic acid formed during this reaction with DIT. Nevertheless, the formation of this complex could not be demonstrated by chemical isolation.

The mechanism of thyroxine formation *in vivo* is unquestionably the key problem in the process of hormone formation. Despite the apparently commonplace nature of the reaction *in vitro*, the mechanism of this process *in vivo* is still far from clear. I have expressed the opinion that thyroxine biosynthesis *in vivo* can take place from free DIT molecules. In previous investigations [526] I described finding ^{131}I-thyroxine in thyroid gland digests and in the blood plasma within 2 h after injecting radioactive iodine into a rat.

On chromatograms of a butanol extract of the medium after incubation of thyroid gland slices for 5 h with radioactive iodine, I demonstrated the presence of T_4 and T_3 bands together with those of MIT, DIT, and iodide. However, under these same conditions neither thyroxine nor triiodotyronine was found in a butanol extract of a digest of thyroid gland tissue. This fact indicates that thyroxine is synthesized (in the presence of thyroid gland tissue) evidently from free iodotyrosine molecules. Recently the synthesis of T_4 from diiodotyrosine has been investigated in our laboratory by Babaev [34] during incubation of thyroid slices with labeled ^{131}I-diiodotyrosine. On the addition of α-ketoglutaric acid and pyridoxal phosphate to the medium, intensive formation of T_4 and T_3 was found both in the thyroglobulin molecule and in the free form. The results confirm the role of transamination of DIT in thyroxine biosynthesis and also, if the mechanism of oxidative condensation described above is accepted, the participation of the peroxidase of thyroid gland tissue in this process.

Biosynthesis of Thyroglobulin and Iodination in the Thyroid Gland

The biosynthesis of thyroid hormones, taking place within the thyroglobulin molecule, has as its essential condition the continuous formation of the protein molecule itself, and the completeness of maturation of the protein is reflected in its adequate iodination. The iodination process, taking place on a polypeptide basis, is the final stage of thyroglobulin biosynthesis, and it creates the conditions required for the formation of iodinated amino acids in its molecule.

Recent autoradiographic and electron-microscopic studies have shown that the biosynthesis of thyroglobulin, an iodinated glycoprotein with complex structure, is a unique process which passes through three independent stages, located in different parts of the follicular epithelial cell: biosynthesis of the protein, addition of carbohydrate components to the polypeptide chain, and iodination.

Biosynthesis of the Polypeptide Chain. This stage of biosynthesis, leading to the formation of the skeleton of the thyroglobulin molecule, takes place in accordance with the well-known general scheme of protein synthesis on the ribosomes and polysomes of the follicular cells of the thyroid gland, on a template of specific mRNA. All the details of formation of the polypeptide chain of the thyroglobulin-like protein have been elucidated in reconstructed systems containing microsomes or polysomes obtained from thyroid gland cells, with the addition of labeled amino acids.

Previous investigations [285, 358, 456] showed that the biosynthesis of thyroglobulin takes place through several consecutive stages.

The process begins with the formation of a polypeptide chain (3–8 S fraction), which evidently must correspond to the product (6 S fraction) obtained by Edelhoch et al. [92, 129] after treatment of thyroglobulin with β-mercaptoethanol. Association of the chains leads to the formation of a 12 S product which, by noncovalent dimerization, yields 17 S prethyroglobulin [285, 359, 455]. This product is converted by halogenation into true thyroglobulin containing on the average 30 atoms of iodine and with a sedimentation coefficient of 19 S [360].

Atakhanova [32], Seitmuratova [535], and Dzhalilova and Saatov [445], in our laboratory, have shown that thyroid slices incorporate ^{14}C-amino acids into proteins which are quarters (3–8 S) and halves (12 S) of the thyroglobulin molecule. These labeled fractions are associated with fractions continuing to be synthesized by incorporation of unlabeled amino acids, and they form small portions of thyroglobulin-like material. These aggregates have a sedimentation coefficient of 17–18 S; they precipitate specifically with antithyroglobulin antibody; and they are converted into substances sedimenting at exactly 19 S by the action of a chemical iodinating system [24, 411, 456, 457, 460]. The interpretation of these results and other similar investigations is that thyroglobulin subunits are synthesized on particulate structures and that iodination takes place primarily after association of the subunits.

During investigation of the biosynthesis of thyroglobulin and its subunits in the rat thyroid gland *in vivo* by administration of ^{3}H-leucine and ^{131}I, it was shown that ^{3}H-leucine is incorporated into 3–8 S, 12 S, and 17–18 S components before it appears in 19 S thyroglobulin [513]. Complete maturation of 19 S thyroglobulin takes 48 h. During prolonged administration of propylthiouracil or perchlorate the protein spectrum changes: 3–8 S is predominant, a 12 S peak appears, and the thyroglobulin peak is shifted to position 17–18 S and 19 S thyroglobulin is never formed. Iodine deficiency accelerates the incorporation of ^{3}H-leucine into thyroglobulin. Small quantities of 12 S thyroglobulin are labeled with ^{125}I in normal rats in the early period, but 24 h is required after administration of ^{125}I for thyroglobulin formation.

Many investigations of the biosynthesis of thyroglobulin-like protein in cell-free systems have been published recently. Ribonucleoprotein particles incorporating labeled amino acids into proteins precipitated by trichloroacetic acid have been isolated from many types of animal tissue.

One of the first investigations of protein synthesis by cell-free systems of the thyroid gland was carried out by Lissitzky's group in Marseille in 1967, and this was followed by other studies [331, 349]. Ribonucleoprotein particles from sheep thyroid gland were prepared with the aid of deoxycholate by centrifugation in a density gradient They consisted chiefly of aggregates larger than 200 S (polysomes) with smaller units forming them. As Kondo et al. [262] showed, the fractions of monomer thyroid ribosomes have a sedimentation constant of 87 S.

Incorporation of ^{14}C-leucine into protein precipitated by TCA, effected by ribonucleoprotein (RNP) particles, required sources of energy and the addition of cell fluid from rat liver or thyroid gland of the medium. Activity of incorporation, calculated per milligram RNA, of RNP-particles from the sheep thyroid gland is analogous to that of protein-synthesizing particles from the liver, but the yield of particles per gram fresh weight of thyroid gland was low. Thyroid polysomes incorporated labeled amino acids more actively than the smaller units. These results were reproduced completely in our laboratory by Seitmuratova et al. [535] with normal and pathological human thyroid glands. This work clearly demonstrated the inhibition of protein synthesis by puromycin and the effect of several coenzymes on the reaction velocity.

Protein newly synthesized on polysomes had no immunological relations with thyroglobulin. Particles extracted with deoxycholate incorporated neither ^{14}C-glucosamine nor ^{14}C-mannose. This important fact was established by other workers using slices [474]. Spiro and Spiro [474] and Allcroft and Salt [25] showed that sugars are incorporated into thyroglobulin by thyroid gland fractions precipitated at 600*g* and 78,000*g* and containing membrane material. Treatment of the RNP-particles with deoxycholate separates them from the membrane material. The important role of membranes in glycoprotein synthesis has also been demonstrated in other tissues.

The inability of the resulting protein to give immunobiological reactions characteristic of thyroglobulin may depend on a number of factors. In the absence of incorporated sugar in the peptide molecule, antigenic properties may be absent. Moreover, the substance synthesized by the polysomes could be a structural protein and not thyroglobulin. If, however, the synthesized protein is the peptide chain of thyroglobulin, it is clear that the sugar component is joined to it at the next stage.

Polyribosomal systems from thyroid gland cells were obtained by Cartouzou et al. [76, 348] who obtained evidence supporting the view of the mechanism based on exchange of newly synthesized subunits of active thyroglobulin. Nunez et al. [360], for instance, reported that thyroid microsomes synthesize thyroglobulin in a cell-free system. These same preparations not only iodinated thyroglobulin but also iodinated all the other proteins added to the incubation medium. In further investigations this group [358] attempted to discover whether thyroid polysomes can carry out the next two processes — synthesis of a protein as complex as thyroglobulin as well as its iodination — in the absence of membranes. They also attempted to answer the question whether the site of synthesis of the polypeptide chain differs from the site of iodination. Experiments were carried out on sheep polysomes obtained by treating subcellular particles with deoxycholate and separated from microsomal and mitochondrial particles on the ultracentrifuge. They showed that thyroid polysomes and microsomes synthesize thyroglobulin (approximately 19 S) in cell-free systems. This is true protein synthesis; membranes are evidently not necessary for this process. The 12 S precursor of thyroglobulin observed in the cellular systems was absent from cell-free systems. This may be because polymerization of the 12 S chain or of the subunit takes place very rapidly and the 12 S fraction formed on the polysomes is quickly hybridized with stable thyroglobulin.

Moralis and Goldberg [331] and Seitmuratova [535], working with preparations of calf ribosomes, observed synthesis as reflected by incorporation of ^{14}C-leucine. Proteins synthesized on thyroid microsomes and ribosomes were similar in their sedimentation and immunochemical properties with thyroglobulin synthesized *in vivo.*

Kondo et al. [262] showed that the intensity of incorporation of ^{14}C-amino acids into thyroglobulin-like protein is higher in heavy polysomes, consisting of 10–35 ribosomes, than in smaller particles. The thyroglobulin in the medium was completely in a bound state, by contrast with cellular systems in which some of the newly synthesized thyroglobulin remains bound to the particles. The RNP-particles contained only a light labeled fraction which evidently does not belong to thyroglobulin. The process of liberation of the chain and polymerization can be observed in both cellular and cell-free systems. In the case of the cell-free system, the newly synthesized chain is liberated in all probability by hybridization with preformed thyroglobulin present in the cell sap.

The specificity observable in cellular systems is lost in cell-free systems. The polysomes have no iodinating activity. Iodinating enzymes are evidently located on the membrane.

Atakhanova [32], in Tashkent, studied the properties of polysomes isolated from the bovine thyroid gland and obtained evidence that 19 S thyroglobulin is synthesized in a polyribosomal cell-free system. As Nayer and Visscher [349] have pointed out, the mechanism of this synthesis may be the result of two consecutive processes. (1) The subunits of thyroglobulin are synthesized on polysomes consisting of approximately 50 ribosomes, possibly containing information for the synthesis of a protein with molecular weight of 150,000, corresponding to the size of the peptide region of the quaternary subunit of thyroglobulin; (2) exchange of these newly synthesized subunits with the subunits of the molecule of native thyroglobulin, which may take place through dissociation and association in the course of formation of the quaternary structure of thyroglobulin.

In connection with this hypothesis it is interesting to examine the latest findings obtained by these workers, for they have described the isolation of polysomes containing 40–60 ribosomes from thyroid glands. These large polyribosomal systems accord well with the predicted molecular weight of the quaternary subunit of thyroglobulin, namely 165,000, and with a ratio of the molecular weight to the ribosomes of 3000, the same as has been established for other proteins.

Atakhanova has also demonstrated the stimulation of protein synthesis *in vitro* by cyclic AMP when a polyribosomal system was used. Under these conditions TSH was ineffective, in agreement with the accepted view of the role of cyclic AMP as the intracellular mediator of hormonal action.

Although Nayer and Visscher [349], working with a cell-free system from the thyroid gland, were able to demonstrate thyroglobulin synthesis by 19 S polysomes, most of the material formed corresponds to 3–8 S subunits. A peak of radioactivity in the 19 S region was found only if the cell-free system contained native thyroglobulin. It is postulated that fragments of thyroglobulin are synthesized in the cell-free system and these are later exchanged with subunits of native thyroglobulin.

In these experiments, on account of the reduced glutathione present in the incubation medium, the 19 S thyroglobulin was reduced to subunits. Reoxidation of the disulfide bonds takes place after dialysis, which removes the reducing agent. As this process comes to an end the newly formed subunits are incorporated into reducible molecules of 19 S thyroglobulin. Thyroglobulin synthesis can also take place in a medium without β-mercaptoethanol. However, the quantity of undissociated thyroglobulin in this case is extremely small. This shows that reduction and uncoiling of the thyroglobulin molecules facilitate covalent association of the thyroglobulin subunits.

Experiments with 6 M guanidine show that aggregation of these new subunits includes the formation of disulfide bonds. In gradient studies conducted under these conditions most of the radioactivity is found in the zone of undissociated 19 S thyroglobulin and in the 12 S zone, which contains six subunits held together by disulfide bonds. Although this reverse organization of S—S bonds must incorporate disulfide-metabolizing enzymes, which exist in the thyroid gland [289], there is as yet no proof that they play a role in cell-free systems.

Foyet and Tixier [151] showed that if thyroid cells obtained from slices by trypsinization are incubated under certain conditions in the presence of TSH, they were reassociated and formed a cell layer similar to the intact gland. The presence of a protein similar to thyroglobulin was demonstrated by microelectrophoresis on agar. The results showed that trypsinized dissociated cell cultures synthesize mature thyroglobulin while monolayer cultures synthesize only a noniodinated thyroglobulin.

In recent years cell cultures obtained from the thyroid gland by trypsinization of slices have been extensively used for studying the individual stages of intrathyroid iodine metabolism and the mechanism of the stimulating effect of TSH. The study of the morphology and function of these cells in culture has shed light on the role of the individual components of the follicles in hormone formation. Research in the author's laboratory has also shown that isolated thyroid cells preserve their ability to concentrate iodine and to incorporate it into organic compounds.

Tong et al. [520] showed that sheep thyroid gland cells in culture are able to take up iodine and incorporate it into iodotyrosines and iodothyronines in amounts comparable with thyroid slices. The cells also preserved their deiodinating activity, and DIT was deiodinated more rapidly than MIT. Consequently, neither the follicular structure nor colloid is essential to the iodine-concentrating function and hormone-forming activity of the thyroid gland. The function of the follicular cavity is essential as a storehouse for the finished hormones and as a means of delivering them into the blood stream under controlled conditions.

Rabin et al. [404] described the growth of thyroid gland cells *in vitro*. They observed that from the second to the fifth day of cultivation the epithelial cells first lose their sensitivity to the specific antibody, the ability to take up iodide from the medium second, and their cytoplasmic thyroid-specific antigen last of all [435].

Pavlovic-Hournac et al. [374] showed that most of the specific protein synthesized in thyroid gland tissue cultures consists of unassociated polypeptide chains. The formation of 19 S and 12 S molecules rapidly declines even after the first day of culture.

The order of incorporation of radioactivity into the individual protein fractions in the course of time was determined by Cavaleri and Serali [77] after injection of labeled ^{14}C-leucine into rats. The radioactivity shifted from 12 S, 1 h after injection, to 16 S 4 h and 18 S 24 h after injection. By 48 h most of the radioactivity was in 19 S protein. The formation of a more stable and compact thyroglobulin molecule is a function of iodination.

Addition of the Carbohydrate Moiety. Cheftel et al. [78] note that synthesis of the polypeptide chain of thyroglobulin precedes addition of the carbohydrate moiety to it, which takes place in intracellular particles. Polysomes, unlike microsomal membranes, do not participate in glycosylation. The progress in our knowledge of the composition and character of binding of the carbohydrate moiety of the thyroglobulin molecule is due primarily to the extensive and systematic researches of Spiro and Spiro. According to data given by Spiro [473] and Cheftel et al. [80], thyroglobulin contains 8.5% of carbohydrates and the linkage of the carbohydrate components to the protein evidently includes N-asparaginylglucosamine bonds. In another investigation using ^{14}C-glucosamine and ^{14}C-leucine as precursors, Spiro and Spiro showed that both the synthesis of the polypeptide of thyroglobulin and the incorporation of the carbohydrate into thyroglobulin take place on the surface of the particles. Experiments with puromycin showed that the peptide part of the molecule is synthesized before the staggered addition of carbohydrates derived from glucose. Activation of monosaccharides into the carbohydrate component of nucleotides and their incorporation into glycoprotein have been observed in the thyroid gland [184].

Cheftel et al. [79] have recently studied the subcellular sites of incorporation of carbohydrate into proteins and thyroglobulin after incubation of sheep thyroid slices with D-(1-^{14}C)-glucosamine and, in some cases, with D-(1-^{14}C)-galactosamine or mannose. By double labeling, using D,L-(4,5-^{3}H)-leucine, these workers were also able to study synthesis of the peptide moiety of the glycoprotein. Analysis of extracts of the microsomes and supernatant on a sucrose density gradient showed that most of the protein, labeled with ^{3}H-leucine and ^{14}C-carbohydrates, synthesized in the system of slices is thyroglobulin.

These results showed that the light precursors of thyroglobulin present in the supernatant were almost unlabeled by ^{14}C-glucosamine, whereas the fraction of almost the same size as thyroglobulin, approximately 18 S, contained appreciable amounts of label. This suggests that the final process in the formation of the molecule is addition of the carbohydrate. The microsomal fractions soluble in deoxycholate (the contents of the vesicles plus the bound membranes) are the site of incorporation of ^{14}C-carbohydrate into the protein, whereas in pure polysomes no such incorporation was observed.

Incubation of slices in the presence of puromycin gave the following results: Incorporation of ^{3}H-leucine was almost completely suppressed whereas incorporation of ^{14}C-carbohydrate was only partially inhibited. These results are further evidence in support of the earlier observation by Spiro and Spiro that glycosylation is observed only after synthesis of the polypeptide and takes place faster on proteins surrounded by microsomal membranes than on the growing peptide chain.

To establish correlation between intracellular protein transport and addition of the carbohydrate, labeled microsomal subfractions of sheep thyroid gland slices in which thyroglobulin was the chief labeled protein were next studied [79]. Intracellular protein transport was found to be of great significance to the addition of carbohydrates to the peptide chain. Rapid transport of protein-bound label from ribosomes to coarse microsomes (including bound membranes and contents of vesicles) was established, but no transfer from these fractions to the smooth microsomes was observed. The results of these experiments also indicate slow secretion of protein from the endoplasmic reticulum into the colloid. On incubation of slices with ^{14}C-glucosamine, incorporation of the label was observed into both the coarse and the smooth fractions of the microsomes. The specific radioactivities of protein-bound glucosamine and sialic acid were higher in the coarse than in the smooth fraction of the microsomes. The results show that glycosylation takes place within the membranes of the intact endoplasmic reticulum rather than only within the Golgi elements.

A slight degree of iodination was later discovered to take place on the surface of the particles, although considerable additional iodination is also found elsewhere.

Iodination of the newly formed glycoprotein molecule is the final stage of thyroglobulin biosynthesis. It is generally accepted that this process does not take place in the course of synthesis of the polypeptide chain of the protein: Iodinated amino acids do not participate in its synthesis, and no direct iodination of amino acids is observed at this stage. Evidence has been obtained that thyroglobulin is iodinated only after aggregation of its subunits [231, 469].

The question of the precise localization of the iodination site has also been debated for a long time. It would logically be expected that iodination takes place intracellularly, for the formation of the iodoprotein is linked with intracellular particles with an active peroxidase mechanism. However, autoradiographic studies have shown that the process takes place at the cell-colloid surface. The apical border of the cells with the membranes of the microvillus is evidently the active region of thyroglobulin iodination. Consequently, iodination must be extracellular. Only completely iodinated thyroglobulin with a sedimentation coefficient of 19 S can exist in the apical part of the cell, so that polymerization of the thyroglobulin precursors must take place continuously during their migration from the rough endoplasmic reticulum to the apical zone of the cells [293].

In the earlier investigations of the anatomical localization of iodide fixation, the chief criterion used was the distribution of radioactivity in the various structural components of the gland at different times after injection of radioactive iodine into the animals. Experiments by Leblond and Gross [267] and Wollman and Wodinsky [558], together with our own investigations [528], showed that radioactive iodine, after injection into animals, appears very quickly in the thyroid gland. Wollman and Wodinsky describe the appearance of radioactive label in the thyroid gland of mice after 11–16 sec and of rats after 30 sec, but only in the colloid, not in the cells. Our own observations [528] showed that radioactive iodine appears within a few seconds both in the colloid and in the epithelial cells; its content in the colloid rises very rapidly so that after 15–30 sec it accounts for 83–85% of the total activity of the gland. Activity in the colloid in the earliest stages after injection of radioiodine is distributed as a narrow band close to the apical end of the follicular cells. However, the problem of the iodination site cannot yet be regarded as finally solved until the precise correlation between this process and biosynthesis and the intracellular migration of thyroglobulin has been established and the role of specific mechanisms and enzyme systems iodinating the protein molecule has been elucidated. Investigations with cell-free systems have recently shown [261] that the iodination of thyroglobulin involves the participation of enzymes obtained from the microsomes of the thyroid gland and that MIT and DIT, connected with thyroglobulin, are formed on the addition of a system generating H_2O_2, i.e., glucose and glucose oxidase. The peroxidase of the thyroid gland is known to be necessary for oxidation of iodide, iodinating tyrosine to MIT and DIT [224, 225]. Direct addition of H_2O_2 to the system also induces iodination, but not for long. Thyroglobulin is iodinated more effectively in this system than free tyrosine or MIT, serum albumin, or egg albumin. These investigations, together with the extensive experiments of Tong et al. [520] with a suspension of thyroid gland cells obtained by trypsinization of slices, showed that the presence of colloid or of a follicular structure is not essential for the iodide-concentrating function or for hormone synthesis. It can be concluded from these and other investigations that iodination, with the formation of iodinated amino acids linked together in the thyroglobulin molecule, can take place entirely within the cell. Croft and Pitt-Rivers [91] have recently made an autoradiographic study of the initial site of formation of protein-bound iodine in the thyroid gland after injection of fixing material into the aorta to allow quicker removal of the thyroid gland and fixation. They found a mainly intracellular accumulation of ^{125}I after 5 and 55 sec. If the perfusion was continued for 2 min or if fixation by immersion was used, the label was found chiefly in the peripheral zone of the follicular surface. These observations confirm the view that the initial site of iodine binding with protein is intracellular, but the nature of the binding protein was not established. If this hypothesis regarding the iodination site of thyroglobulin is accepted, it still remains uncertain how the thyroglobulin molecule penetrates into the colloid, whether any further iodination takes place in the colloid, and what other changes in its structure, if any, take place.

Another aspect of the thyroglobulin iodination problem is the mechanism of the process itself and the participation of cellular components and enzymes in it. The first reactions after the uptake of iodine by the thyroid gland, resulting in its organic combination, require as an essential condition the oxidation of iodide into elementary iodine:

$$2I^- \rightarrow I_2 + 2e^-$$

It has been postulated that this reaction may be catalyzed by the peroxidase found histochemically by Dempsey [108] and also by De Robertis [107] both in the cells and in the colloid. Enzymologic evidence of the presence of peroxidase in the thyroid gland has recently been obtained [21, 224, 487] and, in addition, reports of purification of the enzyme after solubilization from a fraction of the intracellular particles have been published [104, 223, 487]. According to the latest findings of Alexander [22], the peroxidase, being a hemin enzyme, is linked with apoperoxidase by a covalent bond and not by a more labile bond as was hitherto considered.

After the work of Weiss [549] and Fawcett and Kirkwood [150] the impression was obtained that the thyroid gland contains a special tyrosine-iodinating enzyme known as tyrosine iodinase. Subsequent research has conclusively shown that the iodinase activity is linked with peroxidase and that there is no separate iodinating enzyme [291, 487]. Reports on the purification and study of the physicochemical properties of the thyroid gland peroxidase have been published. According to the latest evidence the peroxidase in the thyroid gland participates in several reactions: oxidation of iodide and the oxidative condensation of two iodotyrosine molecules into thyroxine. The presence of deiodination of thyroxine in the thyroid gland and the participation of peroxidase in this process have also recently been demonstrated [44, 98].

According to Bénard et al. [44], in response to stimulation of the thyroid gland with TSH, H_2O_2 formation is intensified, and this leads to an increase in iodination. Morrison and co-workers (cited in [487]) developed an improved method of isolating peroxidase from the thyroid gland with a high yield and investigated the activity of the enzyme in accelerating iodination and oxidation. They found that trypsin reduces the iodinating power of the enzyme by 80%, whereas the oxidative activity is not significantly changed.

Nagasaka and De Groot [337] isolated a peroxidase from coarse mitochondrial-microsomal fractions of calf thyroid gland by trypsinization and studied its molecular structure. Partially purified preparations of the soluble enzyme contained a hemoprotein with an absorption spectrum that differed from that of hemoglobin. Neither hemoglobin nor hematin exhibit iodinating activity in the samples. The enzyme was active in the peroxidase reaction of conversion of I^- into I_3^-. I_3^- or I_2, in equilibrium with I^-, react quantitatively with tyrosine and form iodotyrosine.

If the iodide ion in the thyroid gland is activated by peroxidase by an oxidative mechanism, hydrogen peroxide formation is essential to the reaction. As has already been stated, the ability of homogenates and fractions of subcellular particles of the thyroid gland to form iodotyrosine from free tyrosine and iodide with utilization of hydrogen peroxide has been demonstrated by many investigations *in vitro*. The molecular weight of the enzyme was 80,000; in its structure it was a tetramer, breaking up readily into monomers, each with a molecular weight of 17,000. The iodinating activity of both forms of the enzyme, known as peroxidase-tyrosine-iodinase, was identical. In these experiments artificial systems generating hydrogen peroxide were used, such as glucose + glucose oxidase, FMN + magnesium ions, and magnesium + $NADH_2$ and an $NADPH_2$-generating system.

Taurog [499, 500] has recently obtained pure preparations of peroxidase from pig thyroid glands and has studied their physicochemical properties and the mechanism of iodination and synthesis of thyroxine. The enzyme was a hemoprotein with a molecular weight of 62,000.

Working with partial fractions of organelles of sheep thyroid glands consisting of mitochondria and microsomes, Taurog et al. [502, 504] showed that bound molecules of tyrosine are iodinated and that the addition of a flavin coenzyme considerably increases the activity of the iodinating system. In their opinion, the catalytic oxidation of iodide taken up by the thyroid gland, before its incorporation into tyrosine and protein, is due to the H_2O_2 with the participation of the enzyme iodide peroxidase. This enzyme was found not only in thyroid gland tissue, but also in the salivary glands [17].

Alexander [18] showed that other naturally occurring biological oxidizing agents or electron carriers cannot replace H_2O_2 although flavin coenzymes stimulate the utilization of iodide by thyroid gland preparations. Further research showed that catalase and anaerobiosis prevent the activation of iodide oxidation by flavin. A more detailed study of this problem by the same worker [23] showed that the product obtained by dialysis of a thyroid gland homogenate in phosphate buffer, with the addition of an H_2O_2 generating system (glucose-6-phosphate + glucose oxidase), oxidizes iodide and incorporates it into monoiodotyrosine and protein molecules. On the addition of crystalline catalase the oxidation of iodide was stopped.

Alexander [20] fractionated thyroid gland extracts containing iodide peroxidase into a prosthetic group (hemin) and an apoenzyme. Cytochrome c could not reactivate the apoenzyme after dissociation of the enzyme.

More recently Igo and Mackler [227] have described the isolation of a highly active enzyme preparation from the mitochondrial and microsomal system of thyroid gland homogenates which catalyzes the incorporation of iodide into organic forms in the presence of H_2O_2 and tyrosine. The enzyme activity was completely lost after heating to 75°C for 5 min. The addition of NADP, NAD, ATP, and Mg^{++} did not change its activity. The enzyme not only oxidized inorganic iodide into monoiodotyrosine, but it also catalyzed the formation of diiodotyrosine, thyroxine, and triiodothyronine.

However, the presence and mechanism of formation of the hydrogen peroxide, the essential substrate for the organic fixation of iodide in the intact thyroid gland, has not yet been established.

The sequence of the iodination reactions is illustrated by the scheme

$$AH_2 + O_2 \rightarrow H_2O_2 + A$$

$$H_2O_2 + 2I^- + 2H^+ \rightarrow 2H_2O + I_2$$

$$I_2 + \text{Tyrosine} \rightarrow \text{MIT} + I^- + H^+$$

In the case of thyroid homogenates Shussler and Ingbar [454] showed that reduced pyridine nucleotides stimulate the iodination reaction, and this stimulation was later extensively studied [102] by the use of fractions of particles. Suzuki [487] studied the relations between oxidation of reduced nucleotides and the iodination reactions. The activity of oxidation of reduced nucleotides in cell components and in mitochondrial, microsomal, and soluble fractions, the inhibition of oxidation by various inhibitors, and their relationship to iodination were measured. Removal of $NADPH_2$–cytochrome c reductase from the microsomal fraction by pancreatic lipase had no effect on the iodinating activity. With the use of $NADPH_2$ and

$NADPH_2$—cytochrome c reductase and vitamin K a new system generating hydrogen peroxide was reconstructed. A soluble iodinase, iodinating free tyrosine, highly dependent on oxygen and sensitive to the action of catalase, was prepared from thyroid gland microsomes.

The presence of H_2O_2 in pig thyroid gland and the progressive increase in its content under the influence of TSH on prolonging the incubation were demonstrated by Bénard and Brault [44]. These workers consider that H_2O_2 formation may be the result of solution of lysosomal colloidal droplets in the process of pinocytosis induced in the thyroid gland by TSH.

The process of deiodination of iodotyrosines, also taking place in the thyroid gland, must also be discussed.

Attention to the existence of dehalogenases, removing iodine from the iodotyrosine molecule but not from iodothyronines, in the thyroid gland, liver, kidneys, and salivary glands, was first drawn by Roche et al. [427]. According to Stanbury and Morris [477], deiodinase activity is localized in the microsomes, and $NADPH_2$ is required as coenzyme. However, the presence of a deiodinase of iodotyrosines was established not only in the mitochondria and microsomes of the thyroid gland, but also in its soluble fraction.

A number of papers describing a defect of iodotyrosine dehalogenation in the thyroid gland have been published [48, 103, 475]. This process, taking place under the influence of the deiodinating enzyme, continuously removes the excess of MIT and DIT liberated during proteolysis of thyroglobulin. Absence or a very low concentration of MIT and DIT in the circulating blood, despite their high percentage in thyroglobulin and their liberation during hormonal secretion, is explained by their rapid deiodination in this way. The iodide thus liberated is reused for hormone formation.

Deiodination of iodotyrosines is assumed to take place under the influence of a special deiodinating enzyme or deiodinase. This enzyme evidently utilizes hydrogen peroxide in its action, and it may be identical with iodinating peroxidase [258].

Recent investigations have shown that deiodination of thyroxine takes place in the thyroid gland. Damber et al. [98] investigated the deiodination of thyroxine by thyroid gland homogenates as reflected in the presence of an iodinating system of peroxidase and hydrogen peroxide in the gland. In the presence of glucose oxidase, generating H_2O_2, the gland tissue actively deiodinated thyroxine. The system had many features in common with preparations of peripheral thyroxine-deiodinating tissues. Deiodination was inhibited by PTU, methimazole, and preliminary injection of TSH into hypophysectomized animals. The results showed that the thyroid gland contains a peroxidase which may influence the deiodination of thyroxine.

This problem was also investigated by Haibach [196] who compared the deiodinating activity of the tissues of the thyroid gland, kidney, and skeletal muscle of rats kept on a low iodide diet. The results showed that fresh thyroid gland tissue reduces the quantity of added labeled T_4 and, at the same time, increases the quantity of T_3 in the medium. Liver tissue also increased the T_3/T_4 ratio, but by a lesser degree than thyroid gland. Fresh thyroid gland tissue also deiodinates labeled DIT and MIT. Experiments with inhibition showed, however, that the deiodinating systems for T_4 and the iodotyrosines are not identical. The unsolved problem of the formation of triiodothyronine from thyroxine by deiodination again comes to the fore in these investigations, and the results of the experiments indicate that T_3 and T_4 are formed actually in the thyroid gland itself although, admittedly, in animals on an iodine-deficient diet.

However, the question of deiodination of the iodotyrosines in the thyroid gland cannot be regarded as completely solved as regards either the extent of this process in the gland or the mechanism of the reaction. Deiodination of iodotyrosines also takes place in other tissues, since under normal conditions DIT and MIT are not found in the blood stream or, evidently, in the peripheral tissues. Nevertheless, the presence of an inborn error of iodine metabolism in man, the principal manifestation of which is inability to deiodinate injected MIT and DIT, suggests that the peripheral mechanism of deiodination is also important. The extent of MIT and DIT deiodination in the thyroid gland under physiological conditions was determined quantitatively by Nigmatov [352] in the writer's laboratory. In experiments on dogs, labeled DIT was injected into an artery of the thyroid gland and the composition of the iodized components in the outflowing venous blood was determined for 30 min. Nigmatov found that during the first 15 min after injection of DIT, 47.4 ± 5.6% of the activity left the gland, but only 9.46 ± 1.17% of the injected activity left the gland during the next 15 min. The animals were then thyroidectomized and the total activity and distribution of its fractions were determined in the thyroid gland. These investigations showed that 24.2% of the injected activity is found in the gland after 30 min; 45.9% of the activity is extracted by butanol while the rest remains protein-bound. Chromatographic analysis of the butanol extract of the thyroid gland homogenates revealed 62% DIT, 11% MIT, and 27% iodide, while the corresponding figures for the digest of the gland after hydrolysis were 48%, 32%, and 19%.

An extract of blood plasma collected in the course of 15 min contained 45.8% DIT, 33.12% MIT, and 22.3% inorganic iodine. These results indicate rapid deiodination of iodotyrosines in the thyroid glands on a considerable scale. Nevertheless, some of the iodotyrosines enter the venous blood from the gland and the general circulation, to an extent which depends on substrate saturation of the dehalogenizing system. Part of the iodine liberated is bound by the gland and takes part in the intrathyroid circulation, but in the course of 15 min 22% of the injected activity is excreted from the gland as inorganic iodine. This iodide was evidently eliminated during deiodination of the DIT and was not utilized by the gland. The results indicate the limited capacity of the deiodinating system of the thyroid, although it is sufficient to bring about deiodination of the mono- and diiodotyrosines formed from thyroglobulin under physiological conditions.

Excretion of Thyroid Hormones

In the modern view the thyroglobulin synthesized on the cytoplasmic organelles, when liberated from them, takes part in a continuous migration toward the apical end of the epithelial cells and into the cavity of the follicle, in the course of which the molecule acquires its final structure and becomes mature. Before entering the blood stream, the greater part of the synthesized, hormonally active thyronine structures first enter the cavity of the follicles in the composition of the thyroglobulin, forming, together with the other components, the amorphous mass of colloid.

The thyroglobulin exists temporarily in the colloid as a reserve product containing ready-made hormones in a bound form. When the body needs the hormone, the thyroglobulin is decomposed and the iodinated amino acids enter the blood stream or lymph (Figure 4). As long ago as in 1916 Bensly [46] postulated that normal secretion in the thyroid gland takes place through the basal end of the cell directly into the blood. If the activity of the cells exceeds the body's needs, the cells begin to liberate the secretion into the lumen of the follicle. Other workers [12, 546] have accepted that direct secretion into the blood stream can take place as a normal phenomenon or, perhaps, under exceptional circumstances.

However, in the generally accepted view, direct secretion into the blood is impossible for the further reason that iodination of thyroglobulin and the formation of thyroxine in it, like proteolysis of thyroglobulin, take place at least to some extent in the cavity of the follicle, in the colloid itself [187]. One such scheme, attaching decisive importance to processes taking place in the cavity of the follicle, is based chiefly on histoautoradiographic data for iodine fixation [318, 558] and on the discovery by De Robertis [107] of a proteolytic enzyme in the colloid.

In recent years the process of intracellular migration of thyroglobulin during biosynthesis of the molecule and excretion of the hormones has been thoroughly investigated by electron-microscopic and histoautoradiographic techniques. The results have finally shown that iodination of the protein takes place chiefly in the colloid [41, 247, 293, 479, 546]. Histochemical and autoradiographic investigations [336, 396, 468, 557] have clearly shown that colloid can pass from the cavity of the follicles into the follicular cell by

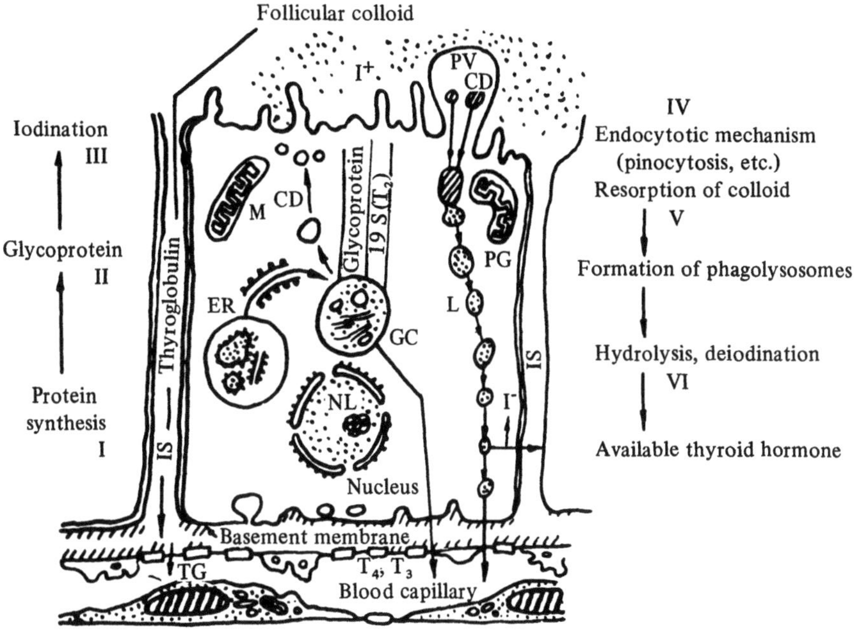

Fig. 4. Diagram showing intracellular migration and proteolysis of thyroglobulin: M–mitochondria, GC–Golgi complex, NL–nucleolus, L–lysosome, ER–endoplasmic reticulum, CD–colloid droplets, PV–pinocytotic vesicles, IS–intercellular space, PG–phagolysosome, TG–thyroglobulin.

pinocytosis as colloid droplets. Wetzil et al. [552] showed by a histochemical method that the fusion of colloid droplets with lysosomes leads to the formation of *secondary lysosomes* [101] in which proteolysis of thyroglobulin evidently takes place [557].

These two types of iodinated particles could in fact be differentiated only by combined electron-microscopic and histochemical studies [552], whereas proteolytic activity was demonstrated only after homogenization of the *mitochondrial fraction*, which may perhaps contain both types of iodinated particles [35].

Recently this problem has been fully investigated by the study of the composition of isolated fractions of lysosomes and phagolysosomes or secondary lysosomes [36] during stimulation of the thyroid gland by injections of TSH. The rapid elimination of iodoamino acid hormones from the thyroid gland after injection of thyrotropin is the result of proteolysis of the follicular colloid. As recent work has shown, hydrolysis of the colloid takes place not in the lumen of the follicle itself, but in the intracellular phagolysosomes, formed by fusion of the colloid droplets and the lysosomes, followed by elimination of iodinated amino acids into the blood stream. This thyroid gland fraction, described by Pick's group (cited in [35]) as P_{15} particles, is obtained by centrifuging at 800–15,000*g*, contains colloid droplets, lysosomes, and phagolysosomes, and accounts for less than 2% of the total protein of the thyroid gland. After injection of TSH the iodoproteins of this fraction are increased by 50–100% through pinocytosis.

Previous investigations [375] showed that reduced glutathione stimulates the elimination of iodoamino acids from thyroglobulin during incubation of both P_{15} particles and of purified thyroglobulin with lysosomal enzymes. In the investigations 15–17 S, 12–13 S, 8–9 S, and 4–6 S intermediates, corresponding to fractions formed after chemical cleavage of the disulfide bonds of thyroglobulin with alkali, were found. The same workers later [376] showed that rupture of the disulfide bond is an important stage in the proteolysis of thyroglobulin and that the particles formed in the phagolysosomes are degraded and not newly formed particles of thyroglobulin.

Trikojus [532] showed that injection of TSH into hypophysectomized animals causes rapid migration of the granules of the lysosomes from the basal part of the thyroid cell to the apical part. During this period colloid droplets from the cavity of the follicle migrate into the cells. More recently Simon et al. [467], after developing a method of rapid fractionation of whole iodinated particles of follicular cells, confirmed that the rat thyroid gland contains more than two distinct populations of iodinated particles. Colloid droplets entering the cells from the cavity of the follicles merge with the dense lysosome-like enzyme granules. As they move toward the base of the cells these mixed granules are believed to undergo disintegration and, as they give up their hormones, they decrease in size and condense again.

Excretion of thyroid hormones into the blood thus assumes their liberation during the proteolysis of thyroglobulin from the intracellular colloid droplets and their penetration from the cavity of the follicles through pinocytosis.

Williams and Wolff [554] investigated the role of microtubules in the secretion of the thyroid gland and showed that colchicine, the fungal metabolite cytocholazine [553], and other agents active against microtubules blocked the liberation of ^{131}I into the incubation medium from previously labeled mouse thyroid glands. In their opinion inhibition of the formation of colloid droplets and the absence of action on adenyl cyclase point to a role of the colchicine-sensitive microtubules in colloid endocytosis in the thyroid gland.

In recent investigations Williams et al. [553] demonstrated a direct correlation between the formation of intracellular colloid droplets in response to stimulation by TSH and dibutyryl-cAMP and the elimination of ^{131}I from the previously labeled thyroid gland. These findings confirm the view that the formation of colloid droplets is the first stage in the secretion of thyroid hormones. Meanwhile the colloid droplets appearing in the cell in response to thyroid stimulation are the result of resorption of colloid from the cavity. There are sufficient grounds for assuming also that intracellular colloid droplets are precursors of the colloid in the cavity of the follicle.

Gorbunova [180], for instance, considers that the dense granules formed in the Golgi zone are thyroglobulin, which becomes less dense as it migrates toward the cavity of the follicle and is converted into large colloid droplets, discharging their contents into the lumen of the follicle. However, it has been postulated [133] that all the populations of colloid droplets are heterogeneous in origin.

So far as the large, dense granules are concerned, most workers consider them to be lysosome-like, for these granules contain enzymes such as acid phosphatase, esterase, and cathepsin [356, 552, 557] and they supply enzymes for the proteolysis of thyroglobulin in phagocytosed colloid droplets. Although it is now generally accepted that the chief site of thyroglobulin proteolysis is the intracellular lysosome granules, the presence of a special protease in thyroid gland tissue, first demonstrated by De Robertis [107] histochemically in the follicular colloid of the rat thyroid gland, has never been disputed. This enzyme has subsequently been studied by several workers. It was extracted from the guinea pig thyroid gland with 60% aqueous glycerol. This extract hydrolyzes edestin at pH 4.0. Consequently, the proteolytic activity disappears at physiological pH values. Roche et al. (cited in [392]) showed that extracts of ^{131}I-labeled thyroid gland liberates ^{131}I-labeled diiodotyrosine and thyroxine during incubation at pH 3.5 and at 37°C. Purified preparations of thyroid protease, hydrolyzing thyroglobulin with the formation of thyroxine and iodotyrosines, as well as an undialyzable iodine-containing residue, were later obtained.

Kobayashi [256] recently investigated the liberation of iodoamino acids from thyroglobulin by various proteinase preparations or by thyroid protease and found that in every case MIT is more easily freed than DIT. Regardless of the degree of iodination, the iodothyronines were more resistant than iodotyrosines. In Kobayashi's opinion, the rapid removal of MIT depends on its structure and not on the quaternary structure of the thyroglobulin.

The purified protease system is complex in character and, besides acting on hemoglobin, when tested on several peptides, splits only one dipeptide, namely cysteinyltyrosine. Later work showed that the cysteinyltyrosine component can be separated from the proteinase, and in the presence of the enzyme hydrolysis of other cysteine-containing peptides readily takes place: L-cysteinyl-L-phenylalanine and L-leucyl-L-cysteine.

An increase in the peptidase activity has also been demonstrated under the influence of thyrotropic hormone, but the concentration of cysteinyl tyrosinase in the gland was reduced although the total activity of the enzyme in the gland or per unit weight of gland was increased. Under the influence of methylthiouracil, the activity of both cysteinyl peptidase and protease was reduced. Talanti and Hopsu [489] demonstrated a decrease in cysteinyl aminopeptidase and leucyl aminopeptidase activity under the influence of methylthiouracil and TSH.

More recently the protease component of the thyroid gland was purified by chromatography on a cellulose column and separated into fractions of two different acid proteases [194]. One fraction has a pH optimum at 3.8 and the other at 5.7.

The presence of a complex system of proteolytic enzymes of the thyroid gland has thus been established, but very little is yet known about its physiological role. Despite much investigation of the properties of the cysteinyl aminopeptidase, it is not yet possible to state whether, in conjunction with protease, it has a proteolytic action on thyroglobulin.

The problem of thyroid secretion has several other aspects. The first of these is the continuity of the secretory process. As Dougherty et al. [114] showed, hormone formation in the thyroid gland takes place continuously and inorganic iodine enters the gland at the same rate as hormonal iodine is liberated from it.

The heterogeneity of the thyroid iodine cycle deserves attention. In recent investigations using double labeling of the iodized components of the rat thyroid gland, first by injection of ^{125}I for 4–6 days, and later by injection of ^{131}I 14–18 h before sacrifice, secretion was studied by perfusion of the gland *in situ*. The results showed that the $^{131}I/^{125}I$ ratio for thyroxine and triiodothyronine is 1.8–2.7 times higher in the venous blood than in a digest of the same glands. After injection of nitrotyrosine, a strong inhibitor of deiodination of the iodotyrosines, these factors were between 1.5 and 2.8 for MIT and DIT. It was accordingly concluded that the ^{131}I of the newly formed iodinated amino acids is eliminated or "cycled" more rapidly than and in preference to the ^{125}I of the iodoamino acids formed previously. These results confirm the existing view that the thyroid gland secretes the iodine arriving later in preference to that arriving earlier, on the principle of "last come, first used."

Another aspect of the problem is concerned with the composition of the iodinated components liberated during proteolysis of thyroglobulin and excreted into the blood stream. Despite the liberation of large quantities of iodotyrosines in addition to hormonally active thyronines during proteolysis of thyroglobulin, only the ready-made hormones and not the iodinated tyrosines enter the blood stream. The absence of appreciable amounts of MIT and DIT in the circulation (about two-thirds of the total organically bound iodine of the gland and liberated by proteolysis of the protein) cannot be explained by their poor penetrating power. It is generally accepted that iodinated tyrosines are rapidly deiodinated in the thyroid gland, so that they do not accumulate in the epithelial cells in the free state and the inorganic iodine liberated as a result of their deiodination is immediately reutilized.

This explanation is supported by the presence of the deiodinating enzymes deiodinase, detaching iodine from the MIT and DIT molecules. However, it is difficult to suppose that the whole quantity of MIT and DIT liberated can be deiodinated so rapidly that they cannot penetrate into the circulation. This is all the more unlikely because we know that the deiodinating enzyme is found in particles of the epithelial cells, while the proteolysis of thyroglobulin takes place in the lysosomal granules in the course of their migration toward the basal end of the cell. These arguments suggest the need for a more thorough investigation of proteolysis and the quantitative description of deiodination of the mono- and diiodotyrosines *in vivo* under physiological conditions.

The results obtained by Torresani et al. [521] are interesting in this respect. During incubation of rat thyroid gland previously labeled with ^{131}I, these workers found progressive liberation of radioactive materials into the medium, so that after 7 h it contained about 64% of the total radioactivity of the gland. According to their observations mainly native thyroglobulin is secreted into the medium. At the beginning of incubation it accounts for 75% of the radioactivity and rises to 95–98% after 7 h. In addition, small quantities of MIT, DIT, T_3, T_4, and iodide are secreted. The addition of TSH, although not increasing the liberation of thyroglobulin, increases the secretion of hormones and iodine.

On the other hand, during the action of large doses of radioactive iodine ^{131}I, large quantities of MIT and DIT enter the blood stream [105, 527]; this possibly reflects a disturbance of the normal course of thyroglobulin proteolysis and, eventually, penetration of iodinated tyrosines through the cell membrane.

According to reports in the literature, certain iodinated compounds of unknown nature, possibly iodinated peptides or an iodinated amino acid with more rapid biological action, appear during the proteolysis of thyroglobulin. However, these reports have not been subsequently confirmed, and there are no grounds for considering that proteolysis of normal thyroglobulin leads to other products being formed during the proteolysis besides MIT, DIT, T_4, and small quantities of T_3.

Evidence has been obtained of differences in the rate of secretion of radioiodine from individual thyroid follicles. Lowenstein and Wollmann [290] showed by autoradiographic investigation of rat thyroid glands 1 and 14 days after injection of radioiodine that the isotope is retained longer in the peripheral follicles and the follicles of the isthmus. Some follicles with an autoradiographic picture of low intensity also were found, suggesting considerable functional heterogeneity in the rate of diffusion of the iodoproteins in the individual cavities and of a reserve of relatively slowly metabolized iodine.

The rate of secretion of the thyroid hormones has been investigated in various species of animals and in man by different methods. The rate of entry of inorganic iodine and of elimination of hormonal iodine has been shown to be constant and equal. The rate of secretion of ^{131}I by the thyroid gland was calculated from the loss of this isotope from the gland after injection of topazole, which blocks the repeated absorption of ^{131}I, and also from the kinetics of distribution of thyroid ^{131}I in the extrathyroid reserves before administration of topazole. The two methods gave equivalent values, namely, about 10% per diem of the total thyroid iodine in thyrotoxic subjects. The use of various methods has shown that euthyroid subjects secrete 115–120 μg of organically bound iodine per diem.

Thyroid Hormones in the Blood

After excretion of the hormones into the blocd stream they are distributed to peripheral organs, then penetrate into the cells, and undergo metabolic conversions in the tissues.

Many years have passed since the discovery of thyroxine, and the nature of the thyroid hormones circulating in the blood has been studied in detail. We now know that the principal circulating thyroid hormone is thyroxine, which accounts for three-quarters of the total blood iodine. Small quantities of a second hormonal principle of the gland, 3,5,3′-triiodothyronine, are also present in the circulating blood. In addition, iodide is constantly present in the blood in an amount equivalent to 21–30% of the total blood iodine, and there may also be negligible quantities of 3,3′,5′-triiodothyronine, as well as 3,3′-diiodothyronine [426], which has no role to play in the hormonal balance of the body.

Besides the hormonal and inorganic iodine, the blood may also contain a certain quantity of monoiodotyrosine and diiodotyrosine, which under certain conditions may reach perceptible amounts. Data in the literature on this problem are extensive but often contradictory. Although fresh research into the presence of iodotyrosines and the changes in their content in the blood stream under special conditions continue to appear, in the writer's view this problem does not play an essential role because free iodotyrosines are unimportant in the iodine metabolism of the body under physiological conditions.

The appearance of iodinated peptides and iodoproteins in the blood has also been reported. This condition occurs after destruction of the thyroid gland with radioactive iodine [528] and in certain forms of congenital diseases of the thyroid gland when abnormal iodoproteins are synthesized in the gland [301, 551]. Under normal conditions thyroglobulin is absent from the blood stream, as Lerman (cited in [387]) showed immunochemically in 1940.

Binding of Thyroxine with the Transport Proteins of the Blood

Electrophoretic studies under various conditions have shown that the thyroxine in the blood serum is combined with three binding proteins, an α-globulin called thyroxine-binding globulin (TBG), thyroxine-binding prealbumin (TBPA), and albumin. In normal human serum containing a normal quantity of thyroxine, at pH 7.5 from 50 to 60% of the hormone is bound with TBG, 30–40% with TBPA, and about 10% with albumin.

Recent investigations of the thyroxine-binding proteins in rat blood serum [100] by electrophoresis on polyacrylamide gel have shown that added radiothyroxine is distributed between three proteins: slowly migrating prealbumin (carrying 55%), albumin (15%), and postalbumin corresponding to thyroxine-binding globulin (18%). This distribution spectrum is qualitatively analogous to the distribution between the protein fractions of human serum, although there are quantitative differences. The principal carrier of T_4 in rat serum is prealbumin, whereas in human serum it is postalbumin — thyroxine-binding globulin. A study of the influence of competitive inhibitors of T_4 binding (D-T_4, tetraiodothyroacetic acid, salicylate, diphenylhydantoin) showed that the combining sites of T_4 on the three proteins are qualitatively different.

All three binding proteins have been obtained in the pure form and characterized [365, 457]. TBG is an acid glycoprotein containing sialic acid, which plays no part in binding the hormone [56]. The concentration of this specific protein in the serum is too low (1 mg/100 ml) to allow it to be localized by any electrophoretic technique. TBPA is also a glycoprotein. Its concentration is 300 mg/100 ml, and it is found before albumin during electrophoresis on starch gel and in other types of electrophoresis. Although TBPA has much less affinity for thyroxine, it is nevertheless an important factor in T_4 transport because of its higher concentration than TBG.

Albumin binds T_4 and T_3 in the same way as many other pharmacological and hydrophobic substances, but without any particularly high affinity. As a result of interaction between binding proteins and thyroid hormones, 99.9% of the thyroxine is in a reversible physical combination with proteins and only 0.1% is in the free state, equivalent to 6×10^{-11} M of free thyroxine.

The generally accepted view of this matter is that protein-bound T_4 is in a state of dynamic equilibrium with the unbound thyroxine, which can diffuse into the peripheral cells [228, 364, 457], and that the unbound thyroxine is responsible for the thyroid state of the body and determines its peripheral effect, the rate of its metabolism, and its influence on the pituitary. However, the association constants are so high that only negligible quantities of thyroxine can be found in the serum in the unbound state.

The results of investigation of the rate of dissociation of T_4 from TBG and TBPA [215] showed that the negligible stocks of free thyroxine in the plasma are cycled more than 100 times every second; two-thirds of this flow is liberated from the combining sites of the prealbumin.

The correct quantitative evaluation of these extremely small amounts of T_4 is an extremely difficult problem which has not yet been satisfactorily solved. Excellent correlation exists between the level of free thyroxine and its stimulant effect, whereas no such correlation is found with the total content of T_4.

In euthyroid persons the ability of the thyroxine-binding proteins (TBP) to accept thyroxine has been estimated at about 0.4 μg thyroxine to 1 ml blood. Free thyroxine remains in the readily metabolized form and in reversible equilibrium with TBP and albumin. The plasma TBP concentration is sufficient to produce complete fixation of endogenous thyroxine. In addition, plasma can bind a certain quantity of the exogenous hormone. It was shown by adding increasing quantities of thyroxine to serum that although a large proportion of indicator concentrations of labeled thyroxine was associated with TBP, with an increase in the hormone concentration more and more of it was fixed with the albumin. It was accordingly postulated that TBP and albumin are primary and secondary carriers, respectively, of thyroxine.

Triiodothyronine is also bound by the blood proteins although rather less strongly. Its behavior in the blood differs greatly from that of L-thyroxine. Conjugation products of L-triiodothyronine with blood proteins are concentrated on globulin glycoproteins and bound together much less strongly than those of L-thyroxine on the same fractions *in vivo*. This phenomenon is of great physiological importance, and it explains the extremely low content of triiodothyronine in the blood despite its continuous liberation from the thyroid gland. The iodine of triiodothyronine corresponds sometimes to 10–15% of the iodine of L-thyroxine in the gland, whereas under the same conditions it never exceeds a few hundredths of 1% of the total plasma iodine. In rats the plasma is sometimes totally without this compound, since the triiodinated derivative diffuses more easily than L-thyroxine and it presumably disappears more quickly from the plasma. In contrast to thyroxine, very little triiodothyronine added to serum combines with prealbumin. Thyroxine, triiodothyronine, and their various analogs differ in their affinity for TSH and TBPA [497].

The bond linking thyroxine with TSH is relatively strong. Triiodothyronine is also fixed by TSH, but its affinity for this protein is much weaker; in the presence of T_4, T_3 is displaced from the complex. McCannon et al.

[298] recently made a simultaneous comparative study of the distribution and the rate of appearance and disappearance of thyroxine and triiodothyronine in healthy subjects and in patients with diseases of the thyroid gland after injection of ^{131}I-T_4 and ^{131}I-T_3. The production of T_4 and T_3 was calculated from this single injection, and their content was found to be 44.75 μg and 97.3 μg, respectively. The production of T_4 and T_3 in most patients was increased equally, while in hypothyroid patients the production of both T_4 and T_3 was reduced, more so in the case of T_4.

It is now accepted, on the basis of much evidence, that the quantity of extrathyroid thyroxine is 1.0 mg and that its rate of degradation is 0.1 mg per diem.

About one-quarter of the iodine excreted by the thyroid gland is in the form of triiodothyronine. However, because its physiological activity is about five times higher than that of thyroxine and because the rate of its turnover and the volume of its distribution are roughly speaking 2.5 times greater, the concentration of T_3 in the serum is only 5% or less of that of T_4 [209, 388, 390]. However, because of these parameters of distribution and turnover, half of the metabolic activity of the thyroid hormones is due to triiodothyronine.

As has already been stated, besides the thyroxine bound with the blood proteins, some of the hormone is present in the *free* state. Free thyroxine is in dynamic equilibrium with protein-bound T_4, which acts as a reservoir. Not unexpectedly, the level of free T_4 is an important factor in the manifestation of its effect, for it seems probable on a priori grounds that free amino acids diffuse and penetrate inside the cells.

The rate of metabolism of T_4 is also evidently determined by the free thyroxine level. As a first approximation, according to Riggs [414] and Berson and Yalow [52], the amount of T_4 degraded daily is proportional to the square of the serum PBI. Presumably, during increased physical exertion, the utilization of free T_4 will be increased, but its level must be maintained by the equilibrium existing between bound and free T_4. However, investigation of the plasma thyroxine and TSH levels in man after submaximal exertion showed an increase of 11% in the total T_4 concentration and of 20% in the free T_4, while the TSH level and the binding properties of TSH and TBPA remained normal (Terjung and Tipton [507]). Terjung and Tipton felt that the increase in free T_4 was due to other factors and not a reflection of concentration in the mass-action equation.

Bekier [43] investigated the effect of hydrogen ion concentration on the dialyzing fraction of the serum T_4 and found an increase in it if the pH of the buffer was changed toward the acid side. The relationships between the serum pH and the binding power of the TBP and free T_4 of the serum show that the hydrogen ion concentration acts as a physiological regulator. In many circumstances (in pregnancy or after administration of methyltestosterone or estrogen, and in rare cases of a congenital increase or decrease in the serum TSH level) the concentration of free thyroxine in the serum and its peripheral metabolism (in μg/day) remain normal [42, 117, 138].

The existence of a reliable system for the regulation and coordination of homeostasis based on reciprocal interaction between nervous and humoral mechanisms unquestionably includes hormones circulating in the blood stream whose participation and activity are determined by the total content and relative proportions of their bound and free forms.

In the complex multicellular organism the endocrine system arises at a certain stage of evolutionary development as an essential component with a regulatory and coordinating function. The nervous system is adapted as the trigger mechanism for predetermined responses. It acts instantaneously and the responses generally terminate rapidly, within a few seconds. By contrast with the nervous system, the endocrine system modifies and regulates activities measured in minutes, hours, or, sometimes, days. Such a system functions very well because of its hormones, the blood level of which changes relatively slowly.

The physiological effects of thyroxine appear a long time after its introduction into the organism, and this slow effect is determined by the fine regulation of the concentration of the thyroid hormones. Rall [407] pointed out that this regulation is achieved through the binding proteins of the blood serum which act as a buffer of free T_4, slowing down and minimizing changes in the free thyroxine level. For instance, if large doses of thyroxine are injected, only a small increase is produced instead of an abnormally high elevation of the free T_4 level. If a large quantity of T_4 is removed, a relatively small decrease in free thyroxine is observed, in harmony with the slow action of thyroxine.

Tissue Metabolism of the Thyroid Hormones

Intracellular Penetration of Thyroxine and the Thyroxine-Binding Proteins of the Cell

An essential condition for the physiological action of thyroxine is its penetration inside the cell. The mechanism of this process continues to attract the attention of the research worker. Intensive absorption of labeled thyroxine in the liver and kidneys after its injection confirms the presence of active transport of T_4, and the accumulation of a large proportion of the injected radiothyroxine (30–50%) is evidently due to the presence of hormone-binding metabolism.

In this connection the presence of cell proteins binding thyroid hormones has been accepted for some time [229, 284, 491]. Unlike the serum thyroxine-binding proteins, they have high specificity for each hormone separately in the soluble liver proteins, but they have much less binding affinity than the serum proteins both for thyroxine and for triiodothyronine [279, 490, 493].

Investigations of the intracellular thyroxine-binding proteins undertaken recently in the writer's laboratory [533], in which ^{131}I-labeled T_4 was added to a protein extract of the liver, revealed two zones of active binding of the hormone during electrophoresis on polyacrylamide gel. Most of the radioactivity was found in the γ-globulin and prealbumin zones of the proteins, which account for 19.7 and 3.9%, respectively, of the total soluble liver proteins and differ completely from the specific hormone-binding proteins of the blood serum. The radioactivity of the bound thyroxine was 59.3% for 1γ-globulin, 6.2% for 2γ-globulin, and 34.5% for 18γ-prealbumin. The remaining 15 fractions of soluble liver proteins isolated by this method of fractionation did not bind the radioactive hormone. In the view generally held, only free thyroxine undergoes intracellular degradation, and the rate of utilization of the hormone is evidently determined by the ratio between the free and bound thyroxine.

Although there is still no clear and unambiguous concept of the role of the thyroid-binding cell proteins, it has been postulated a priori that they are concerned with the intake of hormones inside the cell from the extracellular space and also with the regulation of the rate of their intracellular metabolism. Attention is directed to the paper by Gorski et al. [181], who state that the cell nuclei and extracts prepared from them do not themselves take up the hormone in the absence of cytoplasm. If, however, isolated nuclei and chromatin are incubated with hormones, practically the whole of the hormones is bound with the nuclei; this result points to a role of soluble thyroxine-binding proteins of the liver tissue in the intracellular transport and distribution of thyroid hormones.

Most investigators nowadays accept the view, put forward originally in 1960 by Ingbar and Freinkel [229], that only free thyroxine can be taken up by the tissues. This view, known as the free thyroxine theory, is supported by much direct and indirect evidence [211, 212, 407]. In a series of articles Hillier [213, 214, 215] showed that much of the hormone in the tissues is adsorbed by the surfaces of membranes. Hillier recently gave details of the mechanism of transfer of thyroxine from the plasma to tissue binding sites [214]. By studying the absorption of T_4 by the rat liver perfused with a very dilute solution of TSH and TBPA, he showed that the transfer of T_4 from the plasma to the binding sites of the tissue involves its initial isolation in a free state. Under these conditions there is no direct exchange of the thyroxine bound with the plasma proteins for the other tissue binding proteins. T_4 is evidently transferred inside the cell from one binding surface to another in the same way.

Oppenheimer et al. [365], however, suggested an alternative theory according to which the reserves of free T_4 do not play a role and that the transfer of T_4 takes place by its exchange between the binding surfaces directly, and that the T_4 is never converted into the free state during this process. This *collision theory* lacks direct evidence and none seems likely to be forthcoming. Other investigations have shown that the T_4-binding proteins of the cell compete for T_4 with the intracellular deiodinating system [285, 492] and that only the T_4 which is not bound with the cell proteins is accessible for the deiodinases. However, two alternative points of view have been expressed on the biological significance of this phenomenon. One of them, put forward by Tata [496], postulates that the TBP of the cell is the factor controlling the level of free T_4 inside the cell and that deiodination of free thyroxine by deiodinase may be associated with its hormonal action.

The other view, expressed by Lissitzky [285], is that the complex of thyroxine and the intracellular binding protein is essential to its hormonal action and that deiodination of the free thyroxine is accompanied by its inactivation. The absence of sufficient grounds at the present time for explaining the causative relations between the hormonal action of thyroxine and its deiodination makes an unequivocal solution to this problem difficult. However, T_4 can be bound in the cell with various proteins with different affinities. On the whole it can be accepted that the cell thyroxine-binding proteins perform a function in regulating the quantity of protein available for deiodination; this protein is not metabolized, but in this way it controls the quantity of free T_4. This is a particularly important matter in the liver, where the rate of deiodination is particularly rapid. Without the cell TBP and ascorbic acid, a powerful inhibitor of deiodinase, the T_4 would be lost very quickly.

Intracellular Conversions of the Thyroid Hormones

When thyroid hormones penetrate inside the cells, they undergo various metabolic conversions. Some of these conversions are connected with realization of the hormonal effect, and they evidently take place during interaction with the substrate. Others are connected with the formation of inactive reserve forms of the hormone or with the removal of an excess of hormone from the body. However, sufficient experimental evidence has not yet been obtained for it to be stated with confidence which of the transformations in its molecule are associated with the manifestation of the hormonal effect.

The possible link between the biological activity of thyroxine and its metabolism has aroused great interest ever since the observation that iodide is a metabolic product of thyroxine, but it has attracted particular attention since the discovery of triiodothyronine and its acetic acid analog. Although the biological effects of thyroxine are very clear, as also are the pathways of the metabolic conversions leading to modification of the hormone molecule, the relations of cause and effect between the two series of events have not yet been adequately studied. This problem has been a matter for debate for a long time. The unusual stereochemistry, due to the 110° angulation of the ester oxygen atom first observed by Jörgensen et al. [235], has an important effect on the function of specific substituents in different positions.

The structural formula of thyroxine, showing the bending of the ester bond and the position of the β-ring in the plane of the paper, is given below.

Because of the preference for the perpendicular orientation of the two phenol rings, the 3′ and 5′-iodine atoms are not stereochemically equivalent: one is distal and the other proximal to the ring with the alanine side chain. Whereas 2′,3′-dimethyl-3,5-diiodotyrosine is very active in the prevention of goiter, the 2′,5′-analog has little activity. This suggests that the receptor of the thyroid hormone must conform strictly to its steric demands (limitations). According to this hypothesis the α-ring with the alanine side chain is essential for fixation and the β-ring for the functional receptor. Although the nature of the receptor and the molecular interactions between it and the thyroxine structure are not known, the β-ring is regarded as the functional center of the hormone.

Interaction between the thyroid hormones and their analogs and derivatives with the components of the cell have been the subject of many investigations. These have been confirmed, in particular, with the action of acetic acid analogs of thyroxine, namely tetraiodothyroacetic acid (T_4Ac), and of triiodothyronine, namely triiodothyroacetic acid (T_3Ac), once regarded as the active forms of the thyroid hormones. However, this view, popular some 8 to 10 years ago [148, 165, 511], has now become obsolete because T_4Ac possesses only between 10 and 40% of the activity of thyroxine itself.

Tomita et al. [514] investigated the action of T_4Ac formed, as these same workers showed previously [515], from T_4 by oxidative deamination

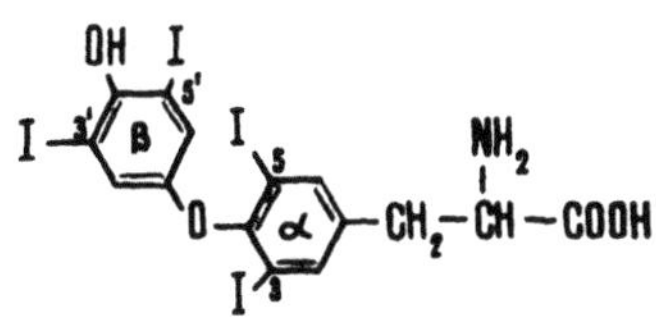

and decarboxylation of the side chain by the mitochondrial enzymes of the kidney. Nevertheless, T_4Ac is not regarded as the end product of conversion of thyroxine, and neither is T_3Ac. Both strongly potentiate the activity of ATPase and possess a shorter latent period when increasing the basal metabolic rate of thyrodectomized rats.

It will be evident from the structural formula given on the preceding page that there are five points in the molecule on which interest is centered from the point of view of the action of thyroxine: (1) the alanine side chain, (2) the α-ring, (3) the ring of the ester oxygen, (4) the β-ring, and (5) the ring of the phenolic hydroxyl group. Many analogs of thyroxine with modifications of the amino acid side chain have been obtained, but none of them possessed greater activity than thyroxine itself.

The biochemical transformations of the molecule of the thyroid hormones affect different parts of the thyronine structure, the alanine chain, and the substituent groups. The following reactions of metabolic conversion of T_4 may be mentioned: deiodination, deamination, oxidation of the phenol, conjugation of the phenol, and rupture of the diphenyl ester bond with decarboxylation. Evidence has been obtained that these conversions take place during investigations *in vitro* with biological material. However, whereas some of them represent the main pathway of metabolism of the thyroid hormones, the others are of secondary importance, and a third group evidently do not take place in the animal organism.

The question of the biochemical conversions of the thyroid hormones and their analogs has been dealt with fully in the monograph by Turakulov [528] and will not be specially considered here with the exception of new data meriting attention.

Deiodination. Deiodination occupies the principal place in the extrathyroid metabolism of the thyroid hormones. From the point of view of possible interaction between the metabolic conversions in the thyroxine molecule and its biological activity, deiodination merits special attention. The initial stages of the deiodination process and its connection with the hormonal activity of thyroxine were examined recently by Barker [38]. He started with the structure of thyroxine postulated by Jörgensen [235], according to which the α- and β-phenol rings lie in two different planes and the ester oxygen forms an angle of 110°. With this stereochemical configuration the 3′- and 5′-iodine atoms in the β-ring are not equivalent. As the experiments of Flock et al. [149] have shown, iodine atoms are removed from the β-ring and an inactive derivative of the hormone is formed during thyroxine metabolism in the liver. Activation of the hormone is connected with removal of the iodine in the 5′ position, in the proximal steric unit. Consequently, a substituent in position 3′ is essential for biological activity, and deiodination in position 5′ enables interaction between the molecule and the active surface of the receptor to take place. According to Barker, the link between the metabolic conversion of thyroxine and its biological action includes the binding of thyroxine to the surface of the receptor protein, accompanied by specific deiodination in the 5′ position, after which the intracellular changes in the hormone molecule soon begin to take place. However, although Barker's concept [38] that the first stage in the realization of the physiological effects of thyroxine is its partial deiodination has many supporters, opposite views based on experimental facts expressed in the literature have not confirmed this concept. Recently Primack et al. [399] concluded from an *in vitro* investigation of the actions of thyroxine and triiodothyronine that the two hormones potentiate protein synthesis in the mitochondria and the absorption of oxygen equally, without undergoing appreciable deiodination.

Despite these contradictory views regarding the importance of deiodination in the manifestation of the biological function of the hormone, it must evidently be recognized that the appearance of a complex of the hormone or of its modified form with the cell protein, even before the atoms of iodine are completely detached from the molecule, is an essential stage along the path of metabolic conversion of thyroxine. Recent investigations have in fact shown that iodinated proteins are formed in the tissues during deiodination [49, 100, 284, 413].

The formation of iodoproteins during the metabolism of thyroxine and triiodothyronine in liver and muscle, after injection of ^{131}I- and ^{125}I-labeled hormones and their derivatives into animals or after their addition to tissue cultures, was demonstrated by Nunez et al. [431, 432], Tata [493], Plaskett [395], Galton and Ingbar [164], Wynn et al. [559], and others. Nunez succeeded in separating the tissue iodoproteins formed during thyroxine metabolism into several fractions differing in their iodine content and in the order of their formation. However, the physiological importance of these stages of deiodination and of the formation of this whole series of iodoproteins, with different degrees of iodination, is unknown. These conversions are evidently directly concerned with the realization of hormonal activity and the mechanism of action of the hormones; they are connected with structural transformations in the molecule of T_4 and its activation and perhaps also with the liberation of an active iodine atom which may be positively or negatively charged [190].

The activated iodothyronine complex formed under these conditions — the specific protein — is considered to exhibit intracellular hormonal action during which further nonspecific degradation takes place with the formation of breakdown products (iodide, tyrosine, thyronine, etc.). Details of the process of intracellular deiodination of the thyroid hormones and the formation of iodoproteins remain favorite topics for research.

Kozyreff et al. [263] recently investigated the distribution of unextractable ^{125}I in liver homogenates formed as the result of metabolism of

^{125}I-labeled thyroid hormones in subcellular fractions 40 h after injection of ^{125}I-triiodothyronine into rats. They found that the unextractable ^{125}I is concentrated chiefly in the microsomal fraction from which it can be transferred to all the other fractions. Most of this iodine was bound with fragments containing soluble membranes and small and large vesicles. Only a little of the unextractable iodine of the microsomes was connected with relatively pure ribosomes. These results show that the unextractable ^{125}I formed in the course of metabolism of the thyroid hormones is associated exclusively with the membranous components of the microsomal fraction. Iodination of the cell proteins can also be considered to take place as a result of interaction between the protein and the surface of the membranes.

To understand the functional significance of the various intracellular iodoproteins, the degree of similarity or difference between the specific thyroxine-binding proteins of the serum and liver and the tissue iodoproteins must also be studied. This problem has been tackled in the writer's laboratory by Mirakhmedov et al. [533] by injecting ^{131}I-thyroxine into rats in a dose of 50 μCi/100 g body weight and fractionating the liver iodoprotein 48 h after the injection by electrophoresis on polyacrylamide gel.

Fractionation of the tissue iodoproteins appearing during peripheral metabolism of the thyroid hormones was carried out by determining the content of the fraction of the radioactive components extractable with butanol and the iodine in the electrophoretic fractions of the soluble liver proteins. Iodinated proteins, both bound with the cell structures and soluble, were detected. From 18 to 25% of the total activity of the liver tissue was accounted for by butanol-extractable iodine, but the content of radioactivity in the soluble protein fractions was much lower (2.4–4%). The iodoproteins formed in the course of metabolism of the thyroid hormones can be presumed to play a specific role by influencing and regulating the course of intermediate metabolism in the cell.

Another aspect of the deiodination process of great physiological importance is the formation of 3,5,3′-triiodothyronine, an analog of thyroxine but with four to five times higher activity then thyroxine itself. The extrathyroid formation of 3,5,3′-triiodo-L-thyronine from L-thyroxine is also important as a means of estimating the balance of thyroid activity and when examining the mechanism of action of thyroxine. However, despite the many investigations carried out on different organs, the possibility of such a conversion and its biological significance still remain in question.

The fact that L-triiodothyronine can be isolated from the thyroid gland is not disputed, and the thyroid is regarded as the main source from which triiodothyronine enters the circulation. In laboratory animals, for instance, the concentration of T_3 in the arterial blood is lower than in venous blood from the thyroid gland, indicating its secretion from the thyroid gland [230, 503]. Alternatively, attention has been directed to the possibility of extrathyroid conversion of T_4 into T_3. The claim that T_4 is converted into T_3 [284] was later withdrawn by some workers [265], and the probability of a metabolic role of the conversion of T_4 into T_3 was generally regarded as of no consequence. Meanwhile, as Barker [38] points out, partial deiodination of T_4 is necessary for its peripheral activity. If it is true that the cellular T_4-binding protein is a receptor for newly formed T_3, the formation of T_3 from T_4 must be accepted as the first stage along the pathway of metabolic conversion of thyroxine.

The possibility that peripheral triiodothyronine may arise through partial deiodination of T_4 has recently been reinvestigated. Sterling et al. [481] and Pittman et al. [389] have recently described the conversion of labeled T_4, injected intravenously into normal volunteers, into T_3. However, the quantitative estimation of this conversion is difficult, especially because the T_3 is determined in the plasma in which the T_4 concentration is many times higher than that of T_3, and T_3 is regarded primarily as an intracellular hormone [364]. For instance, after injection of labeled T_4 in man only 0.5–3.0% of the plasma radioactivity is present in the form of T_3 [389, 481]. Moreover, the possibility of conversion of small quantities of T_4 into T_3 during extraction and chromatography has not been excluded. In this connection Dussault and Fischer [120] described observations which disproved the extrathyroid conversion of thyroxine into triiodothyronine in sheep *in vivo*. The results of this investigation are consistent with those obtained by Primack et al. [399], cited above.

However, Schwartz et al. [455] recently gave what is apparently indisputable evidence of the conversion of T_4 into T_3 in rats. A whole-body rat homogenate was prepared 48, 72, and 96 h after intravenous injection of ^{125}I-T_4 and ^{131}I. The T_4 and the T_3 formed were purified by chromatography repeated several times. Strict control methods were devised to detect the possible conversion of T_4 into T_3 during extraction, chromatography, and determination of the ^{125}I-T_3/^{131}I-T_3 ratio in extracts from the body of the animals at various time intervals. These showed that 17% of the secreted T_4 is converted into T_3. Allowing for the concentration of nonradioactive T_3 in the rat plasma, it can be concluded from these results that about 20% of the total triiodothyronine is formed by conversion of T_4. If it is further assumed that T_3 possesses biological activity from 3 to 5 times stronger than T_4, it can be concluded that the hormonal activity of T_4 is largely dependent on its conversion into T_3.

Similar results were obtained by Rabinowitz et al. [405], who perfused the isolated rat heart with Krebs-Ringer buffer containing thyroxine labeled simultaneously with ^{14}C and ^{125}I. Approximately 5% of the radioactivity with the exact ratio between ^{14}C and ^{125}I was found in the newly formed triiodothyronine molecule in the perfusion fluid.

Finally, the comprehensive and careful investigations of Sterling [480], conducted on healthy, hyperthyroid, and hypothyroid human subjects, in which he determined the thyroxine and triiodothyronine concentration in the serum, the turnover rate, the distribution volume, the 24-hourly clearance of hormones, and the quantitative extrathyroid conversion of thyroxine into triiodothyronine during prolonged administration of ^{125}I-T_4 by mouth to athyroid and hypothyroid patients, confirmed conclusively that under normal conditions thyroxine is converted into triiodothyronine on a considerable scale in the peripheral tissues. The triiodothyronine formed by deiodination of thyroxine is found in the blood and accounts for about one-third of the serum triiodothyronine. If the turnover rate and distribution volume were allowed for, the daily quantities of both hormones utilized were about equal, confirming the great importance of this conversion. However, the question of whether thyroxine acts in the cell by conversion into triiodothyronine or not still remains unanswered.

Thyroxine metabolism linked with conversions of the alanine side chain, including oxidative deamination and decarboxylation, leads to the formation of a series of thyroxine and triiodothyronine analogs with physiological activity. Quantitatively speaking, oxidative deamination of the thyroid hormone is a less important metabolic pathway than deiodination and conversions connected with changes in the phenol group. It is not known whether oxidative deamination of the alanine side chain of thyroid hormones takes place in normal animals. It has been observed under various nonphysiological conditions.

However, the appearance of keto acid, acetic acid, and lactic acid analogs of thyroxine and triiodothyronine has frequently been demonstrated in the bile and in extracts of the thyroid gland, kidneys, liver, muscles, and brain after injection of large doses of thyroxine and triiodothyronine [148, 320, 333, 393, 490, 562].

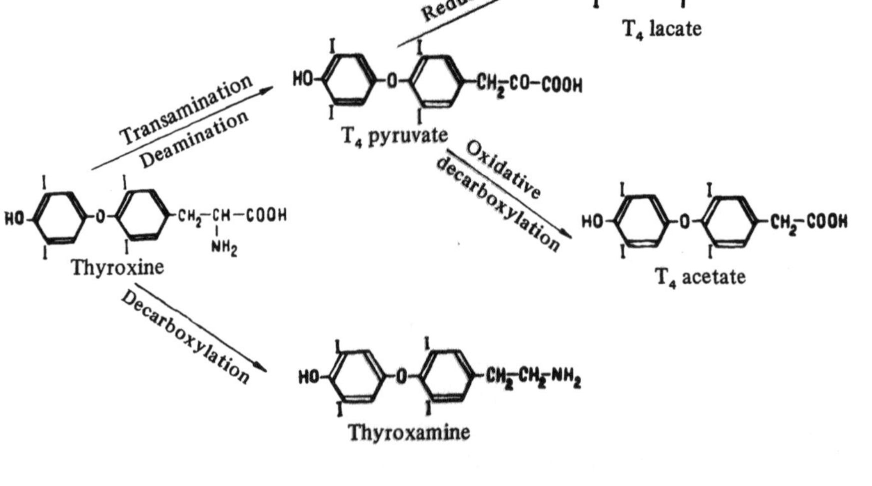

Oxidative deamination or transamination with the corresponding keto acid [494, 562] leads initially to the formation of α-keto derivatives of tetraiodothyropyruvic acid, which can then be reduced to the lactate form [431], or oxidative decarboxylation leads to the formation of the acetic acid analog tetraiodothyroacetic acid. All these transformations in the thyroxine molecule are summarized in the following scheme:

Cleavage of the diphenyl ether bond must evidently be the final process of degradation of the molecule unconnected either with activation or with transport of the hormone in the body. This stage of conversion of the thyronine structure has been inadequately studied, and there are conflicting reports on the appearance of DIT in the human and animal urine after injection of thyroxine.

Careful investigations using suitable systems of solvents have shown that the component taken for DIT consists of pyruvic acid analogs of T_4 and T_3. Fletcher [146] concluded that the DIT appearing in the human urine is formed from circulating thyroglobulin secreted after therapeutic doses of radioactive iodine. The view that DIT is not liberated by the breakdown of T_4 under normal conditions is further confirmed by the fact that if T_4 labeled in the 3,5 or 3′,5′ position is injected, the same metabolites are excreted in the urine. However, the latest research of Roche et al. [280, 431] has convincingly demonstrated DIT formation in experiments *in vitro* when hormones with the double label were incubated with thyroid gland preparations. Although there is no unequivocal evidence in the literature on the appearance of iodinated tyrosines *in vivo* as conversion products of iodothyronines, their formation in experiments *in vitro* is seemingly firmly established.

Conversions of thyroid hormones linked with reaction of the phenolic hydroxyl group. About 30 years ago Nieman [351] put forward the hypothesis that the physiological activity of thyroxine is due to a state of equilibrium between the phenolic and quinone forms of the molecule and to a possible hemiquinone intermediate product. Much later, Lissitzky et al. [285] showed that thyronine and some of its halide derivatives can be oxidized like tyrosine by a system of ascorbic acid–Fe^{++}–O_2. Oxidation is often accompanied by deiodination, but thyroxine itself is not oxidized by this system or by tyrosinase obtained from fungi.

Nevertheless, the fundamental reaction of the phenolic group of the iodothyronines is their binding glucuronic or sulfuric acids with the formation of paired glucuronic or sulfuric esters, utilizable for inactivation and elimination and also for storage and transport. The formation of conjugation products with glucuronic acid is a more important reaction than esterification with sulfuric acid in the iodothyronine series. The conjugation reaction takes place chiefly in the liver, and the conjugation products of T_4 and T_3 appear in the bile.

The binding of thyroid hormones with the formation of glucuronic conjugation products is a mechanism for the removal of excess thyroid gland hormones, but no glucuronoids are found in the feces, for the mucus membrane of the small intestine contains an active β-glucuronidase, capable of hydrolyzing the glucuronic ester rapidly with the liberation of thyroxine. Glucuronic conjugation products of D-thyroxine, L-triiodothyronine, and triiodothyroacetic acid are also found in the bile [422].

The iodine excreted with the feces consists chiefly of the iodine of free T_4, whereas mainly inorganic iodine is excreted with the urine. In fact, less than 10% of labeled iodine is accounted for by organic compounds, but this quantity can be increased if large doses of the hormone are given. In some cases T_4 and other iodized components are found in the urine, but this is observed in disease or after destruction of the thyroid gland with radioactive iodine. As a result of a comprehensive study of the metabolism of the sulfo-derivative of triiodothyronine after its injection, the compound was demonstrated in the bile, blood, and perfusion fluid of the kidneys, but not in the muscles. Gross et al. [187] expressed the opinion that this complex is a transport form of T_3 synthesized in the liver and kidneys. In that case the pathway of T_3 to the peripheral cells on which it acts can be represented as follows:

$$\begin{array}{ccc} \text{Thyroid gland } (T_3) \rightarrow \text{Circulation } (T_3) & \rightarrow & \text{Liver, kidneys (complex)} \\ & & \downarrow \\ \text{Muscles } (T_3) & \longleftarrow & \text{Circulation (complex)} \end{array}$$

However, this is observed only after injection of exogenous triiodothyronine. Since exogenous T_3 is only a small part of the thyroid hormones in the circulation, it is difficult to say whether this pathway in the conversions and transport of T_3 plays a physiological role under normal conditions.

The liver occupies a central position in the metabolism of the thyroid hormones. According to Albert and Keating [11], in the course of a few minutes 30% of the injected T_4 accumulates in the rat liver. The level of radioactivity of the liver then falls sharply but still remains higher than that of other tissues. Deiodination of the hormone, the principal pathway of thyroxine catabolism, takes place most intensively in the liver, after which the liberated iodide is excreted in the urine. However, fecal losses of the hormone are not significant. Thyroxine enters the intestine evidently with the bile, not only in the conjugated form with glucuronic and sulfuric acids. Hillier [215] showed the presence of large quantities of free thyroxine in the bile. His investigation showed that the concentration of free T_4 in the bile was of the same order as in the blood, and active trasnport is not involved in its secretion. Sulfuric and glucuronic conjugation products are hydrolyzed by the β-glucuronidase and aryl sulfatase of the intestine; some of the liberated hormones are returned to the circulation, but most of the thyroxine and triiodothyronine is excreted with the feces. Absorption of the glucuronic conjugation product of triiodothyronine from a loop of small intestine was shown to be slight, whereas absorption from a loop of large intestine was similar to the absorption of free T_3, and it evidently took place after hydrolysis of the contents of the large intestine [89].

Under physiological conditions most of the iodine in the feces consists of thyroxine iodine [209]. In rats kept for a long time on a diet with a low iodine content, however, the ratio of T_3 to thyroxine rose sharply, reaching 7 in the bile and from 4 to 11 in the feces. These results show that in rats with a severe dietary iodine deficiency T_3 can be excreted from the thyroid gland faster than T_4. These results also point to the possibility of rapid conversion of T_4 into T_3 in the body or to T_3 synthesis independent of T_4 synthesis in the stimulated thyroid gland. On a diet with a low iodine content, Middlesworth et al. [322] found a considerable excess of T_3 over T_4 in the bile and in the feces of the rats, whereas in the thyroid gland this ratio was less than 2. These results also point to the possibility of rapid conversion of T_4 into T_3 in the body, or to T_3 synthesis independently of T_4 synthesis in the stimulated thyroid gland. Most of the thyroxine excreted into the intestine enters via the biliary tract [11, 501], and it is excreted as conjugation products with glucuronate and sulfate. In general, thyroxine is conjugated with glucuronate and triiodothyronine with sulfate [421]. Both these esters are found in the large intestine, where they are presumably hydrolyzed by the β-glucuronidase of the intestinal microorganisms and the free T_4 is reabsorbed into the blood stream.

Regulation of Thyroid Function

The problem of the regulation of thyroid function has for a long time occupied the center of attention of physiologists, endocrinologists, and clinicians, and interest in it shows no sign of weakening. The focus of attention in the investigation of these problems has shifted in recent years toward the elucidation of the molecular mechanisms of interaction between thyroid-stimulating hormone and the receptor sites of the follicular cells and to the chemical mechanisms of transmission of nervous signals through hypothalamic neurosecretory processes to the pituitary gland. Together with substantial progress in the study of the neurohumoral mechanisms of thyroid gland regulation, in which a key position is occupied by the hypothalamohypophyseal axis, further evidence has been obtained of the existence of parahypophyseal influences on the thyroid gland via its sympathetic innervation.

The generally accepted view of the existence of control over thyroid function by the cerebral hemispheres, based on numerous indisputable clinical observations [37], is supported by convincing experimental evidence. Changes in thyroid function have been demonstrated during strong stimulation of the central nervous system [26, 243], in response to pharmacological agents stimulating or inhibiting the CNS [136, 259], to a conditioned-reflex increase in the excitability of the higher levels of the CNS [547], and so on. In the recent extensive investigations of Furdui [162] the role of the brain in the production of experimental thyrotoxicosis in dogs was conclusively proved. He developed a reliable method of increasing thyroid function by stimulating the brain centers combined with restricting the movements of the experimental animals.

Although the role of the central nervous system in the regulation of thyroid function is no longer in dispute, the pathways and mechanisms by which this control is effected still remain inadequately explained. The decisive role of the hypothalamus in the nervous regulation of thyroid function, effected through the pituitary by the liberation of a specific substance known as thyrotropin-releasing factor (TRF), is an undisputed fact. However, it has not yet been finally settled whether nervous signals are transmitted in this way from the brain to the thyroid gland or whether there is another direct pathway avoiding the pituitary, a parahypophyseal flow of impulses also playing a role, with the shortest possible pathway, in the regulation of thyroid function and what the physiological significance of this pathway may be. An ardent supporter of the existence of this parahypophyseal mechanism of regulation of thyroid function is Aleshin [15], who, together with his collaborators, has presented fresh experimental evidence in its support in the last few years. These workers have demonstrated increased reactivity of the isolated thyroid gland with respect to thyrotropic hormone under the influence of a sympathomimetic agent (adrenalin) and weakening of its reactivity after the addition of acetylcholine, as the parasympathetic mediator, to the medium. The absence of response to nervous impulses by the thyroid gland *in situ* is explained on the assumption that the possible nervous effects are evidently inhibited by the more powerful hormonal influences of TSH; besides, simultaneous stimulation of the sympathetic ganglia and excitation of the thyroid gland lead to inhibition of the thyrotropic function of the pituitary, which is also innervated by the sympathetic ganglia [12].

On the basis of these arguments the production of TSH in the intact animal was reduced by administration of chlorpromazine, and the direct effect of nervous impulses on the thyroid gland was studied. Under these conditions the thyroid absorbs iodine, and intrathyroid hormonogenesis is stimulated. The liberation of the completed hormones into the circulation is also increased, as reflected by an increase in the blood concentration of protein-bound iodine [16, 82], even if the thyrotropic function is intact. During stimulation of the superior cervical ganglia Churpinova observed a marked increase in size of the thyroxine and triiodothyronine bands on the chromatograms, confirming the stimulant action of nervous impulse on the thyroid gland. The effect of sympathetic impulses on the thyroid gland has also been demonstrated by electron-microscopic investigations after unilateral cervical thyroidectomy. Although the level of iodine absorption was the same by both lobules of the gland, there was a definite decrease in the number and size of the microvilli of the apical surface of the thyrocytes and also a much lower density of the iodothyronine band on chromatograms of hydrolyzates of the sympathectomized side of the gland (cited in [13]). During electrical stimulation of the right cervical sympathetic trunk in mice in which TSH secretion was blocked by exogenous thyroxine, intracelular colloid droplets were formed and the blood ^{131}I level rose. Intravenous injection of noradrenalin led to similar changes [316]. These results show that sympathetic stimulation induces endocytosis of thyroglobulin and liberation of hormonal iodine by a direct action on the α-adrenergic receptors in the follicular cells of the thyroid gland through liberation of noradrenalin from intrathyroid sympathetic nerve endings. In other recent investigations Melander [314, 316] showed that 5-hydroxytryptamine and histamine also play a role in secretion in the thyroid gland. These amines, which, like adrenalin and noradrenalin, are potential inhibitors of TSH, stimulate thyroid secretion by their direct action on the follicular cells in the absence of stimulation by TSH.

The work of Aleshin et al. [15] demonstrated conclusively that, besides humoral regulation, the thyroid gland is under direct nervous control. However, because of the fundamental importance of this concept for the understanding of interaction between nervous and humoral mechanisms of control and because of contradictory facts in the literature [136, 544, 545], for a final solution to this problem confirmation of the role of the sympathetic parahypophyseal regulation of thyroid function ought desirably to be obtained from other laboratories.

The role of the cerebral cortex and of certain other regions of the CNS, as well as the participation of the other endocrine glands in the regulation of thyroid activity, has been discussed in some detail in recent monographs [3, 136, 545]. Since it was also treated at some length by the present writer in an earlier publication [528], this role will not be considered in this book. New information on biochemical aspects of the problem and the molecular mechanisms of regulation can, however, conveniently be mentioned.

It is now generally accepted that the thyrotropic function of the anterior pituitary is under the direct control of the hypothalamus. There is much experimental evidence to show that separation of the pituitary from the diencephalon by division of the pituitary stalk or by injury to or stereotaxic destruction of the anterior hypothalamus is followed by depression of thyroid function [545]. The concept of hypothalamic neurohumoral control over pituitary hormonal secretion has been fully confirmed in recent years as a result of the isolation of a specifc hypophysiotropic factor from extracts of hypothalamic tissue.

As a result of some brilliant research by several groups of workers within a very short time, a new and powerful substance for the control of pituitary function was isolated in a pure form from the hypothalamus of animals, its chemical structure determined, and its biological activity studied; the substance can now be obtained synthetically and is available for experimental and clinical purposes. This substance, one of a group of factors stimulating pituitary secretion, has been called thyrotropin-releasing factor (TRF) or thyrotropin-releasing hormone (TRH) [65, 204, 412].

The analogous substance for corticotropin, known as corticotropin-releasing factor (CRF), was obtained from the pituitary a little earlier [192, 193]. The mediobasal hypothalamus is considered to be the principal site of production of the releasing factors. Akmaev [10] improved the technique of isolating the hypothalamohypophyseal islet and carried out a detailed investigation of the anatomical structures responsible for this function and the neurohumoral interactions involved in the formation and transportation of the releasing factors. He found that axons arising from the basal hypothalamus pass through the median eminence where a hypophyseal trophic neurosecretion is liberated and enters the primary capillaries of the pituitary portal system.

TRF was the first of the hypothalamic releasing factors to have its structure determined. In its chemical structure it is a fairly simple compound. As described by Burgus et al. [63, 64], sheep TRF is a modified tripeptide: L-(pyro)glutamyl-L-histidyl-L-prolinamide
The same workers and others have studied the biological activity of synthetic TRF and other related polypeptide derivatives [65].

Nair et al. [340] studied pig TRF, while Boler et al. [58] showed the chemical and hormonal identity of samples of TRF obtained from several different species of animals. The natural and synthetic TRF are active in mice, rats, and man, and they evidently do not exhibit specificity. TRF is

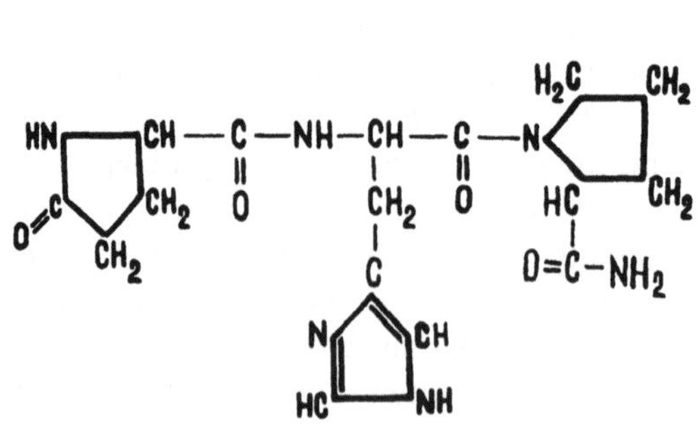

L-(Pyro)glutamyl-L-hystidyl-L-prolinamide

active when administered in various ways, including by mouth. After administration of TRF, the plasma TSH level rises rapidly [60]. Hall et al. [197] investigated the efficacy of synthetic TRF in doses of 1 to 200 μg after intravenous injection into healthy subjects. An increase in the serum TSH concentration occurred 5 min after injection of 50 μg TRF and reached its maximum between 15 and 120 min after the injection. The ready availability of TRF means that it can be used for the diagnosis of lesions of the pituitary and hypothalamus.

In children with idiopathic hypopituitary dwarfism, with a plasma TRF level 2.5–3 times lower than in healthy children or in patients with a deficiency limited to growth hormone but with normal thyroid function, the hypothalamus cannot secrete TRF. As Bruce et al. [62] showed recently, synthetic TRF, injected intravenously in a dose of 500 μg into patients with hypopituitary dwarfism, increases the plasma TSH level for a longer time than in patients of the last two groups. These results serve to distinguish primary hypothalamic TRF deficiency from pituitary TSH deficiency.

A key position in the regulation of thyroid function is unquestionably occupied by the anterior lobe of the pituitary, which exerts its powerful regulatory effect by secreting a special substance—thyroid stimulating hormone (TSH)—into the circulating blood. The action of nearly all, if not all, endogenous regulatory factors, including nervous impulses, on the thyroid gland is also concentrated in the pituitary and is effected through the secretion of TSH. No attempt will be made here to scrutinize the voluminous literature on pituitary-thyroid relationships, and only the results of recent research will be mentioned.

The action of TSH on the assimilation of blood iodide by the thyroid gland is a vital link in the stimulation of hormone formation, and it is very closely connected with the activation of the whole metabolism of the gland. The stimulating action of pituitary TSH on thyroid gland metabolism was first clearly demonstrated by Halmi et al. [199]. They found that a single injection of TSH into a rat leads, after a lag period of about 8 h, to an increase in the absorption of iodine by 50–100% by the thyroid gland. It was suggested that the incubation period for this action of TSH is occupied by the synthesis of new enzymes or iodine carriers.

During the activation of thyroid function by TSH there is an increase in the secretion of iodinated components into the blood and the absorption of iodine by the thyroid gland, an increase in the oxidation of glucose by the phosphogluconate pathway, and the synthesis of phospholipids. Characteristic morphological changes also develop: liquefaction of the colloid, endocytosis (the appearance of droplets of colloid in the follicular cells), and enlargement of the epithelial cells. The increase in the uptake of iodine by the thyroid gland, although the chief factor in the activation of the intrathyroid iodine circulation, is not the initial effect taking place immediately after injection of TSH.

A study of the manifestations of the early action of TSH on the thyroid gland showed that the solution of the colloid and secretion evidently precede hormone synthesis, whereas the increase in the ^{32}P absorption, growth of the cells, and the increase in secretion are observed almost simultaneously with hormone synthesis.

The loss of thyroid hormone following administration of TSH in man was shown to be one of the early features of its action. The blood PBI level is increased and the radioiodine concentration in the thyroid gland reduced under these conditions. This effect is regarded as the result of activation of the proteolytic enzymes of the gland by TSH. The primary action of thyrotropic hormone must therefore be regarded as the liberation of thyroxine from intrafollicular thyroglobulin. Growth of the cells and an increase in the iodine-concentrating function of the thyroid gland take place as a result of liberation of hormonal iodine from the gland. Meticulous investigations of this problem by measuring the concentration of protein-bound ^{131}I have shown that the blood PBI rises 1–1.5 h after intramuscular injection of TSH, whereas the absorption of radioiodine increases only after a latent period of 8 h and reaches its maximum after 15–18 h [132]. Einhorn and Larson [131] also point out that the accumulation of radioiodine by the thyroid gland occurs 8–10 h after a single intramuscular injection of TSH. The radioiodine concentration reached a maximum 18–24 h after the injection and fell to its initial level after 5–6 days. The action of TSH on the secretion of thyroid hormones was manifested after 90 min, and 24 h later they had not yet returned to normal. Although the manifestation of the early action of TSH evidently consists of the proteolysis of colloid, it cannot be assumed that all the other effects are secondary in character.

Taurog et al. [506] stated that the various actions of TSH are manifested independently. The T/S ratio (tissue iodine/serum iodine) is increased in hypophysectomized rats receiving TSH, even if all the hormonal iodine has been eliminated from the gland by preliminary injection of propylthiouracil. TSH also induces growth of the thyroid gland and ^{32}P accumulation in these animals. The effect of TSH on growth can thus be separated from its action on iodine metabolism.

The various parameters of the thyroid gland are altered unequally by an acute fall in the thyrotropic hormone level in the body after hypophysectomy or administration of thyroxine. The most sensitive parameter is the liberation of ^{131}I, followed by its absorption by the thyroid gland, and the weight of the gland is the least sensitive parameter. Hypophysectomy and thyroxine administration produce almost identical effects on the liberation and absorption of ^{131}I by the thyroid [561].

Investigations by Rosenberg et al. [438, 439] on euthyroid and hyperthyroid individuals and on patients with myxedema showed that TSH stimulates the secretion not only of protein-bound iodine, previously labeled with ^{131}I, but also of iodide, from the thyroid gland. Liberation of iodide into the blood stream was observed as early as 30 min after injection of TSH. The iodide liberated under these circumstances is not iodide recently entering the gland from the plasma, but that liberated from iodine-containing precursors, possibly diiodotyrosine, in the gland itself through the action of TSH [439]. Similar results were obtained by Nagataki et al. [338] on dogs kept on a low-iodine diet. In another investigation, Nagataki et al. [339] analyzed arterial and venous blood of the thyroid gland and concluded that, under normal conditions, TSH liberates iodide as well as organically bound iodine from thyroglobulin, but that it is not excreted because the ability of the thyroid gland to bind iodine organically is greater than its ability to form iodide. During the first few minutes of its action TSH accelerates both the proteolysis of thyroglobulin and organic fixation. However, in the early phase of action of TSH, the rate of formation of iodide exceeds the rate of its fixation so that, as a result, iodide is excreted from the thyroid gland. The accumulation of iodide by the thyroid gland begins only after a few hours.

In recent experiments on dogs with the use of ^{131}I, Dobyns and Hirsch [111] demonstrated an increase in the total radioactivity and also in the content of protein-bound iodine in the lymph of a lymphatic vessel located beneath the thyroid gland after injection of thyrotropic hormone. However, radiochromatographic determination of the iodine-containing fractions showed that most activity was present in the stationary component, in all probability in thyroglobulin. No thyroxine or iodide could be found in the lymph. Thyrotropic hormone increased the output of ^{131}I compounds into the blood via the thyroid vein. On the basis of preliminary calculation, these workers suggest that the lymph is a more important pathway for the excretion of ^{131}I from the thyroid gland during thyrotropic stimulation than the blood stream.

It is generally accepted that stimulation of the thyroid gland by TSH is accompanied by changes in the ratio of newly symthesized thyroxine to triiodothyronine. The work of Greer's group [311] has shown that stimulation of the absorption of iodine by the thyroid gland and the morphological and biochemical effects produced by the action of TSH are accompanied by a change in the ratio between newly synthesized thyroxine and triiodothyronine in favor of the latter.

This hypothesis has recently been verified by two groups of workers in two different ways: by endogenous stimulation of the pituitary by keeping rats on an iodine-deficient diet and subsequently suppressing TSH secretion by injection of T_3 [134] and by injecting TSH into hypophysectomized rats kept on diets with different iodine contents [183]. These experiments showed that after iodine deficiency the T_4:T_3 ratio of the newly synthesized hormones changes in favor of T_3, possibly to compensate for the iodine deficiency in the body, whereas after suppression of TSH it changes in favor of T_4. The second investigation confirmed that the T_3:T_4 ratio rises in hypophysectomized rats after injection of TSH if their thyroid glands have lost most of their iodine. Consequently, for the action of TSH on the ratio between the newly synthesized T_3 and T_4 to be effective, it is important that the thyroid gland be emptied of iodine.

The action of TSH on thyroid function, as already stated, is accompanied by stimulation of the metabolism of the gland itself. Freinkel et al. [154, 155] regard the stimulation of thyroid tissue metabolism by TSH as an essential condition for manifestation of the effect of the hormone. The results of their investigations indicate a marked increase in the assimilation of glucose by thyroid slices and the acceleration of lipogenesis from glucose and of the oxidative decarboxylation of glucose following the addition of TSH to the incubation medium. The incorporation of inositol into the lipids of the gland is also stimulated even in a medium not containing glucose. Stimulation of the hexose monophosphate pathway by TSH *in vitro* was also demonstrated by Field et al. [140] in calf thyroid slices. The effect of TSH was specific, and no such action was observed after the addition of other pituitary hormones. Consequently, activation of hormone formation in the thyroid gland by thyrotropic hormone must be considered from the standpoint of an increase in the general level of metabolism and resources of energy in the gland. However, following the discovery of new facts regarding the point of application of TSH, it has only now become possible to determine precisely which process is the trigger mechanism for initiating this complex and varied chain of consecutive reactions. According to the general view of the mechanism of action of hormones by activation of the genetic apparatus of the cell, all effects arising in the thyroid gland after injection of TSH can be assumed to be based on an increase in the synthesis of specific proteins. Much evidence to show that TSH stimulates the incorporation of labeled amino acids into newly synthesized thyroid gland proteins has recently been obtained both *in vivo* and *in vitro*, in slices and isolated cells.

Kondo and Ui [260] showed that TSH, when added to minced bovine and porcine thyroid gland tissue or when administered to hypophysectomized animals, increases the synthesis of iodoproteins. Tong demonstrated a little later that TSH stimulates the incorporation of iodide into iodotyrosines and iodothyronins, linked together in the thyroglobulin molecule, in cells isolated from the thyroid gland of the ox or sheep. The hormone stimulated incorporation of labeled ^{14}C-tyrosine and ^{14}C-phenylalanine into the proteins; iodoprotein formation increased even if iodide transport was blocked by perchlorate. These effects were observed as early as 30 min after the addition of TSH [516]. Iodine transport into the gland and the formation of iodinated components in thyroglobulin take place independently of protein synthesis. For instance, in experiments in which protein synthesis was inhibited by puromycin, stimulation of iodination of thyroglobulin by TSH was dependent neither on an increase in thyroglobulin production nor on an increase in the formation of iodinating enzymes. However, subsequent experiments using 5-deoxyglucose, in which the stimulation of glucose oxidation was inhibited by TSH, showed that incorporation of amino acids into the isolated cells is secondary to the increase in glucose catabolism [517]. The stimulation effect of TSH on protein synthesis in the thyroid gland is also due to an increase in the intensity of nucleic acid formation. The effect of TSH on nucleic acid metabolism in the thyroid gland has attracted the attention of research workers for a long time. As long ago as in 1959, Matovinovic and Vickery [310] reported an increase in the RNA content in the thyroid gland of guinea pigs receiving TSH.

Lecocq and Dumont [268] obtained convincing evidence of stimulation of the incorporation of phosphate, formate, glycine, and adenine into RNA by thyroid slices. As these workers state, intact RNA synthesis is an essential condition for the acceleration of cell and tissue growth in the thyroid gland observed *in vivo* a short time after injection of TSH. Previously it has been postulated that TSH stimulates mRNA synthesis in the nuclei of the thyroid gland. Lecocq and Dumont incubated thyroid slices with uridine-^{3}H and observed incorporation of the uridine chiefly into the polysomal fractions. Actinomycin D suppresses transcription and inhibits the incorporation of uridine-^{3}H into polysomes. Meanwhile TSH induces changes in the ribosomal profile in the cytoplasm: A shift from monosomes toward the formation of polysomes is observed and is evidence of the stimulation of the general synthesis of messenger RNA by TSH. In another investigation these same workers [269] demonstrated that incorporation of uridine-^{3}H into both mRNA and pyrimidine nucleotides is stimulated by thyrotropin.

It was concluded that TSH acts chiefly by accelerating nucleotide synthesis, thereby making mRNA more accessible for the cytoplasmic ribosomes. Proof that increased growth of thyroid tissue is accompanied by stimulation of protein synthesis and of nucleic acid metabolism was obtained in experiments carried out in the writer's laboratory in which experimental goiter was produced in rats and the content and synthesis of nucleic acids were studied in goitrous human tissues.

With an increase in the size of the thyroid gland after prolonged administration of methylthiouracil, which is also accompanied by stimulation of pituitary thyrotropic function, the incorporation of labeled amino

Table V. Incorporation of Labeled Amino Acids into Rat Thyroid Gland Proteins under Normal and Experimental Conditions: pulses/min/100 mg protein

Labeled amino acids	Control, M ± m	Experimental, M ± m
^{35}S-methionine	1163 ± 223.8	3380 ± 540.8 $p < 0.001$
^{14}C-tyrosine	640 ± 103.7	1200 ± 193.1 $p < 0.05$
^{14}C-glycine	2867 ± 467	6200 ± 1100 $p = 0.05$

acids into the tissue proteins of the thyroid gland was sharply increased both *in vivo* and *in vitro* [445]. These experiments showed that in a young growing goiter (administration of MTU for 10 months) the incorporation of amino acids takes place much more intensively than in old goitrous tissue of the gland after the more prolonged administration of the goitrogenic agent. Similar results also were obtained by investigation of the incorporation of glycine-^{14}C in sections of goitrous thyroid gland from animals with goiter of different types and durations (Tables V–IX).

Seitmuratova and Khalikov [529, 535], in investigations using thymidine-2-^{14}C and uridine-2-^{14}C, found an increase in DNA and RNA synthesis; RNA synthesis was much more intensive in goitrous thyroid gland tissue. The intensity of incorporation of various ^{14}C-amino acids into ribo-

Table VI. Incorporation of Glycine-^{14}C into Thyroid Gland Proteins from Patients *in Vitro*: pulses/min/100 mg protein

Nodular goiter		Multinodular goiter	
Nodule	Tissue	Nodule	Tissue
4363 ± 332.6	534 ± 57.7	842 ± 130.8	534 ± 57.7
$p < 0.001$		$p < 0.001$	

Table VII. Incorporation of Glycine-^{14}C *in Vivo* into Rat Thyroid Gland Proteins: pulses/min/100 mg protein

Experiment	Control
35,000 ± 2000 $t = 5.2$	12,900 ± 1000 $P < 0.001$

Table VIII. Incorporation of Tyrosine-^{14}C *in Vitro* into Thyroid Gland Proteins from Patients: pulses/min/100 mg protein

Nodular euthyroid goiter		Multinodular goiter	
Nodule	Tissue	Nodule	Tissue
M ± m			
1038 ± 179.4	533 ± 81.6	450 ± 104.3	533 ± 81.6
$P < 0.05$		$P < 0.1$	

somal proteins of the thyroid also was much higher in the goitrous gland. These results suggest that growth of thyroid gland tissue, accompanied by acceleration of the formation of thyroid proteins, is directly related to the increased RNA synthesis. These experiments clearly showed a more marked increase in the formation of nucleotides from formate-^{14}C, glycine-^{14}C, and other precursors in the goitrous tissue than in normal thyroid gland tissue. In experiments *in vitro* Hall [197] also observed the stimulant effect of TSH on purine synthesis in calf thyroid gland slices. He postulated that the stimulation of purine synthesis is secondary to the increase in glucose oxidation by the phosphogluconate pathway observed in response to the action of TSH.

The effect of TSH on nuclear RNA synthesis in the thyroid gland *in vitro* was studied by Schimada and Yasumasu [451]. Working with isolated nuclei of thyroid gland cells they showed that RNA synthesis is stimulated in the same way as in pig thyroid gland slices. TSH does not increase the template activity of the DNA itself but increases this activity of DNA bound with protein, i.e., in chromatin. The results confirmed the view that TSH can stimulate both the RNA-polymerase activity of the thyroid gland and the template activity of the chromatin. Under these circumstances TSH can abolish the repressive effect of histone by its direct or indirect action on the bond linking DNA to protein.

Table IX. Incorporation of Tyrosine-^{14}C *in Vitro* into Thyroid Gland Proteins from Patients Undergoing Operation for Nodular Goiter (Duration of illness 10-15 years): pulses/min/100 mg protein

Nodule		Tissue
	M ± m	
250 ± 33.3		553 ± 81.6
	$P < 0.05$	

However, there is no evidence that TSH acts directly on the protein-synthesizing system in the cytoplasm of the thyroid gland, whether on the ribosomes or on the enzymes activating the amino acid. TSH added *in vitro* likewise does not increase the incorporation of leucine-^{14}C into proteins of thyroid gland slices obtained from guinea pigs receiving preliminary injections of TSH. Sead and Goldberg [456] stated that thyroglobulin formation is independent of RNA synthesis although the synthesis of other proteins are relatively sensitive to the action of actinomycin D. It is therefore difficult to assess the physiological significance of RNA synthesis in the thyroid gland; perhaps the RNA serves as the template for the synthesis of other proteins than thyroglobulins. This view is indirectly supported by the observations of Saatov [444] and Dzhalilova [124], in the writer's laboratory, who found an increase in certain protein fractions other than thyroglobulin in goitrous human thyroid tissue and in the tissue of a growing experimental goiter in animals.

The action of the thyroid hormones themselves on thyroglobulin biosynthesis in the thyroid gland is interesting. The importance of this problem is explained by the fact that in thyrotoxicosis when thyroxine production is sharply increased, the concentration of the free hormone in the gland itself must also evidently be raised. Experiments in the writer's laboratory [530-532] have shown that mitochondria of the thyroid gland of thyrotoxic patients do not respond to the addition of thyroxine to the medium by an increase in respiration although mitochondria from the thyroid glands of normal and hypothyroid animals and man do respond under the same conditions by a marked increase in oxygen uptake.

The chemical nature of the mechanism of action of TSH and of other stimulators of pituitary thyrotropic function have also been studied from various aspects. Much important evidence of the chemical structure, physicochemical properties, and biological specificity of TSH has recently been obtained by the study of highly purified preparations from the pituitary glands of various species of animals. This work has shown that TSH is in fact a group of similar protein compounds with a molecular weight of 28,000–30,000. There is not a single fixed configuration of amino acids, as is the case with certain other protein and peptide hormones. The amino acid composition of TSH has been determined, and the high concentration of cysteine and, consequently, of disulfide bonds in its molecule has been demonstrated. However, the problem of the terminal amino acids and the primary structure of thyroid-stimulating hormone still await solution.

The TSH molecule has a high content of carbohydrates in the form of monosaccharides and their derivatives. According to some investigators [152] they contain about 3.5% of hexoses and 2.5% of glucosamine, but these figures vary with the purity of the preparations, possibly depending on the presence of gonadotropins as impurities. The carbohydrate moiety of the molecule contains 5–6 mannose residues and one fucose residue. However, these account for only 85% of the total calculated quantity of carbohydrates in TSH with a molecular weight of 28,000 [385, 560]. According to Wynston et al. [560] the chief component of the carbohydrate moiety of the TSH molecule is mannose, but, unlike gonadotropin, it contains no sialic acid. Because of the incomplete information on the primary structure of TSH, there are insufficient grounds at present for predicting the exact localization of the carbohydrate residues and the character of ther bonding in the TSH molecule. Definite information regarding the importance of the carbohydrate component in the manifestation of thyrotropic activity is also lacking. Investigations of the chemical and immunological properties of TSH have shown that it does not possess species specificity in the narrow meaning of this term, as is characteristic, for example, of somatotropic hormone obtained from animals of various species and from man. Pituitary TSH from man, the ox, sheep, and whale differed only slightly in their chromatographic mobility, biological effect, amino acid composition, carbohydrate components, and hydrolysis by proteolytic enzyme. Meanwhile, opposite findings have been described indicating differences between the thyrotropic hormones of different species of mammals in their electrophoretic mobility and the composition of their carbohydrate components. For example, the greater resistance of human thyrotropin to chymotrypsin [276], its more acid character [84], and the higher content of hexoses in its composition [274] have been established. Immunological differences also have been found between human and bovine TSH [536].

Besides this discovery of the heterogeneous chemical composition and electrophoretic mobility of TSH itself, views have already been expressed previously in the literature to the effect that it contains several active principles producing differential effects on the various parameters of thyroid function and on the development of exophthalmos in thyrotoxic patients—a factor inducing exophthalmos, a growth factor, and a metabolic factor. However, later research did not confirm the observations of Dobyns and Wilson [112] on the discovery and chemical isolation of an independent exophthalmic factor. Nor was the view confirmed that there are two different thyrotropins—one stimulating growth of the thyroid gland follicles, the other stimulating the chemical synthesis and secretion of the hormone.

Meanwhile, the suggestion that the serum of thyrotoxic patients contains an agent concerned with stimulating thyroid gland function and the development of exophthalmos has subsequently found much experimental confirmation. In 1958 Adams [5] described the discovery of an atypical TSH in extracts from the pituitary gland and in the serum of certain thyrotoxic patients. When this TSH is injected into guinea pigs receiving thyroxine-^{131}I, the time of excretion of ^{131}I from the thyroid gland and the period of increased concentration in the plasma is prolonged. Adams suggests that this hormone is identical with the exophthalmic factor of Dobyns and Wilson [112], an agent separated from thyrotropin by chemical fractionation and also found in the serum of patients with progressive exophthalmos. This agent, known under several names such as atypical, abnormal, or modified thyrostimulating hormone, and also as abnormal thyroid stimulator, has recently become more generally known as long-acting thyroid stimulator (LATS). It differs from the ordinary TSH in the fact that it induces a delayed increase in the absorption of ^{131}I by the thyroid gland and in the blood PBI level as well as histological changes in the gland. The maximal response to the stimulating agent occurs only 7–9 h after its administration, and it continues to act for a longer time. Comparison of the rate of disappearance of LATS from thyrotoxic patients and of a saline extract of thyrotropin obtained from euthyroid persons, from the blood after injection into guinea pigs, showed that whereas after 1 h only 5% of the injected TSH still remained in the animal's blood, LATS could still be found in the circulation after 7.5 h. Consequently, the prolonged response to LATS is explained by its longer stay in the circulating blood. Adams et al. [6] tested the action of blood serum from patients with exophthalmic goiter, containing high concentrations of abnormal thyroid stimulator, in hypophysectomized mice and concluded that this factor acts not through the pituitary, but directly on the thyroid gland.

LATS increases the absorption of ^{131}I by the thyroid gland and produces changes in its histology similar to those produced by TSH. The character of action of this agent resembles that of low concentrations of TSH maintained for a long time. Recent observations have confirmed that LATS produces all the known effects of TSH and is indistinguishable from it in its mode of action. Like TSH it stimulates the oxidation of 1-^{14}C-glucose and the incorporation of ^{32}P into phospholipids in the thyroid gland. However, as Burke [68] showed recently, iodide (normally inhibiting the oxidation of glucose and phospholipogenesis stimulated by TSH) has no effect or actually potentiates the action of LATS on glucose oxidation and ^{32}P incorporation into phospholipids of the thyroid gland. This is suggestive of qualitative or quantitative differences in the action of TSH and LATS on thyroid metabolism. The question of the site of formation of LATS has still not been settled. In earlier reports an abnormal thyrotropin was described in pituitary extracts, but later sufficient evidence was adduced to prove that the pituitary is not the site of its formation.

It can be concluded from recent investigations that LATS is a hormonally active antibody against certain components of the thyroid gland cells, not found in the blood under normal conditions but appearing in high concentrations in certain forms of thyrotoxicosis [67]. According to the observations of Purves and Adams [401], the quantity of LATS found in the serum of patients corresponds more closely to the degree of exophthalmos than to the severity of the hyperthyroidism. The hypothesis of the immunological nature of LATS is confirmed by the fact that this stimulator is specifically bound by thyroid gland tissue. Glynn et al. [175] showed that thyroid gland homogenates and subparticles isolated from the gland adsorb LATS completely, but the microsomal fraction binds this immunoglobulin particularly well. Kidney homogenates and the fractions of microsomes and light mitochondria prepared from them bound only 30% of the LATS activity. The results confirm that LATS is an antibody, that the site of the antigen is specific for the thyroid gland, and that binding of the added immunoglobulin by kidney homogenates is not an immunochemical reaction.

In a recent investigation of components of the thyroid gland inhibiting LATS [452], the preparation of soluble fractions containing an LATS inhibitor from homogenates of normal human and pig thyroid glands was described. The workers cited conclude, from their discovery of a 5′-nucleotidase normally present in the cell membrane in this fraction, that LATS is microsomal in origin.

Besides LATS, other biological stimulators related to TSH have been described. One of the these is the exophthalmic factor, the discovery of which was first described by Dobyns in 1953 [110]. This factor has been found only in the blood of patients with progressive exophthalmos [252]. In its physicochemical properties it was similar to thyrotropin but by no means identical with it. Later, many investigators also showed that exophthalmic factor is not identical with LATS, as Adams had suggested. It can be separated from TSH by ion-exchange chromatography. The isolation of exophthalmic factor in a purified form by extraction and fractionation of bovine pituitary glands has also been described by Branisch, Hayashi, and Hayashi [61]. These workers stated that the molecular weight of this compound is less than 35,000. Recent parallel investigations by Primstone et al. [400] in various thyroid disorders confirm that TSH, LATS, and exophthalmos-inducing factor are in fact different substances. However, no fresh communications have appeared in recent years confirming the presence of a special factor in the pituitary or in the serum of patients with exophthalmic goiter, with an effect on the orbital tissues [37], or describing the further study of its chemical composition and properties.

The prostaglandins, biologically active lipids with a hypotensive action and causing contraction of the musculature of the stomach, isolated by extraction from human seminal fluid or from the seminal vesicles of sheep [27], are another group of thyroid stimulators.

In his Plenary Lecture at the 7th Conference of the Federation of European Biochemical Societies in Varna in 1971, Bergström described the prostaglandins as a family of bioregulators [51]. In the last ten years many different prostaglandins have been isolated, their structure determined, and the principal reactions of their biosynthesis from C_{20}-fatty acids and of their cell metabolism have been established. The prostaglandins are found in all animals, but in very low concentrations. They have a very powerful influence on physiological reactions, but they are rapidly inactivated metabolically. The prostaglandins stimulate many different parameters of thyroid metabolism, which suggests that they play an important role in the regulation of thyroid function [140]. Proof of the presence of prostaglandins in thyroid tissue gives further support to the hypothesis that they play a role in thyroid function [222].

Of the prostaglandins whose functions have so far been described, prostaglandins E_1 and E_2 have an effect closest to TSH on the thyroid gland [66]. They stimulate oxidation of glucose by thyroid gland slices, endocytosis in the follicles, the assimilation of iodine, and the excretion of radioiodine by the thyroid gland, but they do not stimulate incorporation of ^{32}P into phospholipids. Although the action of the prostaglandins is additive to the action of TSH, they do not potentiate the effect of TSH, and they actually abolish the effects of certain doses on glucose oxidation. Each of the prostaglandins increases the liberation of radioiodine by the mouse thyroid gland *in vivo*. However, in conjunction with a submaximal dose of TSH or LATS, the effect of the hormone is considerably reduced. These results show that different phases of hormone synthesis in the thyroid gland are not necessarily intensified harmoniously and that TSH and, perhaps, LATS and the prostaglandins compete for the common combining sites in the thyroid gland. Similar results have been obtained by the study of the effect of thyrotropin, prostaglandin E, and the prostaglandin antagonist 7-oxo-13-prostinoic acid on iodine transport in isolated thyroid gland cells. The same workers [449], working with isolated bovine thyroid cells and dog thyroid slices, concluded that the thyroid prostaglandins may play an important role in the stimulation of cyclic AMP formation by TSH and, consequently, in the stimulation of hormone formation in the gland.

The various effects of the prostaglandins have been studied intensively in recent years, and the subject has been extensively surveyed [409]. According to many reports, high concentrations of prostaglandins are found in the thyroid gland. The action of prostaglandins in all tissues simulates the effects of tropic hormones by correlating cyclic AMP formation. By modifying the action of phosphodiesterase, responsible for breaking down cyclic AMP in the cell, the prostaglandins can influence the accumulation of this compound.

The isolation of a thyroid-inhibiting factor from the blood serum and adenohypophysis by chromatographic fractionation and the presence of factors inhibiting the thyroid gland in certain fractions of kidney and liver homogenates were reported a few years earlier [294]. However, the chemical nature, mechanism of action on the gland, and biological role of these factors were not explained.

Recently these same workers [141] obtained three fractions with different actions on the blood pressure by fractionation of kidney homogenates with the ultracentrifuge. One fraction (31,500*g*), although neutral in relation to the blood pressure, contained a factor inhibiting the thyroid gland. The experimental results showed that this factor can inhibit thyroid gland function by inhibiting certain stages of the iodine-concentrating mechanism.

In the course of research into the stimulation of thyroid metabolism and of the intrathyroid circulation of iodine by TSH, the need for a detailed study of the initial stage of interaction between TSH and the subcellular and molecular components of the follicular cells became increasingly apparent. Only by explaining the action of TSH on the individual stages of iodine metabolism and of the substrate and energy metabolism of the gland can the fine biochemical mechanism of regulation of the thyrotropic function of the thyroid gland be completely elucidated. This problem has been studied by determining the time of appearance of the individual effects in the thyroid gland after injection of thyrotropin into hypophysectomized animals and studying the fixation and metabolism of ^{35}S-labeled TSH in the thyroid gland [96, 472]. However, this approach did not yield sufficient information to explain the initial effect of TSH and the subsequent development of events in the thyroid gland after administration of TSH.

A new chapter in the investigations of the mechanism of action of TSH on the thyroid gland was begun with the discovery of the effect of 3′,5′-cyclic AMP, hitherto known as a mediator in the action of several hormones or neurohormones [486], on iodine transport in the gland. The cyclic nucleotide adenosine 3′,5′-phosphate, or cyclic adenylate, was found in animal tissues in the course of a study of the mechanism of action of sympathomimetic amines or glucagon [484]. It increases the formation of active phosphorylase in the supernatant fraction of tissue preparations and in the absence of adrenalin and glucagon. Adrenalin and glucagon stimulate the formation of cyclic adenylate.

The hypothesis of Sutherland et al. [485] that cyclic 3′,5′-AMP may be a common intracellular mediator for the action of various hormones on target tissues has recently received abundant confirmation. As a result of research undertaken chiefly by Sutherland's group, it is now firmly established that cyclic AMP, synthesized in the tissues under the influence of hormones, is a *second mediator* between the endocrine gland and target tissue. The hormone itself is regarded in this scheme as the first mediator. The following sequence of reactions is now assumed to take place when a hormone produces its effect at the cell level: The hormone outside the cell binds with the combining site on the outer membrane and activates a special enzyme, adenyl cyclase, which catalyzes the conversion of ATP into cyclic AMP; the newly formed cyclic AMP enters the cell and, in turn, activates other enzymes with which the production of the hormonal effect is connected [370].

Sutherland's hypothesis of the mediator function of cyclic adenylate in the mechanism of action of the hormone evoked an avalanche of new research into the possible role of cyclic AMP in the regulation of other complex intracellular reactions also. It was soon discovered that cyclic AMP is the only known intracellular component to participate in the regulation of such phenomena as the shape of cells and their amalgamation into multicellular structures (aggregation) and the process of secretion. Cyclic AMP was found to be a universal agent concerned with the action of protein-peptide and catecholamine hormones on various target cells leading to a wide range of effects. We now know that cyclic AMP participates in the action of at least 10 hormones or neurohumoral agents and that it plays the part of a key regulator in most mammalian tissues [419].

The activation of adenyl cyclase and the formation of cyclic AMP from ATP by the action of triiodothyronine in spermatozoa has been reported. Besides adrenalin and noradrenalin, glucagon and hydroxytryptamine, TSH, LATS, and prostaglandin, the mediator function of cyclic AMP in connection with corticotropin has also been investigated. As Haynes [205] showed, corticotropin increases the accumulation of cyclic adenylate in slices of adrenal cortex. It was concluded by Grahame-Smith et al. [182] that cyclic AMP not only mediates the effect of ACTH on steroid production, but it may also be an intracellular mediator of the tropic effects of this hormone on adrenalin. The immediate intracellular target system for cyclic AMP is not yet known. The initial experiments of Klainer et al. [253] suggest activation of phosphorylase by cyclic AMP as the trigger mechanism for all subsequent metabolic events.

Cyclic AMP accelerates the accumulation of active phosphorylase from inactive phosphorylase in various tissues. This stimulates glycogenolysis, and every tissue responds by the formation of cyclic AMP to the corresponding hormone. The liver responds to the action of the two catecholamines and glucagon, skeletal muscles respond to catecholamines but not to glucagon, *Fasciola hepatica* responds to 5-hydroxytryptamine but not to catecholamines, the adrenals to corticotropin but not to glucagon and catecholamines, and the thyroid gland to TSH, LATS, and prostaglandin but not to other hormones.

Sufficient evidence has now been obtained to show that TSH exerts its action through cyclic 3′,5′-AMP, with a stimulant action similar to that of TSH *in vitro*. Acording to these views, TSH potentiates the activity of the enzyme adenyl cyclase, which activates the conversion of ATP into cyclic 3′,5′-AMP.

Stimulation of iodide transport by TSH has been shown to be reproduced completely by the addition of cyclic AMP, or its derivative dibutyryl-cyclic AMP, to the medium. This fact can accordingly be interpreted as evidence of the role of cyclic AMP in the mechanism of action of TSH. TSH raises the cyclic AMP level in thyroid slices [171] and homogenates [253]. Cyclic AMP and dibutyryl-cyclic AMP, on the contrary, reproduce some effects of TSH on thyroid gland tissue, such as the stimulation of phospholipid metabolism and glucose oxidation [372], the formation of intracellular colloid droplets [373], the excretion of radioiodine [302], and iodine transport [555] in isolated thyroid gland cells.

It is interesting to note that the action of LATS and prostaglandin E_1, substances of a totally different origin from TSH, on the thyroid gland is also mediated by cyclic adenylate. For this reason, the effects of TSH and other thyroid stimulators on the rate of secretion of thyroid hormones and the accompanying phenomena have been repeatedly compared in recent years to investigate the possible role of cyclic adenylate in this process.

Williams et al. [553] investigated the secretion of ^{131}I from the lobes of previously labeled thyroid glands in rats and showed that the stimulation of excretion of nonprotein ^{131}I after the addition of TSH, cyclic AMP, and dibutyryl-cyclic adenylate is dependent on the dose. This effect of TSH and cyclic adenylate, and also of other thyroid gland stimulators such as prostaglandins and the specific thyroid stimulator, LATS, has been carefully investigated by many workers [8, 172, 244, 273, 371, 372]. These investigations have shown that stimulation of all parameters of thyroid functional activity is observed under the influence of LATS, prostaglandins, cyclic AMP, and its derivatives; the parameters stimulated include the formation of intracellular colloid droplets, the most specific response to the action of TSH.

Macchia and Varrone [299] and Pastan and Katzen [371] showed that TSH exhibits its action on the thyroid gland through cyclic AMP. Dibutyryl-cyclic AMP is as effective as TSH, but cyclic guanosine monophosphate (cyclic GMP) does not affect the formation of intracellular colloid droplets, although AMP, like TSH, has a specific effect on this process. Consequently, cyclic AMP is the intracellular mediator of TSH when stimulating the secretory process. Cyclic GMP does not have this role. Similar results were obtained by Williams et al. [553] in a study of the stimulation of secretion *in vitro* by dog thyroid slices by thyrotropin cyclic 3′,5′-AMP, dibutyryl-cyclic 3′,5′-AMP, and prostaglandin E, by Kendall-Taylor et al. [248] in their investigation of the action of dibutyryl-cyclic 3′,5′-AMP on the mouse thyroid gland *in vitro*, and by Ahn and Rosenberg [9] in a study of the effect of TSH, dibutyryl-cyclic 3′,5′-AMP, and prostaglandin E on proteolysis in the thyroid gland. In this last investigation the principal labeled products of proteolysis were iodide, iodotyrosines, and iodothyronines.

Burke [66] investigated the effect of prostaglandins on the basic and stimulated functions of the thyroid gland and concluded that all four types of prostaglandins studied increase the exretion of radioiodine by the mouse thyroid gland *in vivo*, although if added to a submaximal dose of TSH or LATS they considerably reduce the effect of the hormone. The experiments of Burke and Sato [69] gave additional evidence of the action of these three stimulators on adenyl cyclase activity. By their investigations into the effect of LATS and prostaglandin antagonists on adenyl cyclase activity in isolated cells of the bovine thyroid gland they showed that the immunoglobulin G of LATS stimulates adenyl cyclase depending on the dose of the preparation. The duration of the activation of adenyl cyclase induced by LATS is comparable with that observed under the influence of TSH. Prostaglandin inhibitors appreciably depress the stimulant effect of prostaglandin E_2, TSH, and LATS on adenyl cyclase, although they do not modify the basic cyclase activity. Polyphloretin phosphate, a prostaglandin inhibitor, inhibited the effects of both TSH and LATS on the excretion of radioiodine from the previously labeled mouse thyroid gland, evidently by a competitive mechanism, but did not thereby change the effect of dibutyryl-cyclic AMP on it. These workers conclude that activation of the prostaglandin combining site may be an early stage in the action of both TSH and LATS on the thyroid gland.

Yamashita and Field [564] showed that LATS and TSH stimulate adenyl cyclase activity in plasma membranes obtained from the bovine thyroid gland. LATS depresses the TSH-induced stimulation of adenyl cyclase activity. However, this action of LATS was found not to be completely specific. These workers conclude that the stimulation of the adenyl cyclase of the plasma membranes of the thyroid gland is more likely to be due to changes in the conformation of the membranes than to fixation to a specific combining site.

Some workers suggested earlier that TSH and prostaglandin E_1 compete for a common combining site on adenyl cyclase. Maayan and Ingbar [296] recently reported that adrenalin stimulates the adenyl cyclase activity of isolated thyroid gland cells, although catecholamines mainly increase the organic fixation of iodine rather than its transport inside the cell. These experimental results have shown that the various phases of hormone formation in the thyroid gland are not necessarily stimulated harmoniously and that TSH and also, perhaps, LATS and prostaglandins compete for the common adenyl cyclase combining site in the thyroid gland.

Although LATS and the prostaglandins have an action on the thyroid gland similar to that of the natural thyroid stimulator TSH and although their effect is possibly due to the action of adenyl cyclase and the formation of cyclic AMP, i.e., they have the same mechanism (which is a little unusual considering their different chemical nature), these considerations are important for the elucidation of the nature of the effects observed. Under physiological conditions, the role of TSH in the hormonal secretion of the thyroid gland is incomparably greater, and it is the specific mechanism regulating all aspects of thyroid activity.

Kuchl et al. [264] produced evidence that activation of the combining site by prostaglandin is an essential feature of the action of luteinizing hormone on the stimulation of cyclic AMP formation and of hormone synthesis. They claim that a comparable situation may exist in other glands also. The decisive factor in the stimulant effect of cyclic AMP on the thyroid gland, whether in the case of TSH, LATS, or prostaglandin E, is an intensification of iodide transport.

In a series of experiments Tong et al. [519, 555] demonstrated the stimulant action of TSH on iodide transport by isolated bovine thyroid gland cells. Accumulation of iodine was observed and was expressed as ratios between the cellular (thyroid) concentration of iodide and the iodine concentration in the medium (T/S). After an incubation period of 1–2 h the addition of TSH led to a gradual increase in the value of T/S, and by 6 h it was 50–100% above the control level. This increase in T/S could be blocked by the addition of actinomycin D, puromycin, and cyclohexamide, inhibitors of protein synthesis, thus confirming the view that RNA and protein synthesis participate in this process. Although cyclic AMP participates in the mechanism of the effects of TSH on the thyroid gland, the relationship between activation of adenyl cyclase of the gland and stimulation of iodide transport in it still awaits precise explanation.

On the basis of their initial experiments Klainer et al. [253] postulate the possible action of cyclic AMP on phosphorylase activation, although there is no clear evidence that it can act as a regulator or as an effector of key (allosteric) enzymes or by other mechanisms. An alternative explanation of the action of cyclic AMP is that it can regulate the translation of template RNA in the polysomes.

In recent experiments on bovine thyroid gland cells, Knopp et al. [255] studied the way in which stimulation of iodide transport depends on time in order to identify the period essential for TSH, for cyclic AMP, or for both together and the period essential for synthesis of RNA and protein. They found that the formation of cyclic AMP in thyroid cells rises sharply on the addition of TSH and returns rapidly to its original state after removal of the TSH by treatment with trypsin. These results are in good agreement with the view that the first stage in the action of TSH, in which the hormone is bound to receptor sites on the cell surface, is followed by activation of membrane-bound adenyl cyclase, increasing the formation of cyclic AMP. The increase in accessible intracellular cyclic AMP leads to the cascadelike development of all the metabolic and morphological changes observed in response to the action of TSH.

The third stage in the sequence of reactions initiated by TSH, leading to stimulation of iodide transport, is evidently RNA formation. This stage lasts 1–2 h after addition of TSH and is required for supplying cyclic AMP, a process stimulated by TSH. This is followed by the fourth stage, that of translation, sensitive to the action of cyclohexamide and able to take place even in the absence of TSH.

TSH stimulates protein synthesis both in slices and in isolated thyroid gland cells [518]. However, some of the newly synthesized protein must par-participate in the stimulation of iodide transport. Nucleic acid synthesis is not appreciably changed by TSH in dispersed bovine thyroid gland cells. Knopp et al. [255] consider that specific RNA induced by TSH is concerned with activation of the iodide pump. It is formed in very small quantities and is almost undetectable compared with the large amount of newly synthesized RNA.

Protein induced by TSH also cannot be isolated or its properties determined, and it can be detected only by its single function of stimulating iodide transport. In all probability it is this protein which has the function of limiting the activity of the iodide pump. Lissitzky et al. [282] also showed that cyclic AMP stimulates the protein-synthesizing ability of the polysomes and ribosomes of the thyroid gland. However, this stimulation does not take place by the unmasking of the polysomal template RNA, as happens with ribosomes digested with trypsin. A more likely explanation is that the response of the polysomes to cyclic AMP is nonspecific and leads to a general increase in enzyme synthesis dependent upon the quantity and varieties of mRNA present in the polysomes. Consequently, the nature of the response of thyroid polysomes to cyclic AMP must depend on biochemical differentiation of the thyroid gland cells and the unique properties of its enzymic composition.

Mother–Fetus Relations in the Biosynthesis, Transport, and Distribution of Thyroid Hormones

Hormonal relations between mother and fetus can be examined from the standpoint of the need of maternal hormones by the embryo and fetus during normal organogenesis and the possibibility of mutual compensation of the hormonal function under pathological conditions.

In 1937 Pende [377] wrote: "Functional equilibrium is established between the glands of the mother and fetus in the sense that endocrine hyperfunction of the mother leads to endocrine hypofunction of the fetus, and endocrine hypofunction in the mother leads to compensatory hyperfunction in the fetus."

The first attempts to study the human fetal thyroid gland were nothing more than descriptions of autopsy material and morphological descriptions of the gland in premature infants. The primordial thyroid gland appears early, at the 3rd–4th week of intrauterine life, and the first sign of secretion of thyroid hormones is not observed until the 12th–14th week.

Gudernatsch [191] in 1912 and Laufberger [266] in 1913 gave the first clear demonstration of the importance of thyroid hormones for the metamorphosis of amphibian larvae. Later much work was done on the morphogenetic role of thyroid hormone. Mitskevich [323, 324, 325], Adams and Bull [4], Hageman [195], and Jost et al. [240] showed that blocking thyroid function by some means or other in the embryos of birds and other animals leads to delay in the attainment and a decrease in the value of many growth parameters, lengthening of the incubation period, delay of growth and differentiation, delay in ossification of the skeleton, and inhibition of the appearance of nervous centers. Normal thyroid function of mother and fetus is absolutely essential for adequate intrauterine development of the fetus [189, 254, 303, 335, 434, 565].

Many investigators have shown that the fetal thyroid gland begins to secrete hromonally active compounds long before birth [168–170, 241, 326, 341, 344, 381, 383, 466, 565]. In animals of different species this takes place at different stages of intrauterine development.

The onset of thyroid function *in utero* is identified by the discovery of the first portions of hormonal iodine in embryonic plasma (Table X). However, this moment is preceded by the beginning of iodine absorption and its

Table X. Onset of Thyroid Function in Certain Species of Mammals Based on Observations by Mitskevich [326]

Species of mammals	Duration of pregnancy, days	Beginning of thyroid function, day	Literature cited
Cat	62–65	50	527
Rabbit	32	17	529
Sheep	145	70–130	228
Rat	21	18–19	215, 217, 364, 365
Monkey	164	75–150	399
Mouse	19–20	17	525
Cow	285	85	226, 227
Goat	285	60	537
Pig	114	52	537
Man	280	19–28	544

Note: Lissitzky et al. showed that the ability of the thyroid cells of rabbit embryos to iodinate thyroglobulin starts to appear only on the 22nd day of pregnancy (6th International Conference on the Thyroid Gland, June 22–25, 1970, Vienna).

conversion into organic compounds, first to mono- and diiodotyrosine, later to triiodothyronine and thyroxine. Adolph [7] concluded that iodine is absolutely necessary for the normal intrauterine development of the mammalian fetus in order to maintain homeostasis between mother and fetus.

A certain length of time elapses between the beginning of iodine absorption by the fetal thyroid gland and the appearance of the first portions of thyroid hormones in the plasma [325]. In the rat fetus, for example, the thyroid gland begins to absorb iodine on the 16th day of pregnancy [170, 344]. This order of formation of the various stages of thyroid hormone synthesis during intrauterine development (iodine absorption, formation of MIT, DIT, T_3, T_4) has been established for embryos of different species of animals. Trunnel and Wade [524] showed that the concentration of iodide and its fixation in the chick embryonic thyroid gland take place at different time intervals: Iodide can be found at 7.5 days of embryonic development, MIT appears after 8.5 days, diiodotyrosine after 9.25 days, and thyroxine only after 9.75 days. Thus, the ability to synthesize monoiodotyrosine occurs first, and ability to synthesize diiodotyrosine occurs later. Consequently, in the development of the embryonic chick thyroid gland, there is a period in which monoiodotyrosine is present and diiodotyrosine is not. The calf embryo synthesizes thyroxine in the thyroid gland between the 53rd and 70th days of pregnancy. The thyroid gland of the rabbit fetus begins to concentrate ^{131}I between 15 and 16 days of pregnancy, and it binds iodine in the organic form approximately two days later.

Nataf and Sfez [342] studied the thyroid function in the rat embryo after thyroidectomy of the mother on the 12th–14th day of pregnancy. They found that toward the end of pregnancy the fetal thyroid gland concentrates ^{131}I and metabolizes it, forming the same iodinated compounds as the adult. Often, however, the quantitative relations were different. The MIT/DIT ratio in the embryonic thyroid was 1.4 or more. Under these conditions the ratio between hormone and iodide is lowered. Similar results were obtained in a study of embryonic thyroid function in pregnant rabbits. After removal of the thyroid gland from pregnant females the embryonic gland functioned qualitatively as the adult gland but its activity was lower.

In another paper Nataf and Sfez [343] gave evidence that the thyroid gland of rat embryos fixes very small amounts of radioiodine before the 19th day of pregnancy, although both MIT and DIT were found in the glands on the 17th day. After 17.5 days of pregnancy thyroxine begins to be synthesized and can be found in both the gland and the plasma of the fetus. Starting from the 18th day, the fetal gland functions in the same way as in the mature fetus. Pickering and Kontaxis [382] studied the chemical and morphological characteristics of the thyroid gland in monkey fetuses and found that radioiodine, injected into the mother on the 75th day after conception, was actively assimilated by the gland and converted into organic forms. By this time follicles are present in the gland, where not only iodotyrosines but also thyroxine and triiodothyronine are synthesized.

The thyroid gland of the human fetus begins to function in the early stages of pregnancy. In the 12th week of development this gland can assimilate iodine, and it contains thyroxine [220, 369]. According to Yamasaki et al. [563] the thyroid gland of the human fetus becomes capable of concentrating iodine at the age of 14 weeks and of converting it into the organic form with the formation of thyroxine between 15 and 19 weeks. Recent research into this problem by Lenart [272] showed that ^{131}I accumulates in large quantities in the thyroid gland of the human fetus with effect from the 13th week of pregnancy; in this investigation 50 mCi ^{131}I was injected 24 h before the termination of pregnancy.

Chromatographic studies showed that only inorganic iodine accumulates in the fetal gland before the 14th week, but later organic iodine also accumulate. The quantity of iodine in the fetal gland was 1 μg at the beginning of the 4th month, 3 μg at the end of the 4th month, 6 μg at the end of the 5th month, 20–40 μg at the end of the 6th month, and 350 μg at birth. The dynamics of iodine accumulation and metabolism in the human fetus can be studied with the aid of ^{131}I.

Costa et al. [88] investigated thyroid function in the human fetus in connection with the placental factor and found that the weight of the thyroid and weight of the pituitary glands remain constant relative to the length of the fetus and its degree of maturity. The fetal thyroid gland accumulates iodine administered to the mother, and it contains stable iodine by the 80th day of gestation; accumulation of ^{131}I in the fetal thyroid gland takes place much faster per unit weight of gland than in the mother.

In a study of 19 fresh fetal human thyroid glands Hodges et al. [220] and Shepard [462] found by biochemical and autoradiographic methods in organ cultures that active differentiation and hormonal activity of the thyroid gland begin in the fetus 65–80 mm long, corresponding to the 73rd–80th days of pregnancy. These workers distinguish three stages in the development of the human thyroid gland: a precolloid stage, commencing colloid, and growth of the follicles of the gland.

Since triiodothyronine possesses the greatest hormonal activity, Abbott et al. [1] studied the relationship between the elimination of radioactive triiodothyronine and the physiological state of the thyroid gland in each successive 3-month period of pregnancy. Blood tests for this purpose were carried out during each 3-month period of normal pregnancy and also in women with incomplete abortion 12–24 h after it began. The results showed that in the first 3-month period the blood triiodothyronine concentration falls and the decrease is more marked in the second and, in particular, in the third 3-month period. During the 6 weeks after delivery the blood triiodothyronine level returns to normal. Fluctuations in its level were not observed after abortion. Abbott describes considerable individual variations in the triiodothyronine level, and these must inevitably make it difficult to assess the state of the thyroid function.

Just as in the adult, 19 S thyroglobulin is the main iodinated protein in the fetal thyroid gland. As long ago as in 1952, Gorbman et al. [178] obtained fetal thyroglobulin from the thyroid glands of calves and described some of its properties. Until 1970, however, the presence of thyroglobulin in the human fetal thyroid gland could only be postulated on the basis of the results of immunological tests [174, 440] or following the enzymic hydrolysis of thyroid tissue [462, 463], indicating that it contained iodinated amino acids. This indirect evidence did not permit definite conclusions to be drawn regarding the time at which this protein molecule first appears during intrauterine life. Further, the discovery of a substance reacting immunologically with antithyroglobulin antibodies is not itself sufficient to identify it as a molecule of 19 S thyroglobulin.

Olin [362, 363], using incubation *in vitro* in the presence of $Na^{125}I$ and leucine-^{3}H, succeeded in demonstrating the existence of human fetal thyroglobulin and described some of its properties and those of other thyroid proteins. He detected the presence of thyroglobulin on the 77th day of pregnancy, i.e., at the time when iodine begins to accumulate. Human fetal thyroglobulin was obtained from the thyroid glands of fetuses aged between 77 and 148 days. It was identical to the thyroglobulin of adults in its immunological reactivity with adult human antithyroglobulin antibodies and in the presence of iodinated amino acids, including thyroxine. It was also shown that the 47-day fetus synthesizes uniodinated prethyroglobulin. Olin considers that during normal intrauterine development of the human fetus the synthesis of the protein matrix (molecule) of thyroglobulin precedes the iodination of the molecule. Before the 77th day of intrauterine life (65-mm fetus) the thyroid gland cannot accumulate iodine (Olin [362, 363]). These observations are in agreement with the results obtained by Shepard [462], who was unable to find evidence of thyroglobulin synthesis by the use of isotopes (^{131}II and ^{3}H) in fetuses from 30 to 55 mm long. He likewise could not demonstrate it in a fetus 60 mm long after incubation for 4 h in medium containing a high concentration of radioiodine.

Grigor'eva [185] recently studied thyroglobulin formation by the fetal thyroid gland of three species of animals by an immunofluorescence method. She found that iodinated thyroglobulin is present on the 17th day of intrauterine development of the rat, the 28th day of intrauterine development of the guinea pig, and the 10th day of incubation of chick embryos, i.e., at times when the fetal thyroid gland is beginning to function. In these experiments, when the follicles were still only beginning to be formed, thyroglobulin was found between the epithelial cells. With the appearance of colloid spaces bright specific fluorescence was observed chiefly at the boundary between the cell and the colloid.

The plasma PBI level of the fetus reflects the hormonal balance, itself an expression of the function of the thyroid gland, i.e., the ability to secrete thyroid hormones. However, it gives no idea of quantitative correlations between mother and fetus, although it does reflect the very important ability of the gland to absorb iodine and synthesize thyroid hormones.

In defects of thyroid hormone synthesis, the PBI level may fall sharply although the thyroid gland is hypertrophied and assimilates large quantities of iodine. Despite these defects, determination of the fetal plasma PBI simultaneously with other functional and morphological indices is an essential part of the evaluation of the state of thyroid function.

The ability of fetal blood proteins to bind thyroxine increases as pregnancy advances. However, near the time of birth the concentration of proteins binding thyroid hormones (TBP) is lower than in the maternal blood; this may explain the low values of PBI in the fetal blood [115, 158, 250, 308, 309, 379, 417, 436, 442].

In 1951, Danowski et al. [99] first reported that the PBI concentration in newborn infants rises to the hyperthyroid level during the first few hours and days of extrauterine life. This observation was fully confirmed later by other workers [144, 145, 304, 305, 308, 309, 379, 383]. During the first 1–2 months of pregnancy an increase in the PBI level in the maternal blood serum above the normal 3.5–8 $\mu g\%$ is observed [508]; later it remains more or less constant [394, 442] although the basal metabolism starts to rise only after the middle of pregnancy, increasing steadily until its end. During the first weeks of pregnancy the TBP level rises to 2–2.5 times its normal value, at which it remains until the end of pregnancy. The TBP level in newborn infants is 1.5 times higher than in unweaned infants [313].

Pitt-Rivers and Trotter [394] injected radioiodine into the maternal blood stream and observed the liberation of radioactive thyroxine into the blood starting from the end of the 16th week of pregnancy. They regard this as evidence of a connection between the pituitary and thyroid glands at this period. Since the degree of thyroxine binding by the protein carriers of maternal blood is sharply increased during pregnancy, the quantity of free thyroid hormone may be reduced below its level before pregnancy despite the frequent occurrence of hypertrophy of the thyroid gland or increased affinity of the thyroid gland tissue for radioactive iodine.

According to Berger and Nelken [50], Dowling et al. [117], and Tervilla [508] the mean PBI level in maternal blood is comparatively high but in umbilical blood it is lower; on the whole the maternal blood levels were much higher than the fetal (the difference amounts to 2–4 $\mu g\%$).

The author [447] has investigated thyroid function of the mother and fetus in rabbits as reflected in the PBI level in the blood and in the thyroid gland tissue of mother and fetus at different periods of pregnancy. The PBI level in maternal blood was determined from the 10th day of pregnancy until parturition and on the first day thereafter. The results showed that the

PBI level in the maternal blood rises considerably toward the end of pregnancy, when it is 8–9 μg% compared with the normal 2.4 μg%. On the second day after parturition the PBI level falls to 3.6 μg%. It is practicable to determine the fetal blood PBI level from the 21st or 22nd day of pregnancy.

According to data in the literature, the thyroid gland in 18-day-old rabbit embryos synthesizes chiefly a low-molecular-weight thyroglobulin with a sedimentation coefficient of 12 S. This polymerizes with the formation of thyroglobulin with a sedimentation coefficient of 19 S only after the 22nd day. Further, the ability of thyroid cells of rabbit embryos to iodinate thyroglobulin is closely linked with the appearance of the endoplasmic reticulum and the beginning of follicle formation on the 22nd day.

Investigations have shown that the PBI concentration in fetal blood rises steadily from the time when the fetal thyroid gland begins to function until the end of pregnancy, when it is 6.3 μg%. The low fetal PBI levels can evidently be explained by the lower thyroxine binding power of fetal than maternal TBP [313]. A tendency for the PBI to increase with an increase in the duration of pregnancy was observed. The PBI level in the maternal thyroid gland tissue rises sharply toward the end of pregnancy (50.7 μg% compared with 7.3 μg%/100 mg weight of tissue). With the approach of parturition the functional activity of the fetal thyroid gland also increases.

It must not be forgotten that the PBI level can be raised by an increase in the estrogen concentration in the blood of pregnant women. This has been established by both clinical and biochemical investigations [117, 135, 508]. Pregnancy stimulates the activity of many endocrine glands, including the thyroid. According to Tsarikovskaya and Miloslavskii [525] in the early stages the thyroid gland increased in size and weight and developed hyperplasia and proliferation of the epithelium, with the formation of new follicles. In the second half of pregnancy the basal metabolic rate increased by 10–20%. The blood thyroxine concentration rose at the same time, evidence of an increase in the concentration of hormonal iodine in the blood serum.

From the 16th week of pregnancy until term the PBI concentration rises steadily to reach 7–12 μg% at the end of pregnancy compared with the normal 4–7 μg%. Pregnancy also increases the degree of uptake of radioactive iodine by the maternal thyroid gland [81, 251]. Sircar and Chaterjee [470] observed a gradual increase in the PBI level in the early stages of pregnancy, a sharp increase toward the end, and a rapid decrease after parturition.

Mestman et al. [319] studied thyroid function in 24 healthy women between the 23rd and 40th weeks of pregnancy and also 4–8 weeks after parturition. They found that the PBI level in nonpregnant women varies from 4 to 8 μg%. During pregnancy its mean value is 7.6, and in the postnatal period, 5.1 μg%. The iodothyronine concentration in the blood of healthy nonpregnant women is 2.9–6.4 μg%. It increases during pregnancy (6.8 μg%), and is somewhat lower after parturition (4.3 μg%).

Costa et al. [88] studied the concentrations of PBI, TBP, proteins, and some inorganic substances (nitrogen, sodium, potassium, iodine salts) in the serum of pregnant women and human fetuses and also in the amniotic fluid during the second 3-month period of pregnancy and during labor. They found that the fetus obtains a small quantity of thyroxine from the mother until birth, i.e., long after the fetal thyroid gland has attained complete functional maturity. They found larger quantities of iodides in the fetal than in the maternal serum. Together with the increased uptake of iodine by the fetal thyroid gland compared with the maternal gland, this stimulates hormone production by the fetal thyroid gland, which is in a state of disturbed equilibrium because of the presence of a large quantity of thyroid iodine not utilizable for hormone synthesis [87]. By the third trimester of pregnancy, iodides and organic iodine are found in the amniotic fluid. The amniotic fluid plays no part in the synthesis of thyroid hormone, which is confirmed by the fact that the iodine level in the amniotic fluid and the TBP remain constant throughout pregnancy. On the other hand, the fetus quickly acquires some degree of independence; as pregnancy develops the protein and PBI concentrations in the fetal serum gradually approach those of the adult, diverging further and further from their concentrations in the amniotic fluid. Toward the end of pregnancy the fetus receives a powerful stimulus in the form of the discharge of large quantities of thyrotropin into the blood stream. This acts as a powerful stimulus to the thyroid gland and prepares the fetus for its departure into the external environment and its conflict with harmful exogenous influences.

Many investigations have shown that, if maternal thyroid hormones are deficient, the mammalian fetus is retarded in its development; children of mothers with hypothyroidism are underdeveloped mentally as well as physically [240, 271, 305, 415]. Maternal hormones are essential for the fetus until a certain stage of its intrauterine development. When the endocrine glands of the fetus itself begin to function, they are able to supply the corresponding hormones to the mother as well as to the fetus. Information on the effect of thyrotoxicosis on fetal and neonatal development is very scanty, although, according to some figures, this condition is found in 2.8% of all pregnant women [208].

Thalhammer [509] described several cases of congenital thyrotoxicosis in newborn infants of mothers with diffuse toxic goiter. Barkhatova [39] found various disturbances, more frequently affecting the central nervous and cardiovascular systems, less frequently the reproductive, endocrine, and musculoskeletal systems, in one-third of children of mothers with moderately severe toxic goiter. Offspring from untreated mothers were affected more often and more severely, while vigorous treatment of the goiter greatly improved the condition of these children. The severe late sequelae must be specially mentioned. During the first year of life, various disturbances of the CNS were found (increased excitability, hyperkinesia, disturbances of sleep). In three children organic lesions of the nervous system were present (microcephaly, hydrocephalus, Down's syndrome). Congenital heart defects were diagnosed in 5 children; 13 boys had disturbances of the reproductive system (cryptorchidism, phimosis, hydrocele); and in some children changes in the skeletal system were found. In most cases an increased predisposition to allergic and infectious diseases was observed.

Barkhatova [39] also found that pregnancy occurs in 0.4–3% of cases in patients with toxic goiter. In severe forms of the disease and if, as frequently happens, amenorrhea is present, pregnancy does not develop. Pregnancy terminated prematurely in 33–50% of the pregnant women. Farrehi [139] mentions accelerated maturation of a thyrotoxic fetus born after 33 weeks of pregnancy. In an attempt to explain this phenomenon he concludes that the long-acting thyroid stimulator discovered in the maternal blood serum penetrates into the fetus and causes hyperfunction of the fetal thyroid gland. Sunshine [482] described a case of congenital thyrotoxicosis in a child of a healthy mother with long-acting thyroid stimulator in her blood stream. The same stimulator was found in the blood of the newborn infant. After birth of the child the LATS soon disappeared from its blood but persisted in the maternal blood. This is evidence of the transplacental transmission of this biological thyroid stimulator from mother to fetus.

Khomasuridze [251] studied the thyroid function in the progeny of hypothyroid rats. His investigations showed that the reproductivity of the rats depends essentially on the level of thyroid function. Thyroid hormones are evidently essential for conception and for the intrauterine development of the fetus.

The decrease in the level of thyroid function in hypothyroid female rats during pregnancy caused not only an appearance of morphological evidence of hyperactivity of the fetal thyroid but also a sharp increase in the indices of fetal thyroid function. Khomasuridze also states that the intensity of absorption of ^{131}I, the PBI concentration in the plasma and thyroid gland, and the absolute and relative weight of the gland in young rats born from thyroidectomized females are considerably greater in the early stages of postnatal development than in rats born from intact mothers. The results of histological investigations agree with these findings.

The increase in thyroid function in newborn rats born from thyroidectomized females is evidently based on the fact that if the maternal thyroid hormones are absent or deficient, the thyroid-stimulating function of the fetal pituitary is *disinhibited.* Larger amounts of TSH are then secreted, and functional hyperactivity of the fetal thyroid gland results. The possibility likewise cannot be ruled out that the mother is also supplied with thyroid hormones by the fetus [198, 345, 346, 565].

In the author's laboratory the PBI levels in the blood and thyroid gland tissue were investigated in a group of female rabbits undergoing thyroidectomy on the 10th–12th day of pregnancy and also in their fetuses in order to discover whether the fetal thyroid gland is capable of independent function as soon as the fetus attains functional maturity. The results [446] showed that the dynamics of changes in PBI in thyroidectomized females confirms the hypothesis that the fetal thyroid gland can compensate for a deficiency of maternal thyroid hormones.

Transplacental transmission of maternal hormones and the character and mechanisms of their effects on development of the fetus and modifications of the maternal hormonal status by the fetal endocrine function differ according to the permeability of the placenta for the particular hormones under normal physiological conditions.

According to Mitskevich [326, 327] different types of hormonal compensatory relationships exist between mother and fetus: In some, endocrine factors (thyroid hormone, sex and adrenocortical hormones) can pass through the placental barrier in both directions, i.e., from mother to fetus and from fetus to mother, while transmission of the polypeptide trophic hormones of the anterior pituitary gland is impossible or improbable. The effects of these trophic factors on the fetus are brought about through their stimulation of maternal endocrine organs producing hormones that are capable of transplacental transmission. A third group of hormones (insulin, adrenalin, parathormone) likewise cannot pass through the placental barrier, although these hormones can exert their effect on the fetus and mother through changes in carbohydrate and calcium metabolism. With respect to the first group of hormones, Mitskevich describes them as giving rise to direct hormonal compensation; in the second case, indirect hormonal compensation takes place; in the third case, compensation is the result of regulation of metabolism.

Courrier and Aron [90] produced the first evidence, admittedly indirect, that thyroxine can penetrate through the placenta of dogs and guinea pigs in the last days of pregnancy. After injecting thyroxine into the blood stream of pregnant animals, they observed a decrease in function of the fetal thyroid gland and further concluded that proteins did not pass through the *placental filter.*

In their fundamental investigations Arshavskii and co-workers [29] found that, irrespective of the ratio between the concentrations of a particular substance in the mother and fetus, the molecular weight of the compound (within certain limits) and the structure of the placenta determined whether the compound could pass through the placenta in either direction, depending on the needs of the mother and fetus. They further concluded that this relationship was associated with the *gestation dominant*, which can regulate the acid-base balance in the mother and thereby influence the permeability of the placenta. They also showed that acidosis in the mother increases the permeability of her placenta. However, MacClendon and Maclennan [300], who investigated this problem 10 years later, concluded that the placental barrier is essentially impermeable to thyroid hormones. If any hormone did pass through the placenta, it was only in extremely small quantities. More recent investigations [50, 313, 394] also adhere to the view that under normal conditions thyroxine and triiodothyronine can pass through the placental barrier, but only in extremely small amounts. These amounts, in their opinion, are unlikely to be of any physiological significance.

The permeability of the placenta for thyroid hormones has since been investigated by many workers. Definite species differences in placental permeability for thyroid hormone have now been established. In particular, the highest degree of permeability of the placenta for triiodothyronine is observed in rats [345, 346]. Thyroxine passes through the placenta with considerable difficulty, especially in the early stage of pregnancy, in man [189] and the rabbit [244], while triiodothyronine passes with difficulty in the guinea pig [397]. Evidence of the passage of thyroid hormones through the placenta is fully convincing only if large doses are given—not less than 300 μg for triiodothyronine [406]. It has been shown quantitatively that the permeability of the placenta increases considerably in the later stages of pregnancy. After injection of labeled thyroxine into pregnant rats, hormonal iodine was found to be present in the fetal blood stream in an amount of less than 3% on the 17th day of pregnancy. Its level in the fetal blood rose as pregnancy continued, and at the end of pregnancy was over 30%. The fetal pituitary played virtually no part in this distribution for the intake of hormonal iodine into the fetus continued at the same level even after its decapitation. After injection of labeled triiodothyronine into the mother, the ratio between the fetal and maternal hormonal iodine concentrations was higher than that obtained for thyroxine; just as with thyroxine, the amount which passed increased during pregnancy. The concentration of labeled thyroxine in the fetal part of the placenta was 2.5 times greater than in the maternal blood plasma [334]. In addition, as shown by Nataf et al. [345], triiodothyronine passes more readily from mother to fetus than in the opposite direction.

In experiments on guinea pigs [288] the umbilical cord of a fetus taken from the uterus was clamped at its origin, cannulas were inserted into the umbilical artery and vein, and the placenta was perfused with a mixture of guinea pig blood plasma and physiological saline. After injection of ^{131}I-labeled triiodothyronine and thyroxine into the fluid perfusing the placenta or into the maternal blood stream, the passage of hormones from mother to fetus and vice versa was established. Chromatography of the outflowing perfusion fluid revealed that it contained about 50% of the thyroxine. Very little thyroxine passed from fetus to mother. Conversely, labeled triiodothyronine was found in the outflowing perfusion fluid, but its passage through the placenta from mother to fetus could not be demonstrated. Since chromatography revealed undegraded triiodothyronine in the perfusion fluid, it can be assumed that it does not undergo deiodination in the placenta.

The recent work of Dussault et al. [122] on triiodothyronine metabolism in maternal and fetal sheep is most interesting. These workers obtained serial blood samples through catheters introduced into a maternal artery and fetal vein on the 98th and 125th days of pregnancy. Blood sampling was carried out 48 h after injection of $^{125}I\text{-}T_3$ and $^{131}I\text{-}T_3$ into mother and fetus, respectively. They determined the quantitative levels of passage of triiodothyronine through the placenta; in particular the absolute passage of triiodothyronine from mother to fetus was 2 μg per diem and from fetus to mother about 1.2 μg per diem. The resultant passage of triiodothyronine from mother to fetus was thus approximately 1 μg daily.

During pregnancy some of the thyroxine is bound with albumins, some with a_1-and a_2-globulins, and only 0.1% of the total circulating thyroxine is in a free state in the blood stream [100, 101, 308]. Theoretically, the maternal proteins, for various reasons, cannot pass through the placental barrier to the fetus [2, 71, 102].

Experiments on rats have shown that the level of metabolism and conversion of thyroid hormones in the mother and also the degree of their binding by the maternal serum proteins depend on the intensity of deiodination of the thyroid hormones entering the fetal tissues from the mother, which is itself evidently connected with their utilization in the prenatal period of development [163].

The fetal thyroid hormones are also bound by plasma proteins, but not by the same fractions as in the maternal plasma. Fetal thyroid hormones bound with proteins migrate during electrophoresis between the a- and β-globulins [102]. A study of the properties of the fetal protein binding thyroxine in rabbits (fetal TBP) shows that on the 19th day of pregnancy the total volume of maternal TBP is 10 times greater than the volume of fetal TBP but the binding capacity of the latter is about five times greater than that of the maternal plasma.

Abdul-Karim [2] found that free thyroxine passes easily through the placental barrier in both directions, but despite this fact the quantity of maternal thyroxine entering the fetus and of fetal thyroxine entering the mother was unknown. Meanwhile, Gimbette and Piffanelli [173] consider that the free thyroxine level in the blood is the most reliable indicator of the state of the thyroid gland. Regardless of the fact that the concentration of TBP and of total thyroxine in the fetal plasma is lower than in maternal plasma [158], the quantity of free thyroxine in the fetus is equal to that in the mother [102] or may even exceed it [143, 156]. With an increase in age of the fetus, the concentration of free and bound thyroxine in the fetal plasma rises.

Investigations with radioactive thyroxine and triiodothyronine yielded fresh results, but the disagreements continued. Iodine ions are known to pass readily through the placenta [50], but this passage is extremely selective: only mineral iodine and only from mother to fetus [345].

In the monkey *Macaca mulatta*, labeled thyroxine injected into the mother in the second half of pregnancy was found in the placenta and the fetal blood serum and tissues. Comparison of its specific activity in the fetal tissues and fluid with its specific activity in the maternal blood showed that this hormone was maternal in origin. This conclusion is also supported by the fact that the specific activity of thyroxine in the fetal thyroid gland was always lower than in the fetal blood serum [381].

Comparison of the fetal and maternal plasma showed that iodinated compounds pass through the placenta, but the ratio of hormones to iodide in the fetal plasma is much higher, evidence of the important role of the placenta in the exchange between mother and fetus. According to Nataf et al. [345, 346], by the end of pregnancy ^{131}I, L-3,3′-diiodothyronine and L-3,5,3′-triiodothyronine pass readily through the rat placenta, ^{131}I by free diffusion but DIT and T_3 only along the *biological gradient*. These compounds can also pass from fetus to mother, but less than in the opposite direction.

Nataf and Sfez [343] injected ^{131}I into a thyroidectomized pregnant rat and found extremely small quantities of thyroxine in the placenta by a radiochromatographic method. This thyroxine was evidently formed in the fetal thyroid gland, for thyroid hormones are not synthesized in the placenta itself. This fact also confirms the possibility of an exchange of thyroxine between mother and fetus through the placenta.

More recent investigations have not settled the disagreements regarding the passage of thyroxine and its derivatives through the placental barrier. Grumbach and Werner [189], for instance, injected ^{131}I-labeled L-thyroxine a few hours before parturition and found that after 79 h, 49% of the radioactivity was in the maternal blood. The radioactivity in the fetal blood 10 h after injection of labeled triiodothyronine was 20% of the radioactivity of the maternal blood. These workers accept that the hormone found in the fetal blood is a metabolite of the hormone injected into the mother and not the hormone itself.

Postel [397] also observed the passage of very small quantities of labeled triiodothyronine through the guinea pig placenta 24 h after its injection. The results of a radioisotopic investigation of placental permeability in pregnant cows [347] show that the concentration of unbound iodine in the circulating fetal blood is five times higher than in the maternal blood. In the amniotic fluid, according to these workers, the iodine content is higher than in the fetal plasma. The iodine content in the chorionic fluid was midway between that in the maternal and fetal plasma. Evidently the inability of the fetus to excrete iodine in the urine is the main reason why the iodine concentration in the fetus is so much higher than that in the maternal blood plasma. After birth the rate of disappearance of unbound iodine in the calf is much greater than that in the cow during the first two days after injection of iodine. So far as the percentage of iodine absorbed by the thyroid gland and the changes in the general metabolism of radioactive iodine in the plasma immediately or 24 h after birth are concerned, these were similar in cow and calf.

Hopkins and Thorburn [221] determined the placental permeability of lamb fetuses after thyroidectomy of the mothers on the 110th day of pregnancy. After the operation the thyroxine concentration in the fetal blood plasma fell to zero and did not increase until birth even after injection of exogenous thyroxine into the mother; this result is evidence that the placenta is impermeable to thyroxine in the late stage of pregnancy in sheep.

There is evidence in the literature that in some laboratory animals iodine can pass through the placental barrier and that a concentration of iodine several times greater than that in the mother may develop in the fetal blood plasma [86, 198, 287]. However, information on this question is also contradictory. For instance, according to Gorbman [178], the ratio between the radioactive iodine in the fetus and mother 24 h after injection is 1:3. Meanwhile Monroe [330] found that the concentration of labeled iodine in the fetus 7 days after injection was 5–20 times higher than in the maternal plasma. A similar observation is described by Bustad et al. [70].

Studies with labeled preparations also revealed that the human placenta is permeable to thyroxine and triiodothyronine. However, these substances reach the fetus only with difficulty: The concentration of organic iodine in the fetal serum 14–53 h after injection of labeled thyroxine was only one-tenth that in the maternal serum. After injection of labeled triiodothyronine, its concentration in the fetal blood was also much lower than in the maternal blood [334].

Dyer et al. [123] determined the permeability of the placenta for radioactive ^{131}I and Fe^{99} in mothers undergoing therapeutic abortion. The ^{131}I was given by mouth in a dose of 50 μCi 12 h before the abortion; absorption of ^{131}I was measured in the fetus as a whole and in its organs separately. The fetal thyroid gland was found to have accumulated the greatest quantity of ^{131}I, 3000 times more than the other organs.

After intravenous injection of the sodium salt of thyroxine, the concentration of iodine extractable with butanol and the absorption of thyroxine in the newborn infants increased in accordance with the dose of the compound injected and the duration of the infusion. However, even with a dose of 8000 μg of sodium L-thyroxine and with a suitably prolonged infusion, this increase was much less marked than in the mother [144]. With an increase in the period between injection of labeled thyroxine into women and the onset of labor, the quantity of protein-bound ^{131}I in the maternal blood became relatively smaller, and there was a corresponding increase in its content in the neonatal blood. This indicates the relative slowness of passage of thyroxine through the placenta. Labeled triiodothyronine disappeared faster from the maternal blood than thyroxine, from which it can be concluded that it passes more rapidly through the placenta than thyroxine. This quicker transplacental passage may be due to the less strong binding of triiodothyronine with the plasma proteins [189].

The problem of placental permeability for iodinated compounds and, in particular, for thyroxine has been investigated in the author's laboratory by Salakhova and Saipov by injecting T_4-^{131}I and DIT-^{131}I into pregnant rats and also into their fetuses at different times of pregnancy and by determining the activity and composition of the iodinated components in the maternal and fetal blood. These investigations showed that 1 and 4 h after injection of the labeled hormone or of DIT-^{131}I into the mother, very slight activity was found in the fetal blood and liver, none of which was thyroxine. All activity was concentrated in the mother, most of it as T_4-^{131}I. After injection of the labeled hormone and DIT into the fetus, most activity and all of the T_4 and DIT were found in the fetus. These results confirm data in the literature on the impermeability of the placenta for thyroxine and other iodinated components both from mother to fetus and vice versa.

It has been stated in the literature that the placental barrier is permeable to endogenous or exogenous TSH in the direction from mother to fetus [236], but this is not supported by the results of other experiments [355]. Experiments on rats showed that, although these animals have a comparatively simply organized placenta (of hemochorial type), it is imppermeable to thyrotropic hormone. The guinea pig placenta also appears impermeable to the trophic hormone [97].

It can be concluded from the data described above that the question of permeability of the placenta for thyroid hormones still remains open. It is evidently impossible to state categorically whether the placental barrier is permeable or impermeable for thyroid hormones. The species of mammal, the requirements of thyroid hormones of the mother and fetus, the concentration and binding activity of the TBP, and also the state of the central nervous system must be taken into account in each individual case. In most mammals movement of the thyroid hormones takes place from mother to fetus, for the fetus usually is deficient in them [137, 163, 170, 321], although, according to Fisher and Oddie [144] and other workers [156], movement of the thyroid hormones must take place from fetus to mother toward the end of pregnancy, for a high concentration of free thyroxine is present in the fetal plasma. Before any firm and reliable conclusions can be reached on this question, further evidence must be obtained, especially quantitative evidence on the form and composition of the iodine compounds in the thyroid gland and peripheral organs at the various stages of pregnancy and after administration of radioactive iodine or of ^{131}I- and ^{125}I-labeled thyroid hormones.

Pituitary–Thyroid Correlation in Man and Animals during Ontogeny

Research in the field of hypothalamohypophyseal regulation of the endocrine glands owes its importance to the correlations which exist in the prenatal period of development of man and animals. Normal ontogeny in the early period depends on the coordinated activity of all levels of endocrine regulation. Whereas the thyroid hormones themselves are essential for hypothalamic differentiation, the development of the thyroid gland starting from a certain period is, in turn, under the control of its own hypothalamohypophyseal system.

Much has been written on the hypothalamic neurosecretion in the fetus [40, 45, 161, 210, 433, 450]. Denis'evskii [106] studied the functional differentiation of the adenohypophysis in 13- to 16-day Pekin duck embryos and found that the hypothalamic factor is essential for the appearance of the anlage of the anterior lobe of the pituitary in these birds. Cells of the adenohypophysis become specifically sensitive to hypothalamic-releasing factors during fetal development before these factors begin to enter the portal blood system of the pituitary in sufficient quantity.

Rumyantseva et al. [441] investigated the hypothalamic regulation of thyrotropic function by comparing the degree of development of goiter in response to administration of antithyroid agents to control and encephalectomized rat, rabbit, and guinea pig embryos. Weakening of the goitrogenic response occurred only in the encephalectomized guinea pig embryos as compared with the intact animals. It was concluded that in animals born immature (rat, rabbit), their thyroid gland is under only pituitary control during prenatal development, whereas in species born mature (guinea pig), some degree of hypothalamic control over thyrotropic function is exhibited. The preliminary results obtained by workers who injected synthetic thyrotropin-releasing factor into pregnant guinea pigs showed that the TRS does not pass through the placental barrier.

The state of function of the thyroid gland is directly connected with pituitary TSH and is, at the same time, more independent of the hypothalamic regulatory mechanism. The thyrotropic function of the anterior pituitary is activated in early ontogeny. TSH is found in the anterior lobe of the pituitary gland of the human fetus after 12–14 weeks [232].

According to Maraud and Stoll [307], the development of the fetal thyroid gland passes through two stages. In the first stage the fetal pituitary gland does not regulate thyroid function. Thyroid function is regulated by the iodide concentration, blood pressure, temperature, and so on. At this time the follicles of the thyroid gland are formed, but thyroid hormones are not liberated into the blood stream. In the second stage the thyroid gland comes under the control of the pituitary, and later this becomes the chief regulator of its activity.

Experiments on the decapitated fetus *in utero* at various stages of antenatal development revealed definite changes in thyroid function and structure [167, 170, 236, 384]. However, some workers do not consider that TSH is essential for the formation of the fetal thyroid gland. In their opinion the pituitary is important only for normal thyroid function. Evidence has in fact been obtained to show that the thyroid gland can develop in a fetus without its pituitary [109, 160, 170, 420, 563].

Jost [238] hypophysectomized rabbit fetuses by decapitation *in utero* and showed that the absorption and excretion of ^{131}I by the fetal thyroid gland was suppressed under these conditions; however, neither hypophysectomy nor thyroidectomy had any effect on development of the fetus. Trunnel and Wade [524] found that administration of TSH increases the amount of iodine fixed by the chick embryonic thyroid gland but does not affect the time when iodide fixation begins. Sobel et al. [471], in experiments on intact and hypophysectomized pregnant rats, studied whether maternal TSH and T_4 are essential for development of the fetal thyroid gland. The rats were hypophysectomized on the 12th day of pregnancy. Development of the fetal thyroid gland took place normally after hypophysectomy; this indicates that the maternal pituitary is not essential for the development of fetal thyroid function. Injection of large doses of thyroxine into the pregnant animals reduced the weight of the fetal thyroid gland by 50% and disturbed its follicular structure, as a result of inhibition of the fetal pituitary by thyroxine.

After injection of perchlorate and propylthiouracil into the mother, the fetal thyroid increased in weight, and its follicular structure was disturbed as a result of stimulation of the fetal pituitary in response to inhibition of the thyroid gland. These results point to functional interaction between the fetal pituitary and thyroid glands during development [327]. The experiments of Sobel et al. also demonstrated that the fetus can utilize thyroxine injected into the mother, indicating that excess thyroxine can pass through the placenta into the fetus.

These observations on function of the pituitary–thyroid system in the rat fetus at the end of intrauterine development were confirmed by Hwang and Wells [226] who found that injection of T_3 or T_4 into rat fetuses *in utero*, like decapitation, retards the development of their thyroid gland. These effects were abolished if TSH was injected at the same time into the fetuses.

Jost [237] observed hyperplasia of the thyroid gland in rat fetuses if methylthiouracil was given to the mothers during pregnancy. The goitrogenic effect of methylthiouracil on the fetal thyroid gland was reduced if the fetuses were decapitated. Jost explains this result by the maturity of the pituitary–thyroid system of rat fetuses toward the end of pregnancy.

Interdependence of the fetal and maternal pituitary–thyroid systems can be studied to some degree by direct determination of thyrotropin secretion in the mother, the fetus, and the newborn animals. Simultaneous determination of thyrotropin in the blood and pituitary under these conditions is an ideal method not only during pregnancy but also in the prenatal period. D'Angelo [96, 97] carried out experiments on guinea pigs to evaluate the secretion of TSH by the pituitary in mother, fetus, and newborn animal immediately after providing propylthiouracil or thyroid hormone during and after pregnancy. His most important conclusions were: Injection of propylthiouracil (PTU) in the last few weeks of pregnancy led to a 13- to 50-fold increase in size of the thyroid gland, and at the same time the TSH concentration in the plasma and pituitary gland was considerably increased in the *goitrous* progeny. The increase in TSH concentration correlated closely with the appearance of numerous large granular basophils in the pars distalis of the adenohypophysis. The TSH titer in the maternal plasma also was raised, but structural changes in the thyroid gland were negligible during continued treatment with the goitrogenic preparations. These experimental results are conclusive evidence that the pituitary–thyroid system functions more intensively in the late period of intrauterine development than in the immediate postnatal period.

The study of hypophysectomized embryos indicates that if the anlage of the thyroid gland is undifferentiated, it retains its ability to differentiate and to develop morphogenetically without abnormality even in the absence of the pituitary [76, 239, 270]. Pituitary hormone begins to exert its stimulant action in the rabbit, for example, on the 22nd day when it accelerates differentiation and growth of the gland and stimulates its function.

In embryos hypophysectomized by decapitation, the discharge of thyroxine into the blood stream is sharply reduced. Geloso [169] showed by radiochromatography that the thyroid gland of rodent fetuses synthesizes and liberates iodothyronines in the late stages of pregnancy. These results are evidence that thyrotropin secretion from the fetal pituitary is necessary for synthesis of thyroid hormones and that negative feedback between thyroid and pituitary appears and becomes firmly established before birth.

After hypophysectomy by subtotal decapitation of rabbit or rat fetuses, according to Geloso [169] and Wells [550], the histological differentiation and growth of the thyroid gland are inhibited [226, 236, 355] and the accumulation of iodine and the secretion of thyroid hormones are sharply reduced. The resulting deficiency is easily corrected by injection of TSH, and, conversely, injections of thyroxine into intact fetuses inhibit growth of the thyroid gland and the secretion of thyroid hormones, although this does not happen if TSH is injected at the same time.

The possible influence of maternal hormones on functional development of the pituitary–thyroid system has been studied in detail with the aid of antithyroid agents administered to pregnant rats [176, 206, 353, 355], rabbits [238], and guinea pigs [97, 326, 380, 398]. They give rise to hyperplasia of the thyroid gland in the fetuses, from which it can be concluded that antithyroid agents pass through the placental barrier, block the synthesis of thyroid hormones by the fetus, and increase the secretion of TSH.

A group of investigators [122, 413] studied the question of thyroxine secretion in mother and fetus during pregnancy in sheep. They inserted catheters into the fetus and mother, injected trace doses of ^{125}I-thyroxine and ^{131}I-thyroxine into the mother and fetus, respectively, and then took serial blood samples from mother and fetus for 96 h while injecting perchlorate simultaneously into the mother. These workers conclude that the pituitary–thyroid system of the fetus is independent. They found a high rate of secretion of thyroxine by the fetus during the last three months of pregnancy, five times greater than the maternal rate.

However, it has not yet been settled whether the maternal pituitary gland has any role to play in the formation of goiter in the fetus. Injection of antithyroid agents into hypophysectomized or thyroidectomized mothers can induce hyperplasia of the thyroid gland in their fetuses provided that the fetal pituitary gland is intact [206, 238, 353, 355]. The development of a goiter in adult guinea pigs was delayed following PTU treatment [D'Angelo, 97]. This was also observed in normal newborn animals. Injection of PTU during the first two weeks of life did not cause any considerable histological changes in the thyroid gland, nor did it alter the TSH level in the blood and pituitary. Daily subcutaneous injections of thyroxine or triiodothyronine in massive doses for 3–9 days into pregnant guinea pigs considerably reduced the TSH reserves in the adenohypophysis but had no appreciable effect on the pituitary–thyroid system of the newborn guinea pigs. Injection of thyroxine into normal newborn animals during the first weeks after birth effectively suppressed TSH secretion, as shown by a decrease in weight of the thyroid and pituitary glands and a decrease in the TSH concentrations.

D'Angelo concludes that in guinea pigs a deficiency of thyroid hormone or excess of TSH in the mother has little effect on the pituitary–thyroid system of the fetus. The fetal pituitary can increase TSH secretion in response to chemical thyroidectomy produced by administration of antithyroid drugs. The results are convincing evidence that the pituitary–thyroid system functions more actively in the later stages of intrauterine fetal development than in the early stages after birth.

Geloso [170] considers that two sources of thyroid hormones are necessary for intrauterine development of rats: fetal and maternal. As Picon [384], Man et al. [305], and others have shown, absence of the thyroid or pituitary gland in the developing fetus leads to an increase in the supply of maternal thyroid hormones to the fetus [170, 242].

In connection with the widely known concept of possible regulation of thyroid function by TSH through the adenyl cyclase-cyclic AMP mechanism, Nataf et al. [343] investigated the action of dibutyryl-cyclic AMP (DB-cAMP) and TSH on the thyroid gland of fetal rats in culture. They found that TSH and DB-cAMP quickly increase the incorporation of ^{32}P and uridine-^{3}H into RNA of the rat fetal thyroid gland. However, the action of DB-cAMP was somewhat weaker than that of TSH. These stimulating agents, when added to the medium, increase the fixation of iodine and its incorporation into soluble iodoproteins and, in particular, into thyroglobulin. In this case, also, however, DB-cAMP was less active than TSH. These results show that the stimulant action of TSH is probably effected through a mechanism of adenyl cyclase activation in the fetal thyroid gland just as in the adult animal.

The results described above show that intrathyroid metabolism in the fetal thyroid gland is qualitatively indistinguishable from the corresponding metabolism in the thyroid of the adult animal, but its regulation during intrauterine development depends on the hormonal balance of the mother and the conditions of development of the fetus itself, it is established at different times in different animals, and it acquires its final features primarily at the time of birth.

REFERENCES FOR PART I

1. Abbott, P., Kantor, H., and Rember, H. *Am. J. Obstet. Gynecol. 98*(6):818, 1967.
2. Abdul-Karim, R. *J. Med. Livan 20*(3):201, 1967.
3. Aber, V., Aleshin, B., Astapenko, V., Mishenin, M., and Gnilorybov, T. *Diseases of the Thyroid Gland* (in Russian), Minsk, 1970.
4. Adams, A. E., and Bull, A. L. *Anat. Rec. 104*:421, 1949.
5. Adams, D. D. *J. Clin. Endocrinol. Metabol. 18*:699, 1958.
6. Adams, D. D., Purves, H. D., and Strett, N. E. *Endocrinology 68*:154, 1961.
7. Adolph, E. P. *Growth 34*(1):113, 1970.
8. Ahn, C. S., and Rosenberg, I. N. *Endocrinology 86*:396, 1970a.
9. Ahn, C. S., and Rosenberg, I. N. *Endocrinology 86*:873, 1970b.
10. Akmaev, I. T. in: *Neurosecretory Elements and Their Importance in the Body* (in Russian), Moscow, 1964, pp. 141–143.
11. Albert, A., and Keating, F. R., Jr. *Endocrinology 51*:427, 1952.
12. Aleshin, B. V. *Development of the Thyroid Gland and the Pathogenesis of Goiter* (in Russian), Kiev, 1954.
13. Aleshin, B. V. *Dissertation* (in Russian), Khar'kov, 1971.
14. Aleshin, B. V. *The Histophysiology of the Hypothalamo-hypophyseal System* (in Russian), Meditsina, Moscow, 1971.
15. Aleshin, B. V., Demidenko, N. S., and Mamina, V. V. in: *Transactions of the Institute of Regional Experimental Medicine* (in Russian), Tashkent, 1961.
16. Aleshin, B. V., and Chuprinova, S. I. *Probl. Éndokrinol. Gormonoter. 13*:63, 1967.
17. Alexander, N. M. *J. Biol. Chem. 234*:1530, 1959.
18. Alexander, N. M. *Excerpta Med. Int. Congr. Ser. 26*:62, 1960.
19. Alexander, N. M. *Biochem. Biophys. Res. Commun. 4*:248, 1961.
20. Alexander, N. M. *Abstracts of Proceedings of the Fifth International Biochemical Congress* (in Russian), Vol. 1, Moscow, 1961, p. 519.
21. Alexander, N. M. *Endocrinology 76*:737, 1965.
22. Alexander, N. M. *Endocrinology 82*:925, 1968.
23. Alexander, N. M., and Corcoran, B. J. *Biochem. Biophys. Res. Commun. 4*:248, 1961.
24. Alexander, R. W., and Marmarston, J. *J. Clin. Endocrinol. Metabol. 21*:243, 1961.
25. Allcroft, R., and Salt, F. G. *Excerpta Med. Int. Congr. Ser. 26*:2, 1960.
26. Althausen, T. L. *J. Am. Med. Assoc. 115*:101, 1940.
27. Ambache, N. in: *Comparative Endocrinology,* Vol. 2, Academic Press, New York, 1963, p. 130.
28. Andreole, M., Sena, L., Edelhoch, H., and Salvatore, G. *Arch. Biochem. Biophys. 134*: 342, 1969.
29. Arshavskii, I. A. *The Physiology of the Circulation in the Intrauterine Period* (in Russian), Medgiz, Moscow, 1960.
30. Atakhanova, B. A. *Dokl. Akad. Nauk Uzb. SSR 1967*(4):58.

31. Atakhanova, B. A. *Nucleic Acids of the Thyroid Gland under Normal Conditions and in Nodular Euthyroid Goiter*. Author's abstract of dissertation for the degree of Candidate of Medical Sciences, Tashkent, 1967.
32. Atakhanova, B. A., and Turakulov, Ya. Kh. *Dokl. Akad. Nauk Uzb. SSR 1971*(6):6.
33. Azyavchik, A. V. *Biokhimiya 14*:405, 1949.
34. Babaev, T. A. *Abstracts of Sectional Proceedings, Second All-Union Biochemical Congress* (in Russian), No. 5, Tashkent, 1969.
35. Balasubramaniam, K., and Deiss, W. P., Jr. *Biochim. Biophys. Acta 110*:564, 1965.
36. Balasubramaniam, K., Deiss, W. P., Tan, W. C., and Powell, R. C. *Endocrinology 77*: 54, 1965.
37. Baranov, V. G. *Diseases of the Endocrine System* (in Russian), Moscow, 1966.
38. Barker, S. B. *Gumma Symp. Endocrinol. 3*:181, 1966.
39. Barkhatova, T. P. *Akush. Ginekol. 1968*(12):62.
40. Bashore, R. A., Jafek, B., and Goblence, C. *Obstet. Gynecol. 36*:391, 1970.
41. Bauer, W. C., and Meyer, J. S. *Lab. Invest. 14*:1975, 1965.
42. Beierwaltes, W. H., and Robbins, J. *J. Clin. Invest. 38*:1683, 1959.
43. Bekier, A. *Nucl. Med. 10*:1, 1971.
44. Bénard, B., and Brault, J. *Union Med. Can.* (*Bull.*) *100*(4):701, 1971.
45. Benirschke, K., and Mackay, D. G. *Am. J. Obstet. Gynecol. 1*:638, 1953.
46. Bensly, R. R. *Am. J. Anat. 19*:57, 1916.
47. Béraud, T. *Acta Endocrinol. 35*:65, 1960.
48. Béraud, T., and Vannotti, D. *Schweiz Med. Wochenschr. 89*:980, 1959.
49. Berger, S., Goldstein, M. S., and Meizoez, B. E. *N. Engl. J. Med. 267*:801, 1962.
50. Berger, M., and Nelken, S. *Presse Med. 4*:62, 1958.
51. Bergström, S. *Abstracts of Communications of the Seventh Meeting of FEBS.* Plenary lectures, abstracts 1, Varna, 1971.
52. Berson, S.A., and Yalow, R. J. *Clin. Invest. 33*:1533, 1954.
53. Berzin, T. *The Biochemistry of Hormones* (Transl. from Russian), Mir, Moscow, 1964.
54. Blasi, F., Fragomele, F., and Cavelli, I. *Eur. J. Biochem. 5*:215, 1968.
55. Block, R. I., Werner, S. C., Mandl, R. H., Row, V. V., and Radichevich, I. *Arch. Biochem. Biophys. 88*:98, 1960.
56. Blumberg, B. S., and Warren, L. *Biochim. Biophys. Acta 50*:90, 1961.
57. Bois, I., and Larsson, L. G. *Acta Endocrinol. 29*:102, 1958.
58. Boler, J., Enzmann, F., Folkers, K., Bowers, C. Y., and Schally, A. V. *Biochem. Biophys. Res. Commun. 37*:705, 1969.
59. Bouchilloux, S., Rolland, M., Torresani, M., Roques, M., and Lissitzky, S. *Biochim. Biophys. Acta 93*:15, 1964.
60. Bowers, C. Y., Redding, T. W., and Schally, A. V. *Endocrinology 77*:809, 1965.
61. Branisch, Hayashi, and Hayashi, *5th Intern. Biochem. Congr., Abstracts* (in Russian), Vol. 1, Moscow, 1961, p. 527.
62. Bruce, C. H., Melvin, G. M., and Selna, K. L. *J. Clin. Invest. 50*:2219, 1971.
63. Burgus, R., Dunn, T. F., Desiderio, D., and Guillemin, *R. C. R. Acad. Sci. 269*:1870, 1969.
64. Burgus, R., Dunn, T. F., Desiderio, D., Ward, D. N., Vale, W., and Guillemin, R. *Nature* (London) *225*:321, 1970.
65. Burgus, R., and Guillemin, R. *Ann. Rev. Biochem. 39*:499, 1970.
66. Burke, G. *Am. J. Physiol. 218*:1445, 1970.
67. Burke, G. *Acta Endocrinol. 66*:558, 1971.
68. Burke, G., Kowalski, K., and Babiarz, D. *Life Sci. 10*:513, 1971, Part 2.
69. Burke, G., and Sato, S. *Life Sci. 10*(17):969, 1971, Part 2.
70. Bustad, L. K., Barnes, C. M., and George, L. A., in: *Use of Radioisotopes in Animal Research and the Medical Sciences,* Academic Press, New York, 1962, p. 401.
71. Bustad, L. K., and Fuller, J. M. *Lab. Anim. Care 20*(3):561, 1970.
72. Cahnmann, H. J., and Funakoshi, K. *Biochemistry 9*:91, 1970.

73. Cameron, A. T. *Recent Advances in Endocrinology*, London, 1940.
74. Carpenter, E., and Rondon-Tarchetti, T. *J. Exp. Zool. 136*:393, 1957.
75. Cartouzou, G., Aquaron, R., and Lissitzky, S. *Biochem. Biophys. Res. Commun. 15*(1): 82, 1964.
76. Cartouzou, G., Greif, R., Depieds, R., and Visscher, M. *Biochim. Biophys. Acta 138*:80, 1967.
77. Cavaleri, R. R., and Serali, G. L. *Biochem. J. 162*:279, 1967.
78. Cheftel, C., and Bouchilloux, S. *Biochim. Biophys. Acta 170*:15, 1968a.
79. Cheftel, C., Bouchilloux, S., and Chabaud, O. *Biochim. Biophys. Acta 170*:29, 1968b.
80. Cheftel, C., Bouchilloux, S., and Lissitzky, S. *C. R. Soc. Biol. 259*:1458, 1964.
81. Chiladze, Z. A. *Abstracts of Proceedings of the Institute of Obstetrics and Gynecology*, Ministry of Health of the USSR, Vol. 3, 1957.
82. Chuprinova, S. I. *Byull. Éksp. Biol. Med. 64*(9):21, 1967.
83. Clever, U. *Chromosoma 12*:607, 1961.
84. Condliffe, P. G. *Endocrinology 72*:893, 1963.
85. Condliffe, P. G., Bates, R. W., Garrison, M. M., and Howard, T. B. *Biochim. Biophys. Acta 37*:150, 1960.
86. Contopoulos, A. N., Ryan, M., and Contopoulos, C. R. *Proc. Zool. Soc. London 142*: 699, 1964.
87. Costa, A., Cottino, F., and Dellepiane, M. *Acta Endocrinol.* p. 107, 1964.
88. Costa, A., Cottino, F., Dellepiane, M., Ferraris, G. M., Lenart, L., Margo, G., Patrito, G., and Zoppetti, G. *Fifth International Thyroid Conference,* 1965, p. 738.
89. Cottle, W. H., and Veress, A. T. *Endocrinology 88*:522, 1971.
90. Courrier, R., and Aron, M. *C. R. Soc. Biol. 100*:839, 1929.
91. Croft, C. J., and Pitt-Rivers, R. *Biochem. J. 118*:311, 1970.
92. Crombrughe, B. de, Edelhoch, H., Beckers, C., and Vissoher, M. de *J. Biol. Chem. 242*: 5681, 1967.
93. Crombrughe, B. de, Pitt-Rivers, R., and Edelhoch, H. *J. Biol. Chem. 241*:2766, 1966.
94. Crombrughe, B. de, and Vesscher, M. de *Ann. Intern. Physiol. Biochem. 77*:150, 1969.
95. D'Angelo, S. A. *Endocrinology 56*:37, 1955.
96. D'Angelo, S. A. *Proc. Soc. Exp. Biol. Med. 121*:555, 1966.
97. D'Angelo, S. A. *Endocrinology 81*(1):132, 1967.
98. Damber, N. A., Galton, V. A., and Ingbar, S. H. *Endocrinology 88*:144, 1971.
99. Danowski, T. S., Johnson, S. Y., Price, W. C., McKelvey, M., Stevenson, S. S., and McCluskey, E. *Pediatrics 7*:240, 1951.
100. Davis, P. J., Spaulding, S. W., and Gregerman, R. I. *Endocrinology 87*:978, 1970.
101. De Duve, C. *Fed. Proc. 23*:1431, 1964.
102. De Groot, L. J., and Davis, A. M. *J. Biol. Chem. 236*:2009, 1961.
103. De Groot, L. J., Postel, S., Litvak, J., and Stanbury, J. B. *J. Clin. Endocrinol. Metabol. 18*:158, 1958.
104. De Groot, L. J., Thompson, J. E., and Dinn, D. *Endocrinology 76*:632, 1965.
105. De Luca, F., Girolamo, M. D., Menzinger, G., and Baschieri, L. *Ann. Endocrinol. 20*:447, 1959.
106. Denis'evskii, A. V. *Proceedings of a Symposium on Hormonal Factors in Individual Development* (in Russian), Moscow, 1971, p. 32.
107. De Robertis, E. *Ann. N. Y. Acad. Sci. 50*:317, 1949.
108. Dempsey, E. W. *Endocrinology 34*:27, 1944.
109. Derrien, I., Michel, R., and Roche, J. *Biochim. Biophys. Acta 2*:254, 1958.
110. Dobyns, B. M. *Endocrinology 52*:705, 1953.
111. Dobyns, B. M., and Hirsch, E. L. *J. Clin. Endocrinol. Metabol. 16*:153, 1956.
112. Dobyns, B. M., and Wilson, L. A. *J. Clin. Endocrinol. Metabol. 14*:1393, 1954.
113. Dopheide, T. A. A., and Trikojus, V. M. *Nature 201*:1128, 1964.
114. Dougherty, I., Gross, I., and Leblond, C. P. *Endocrinology 48*:700, 1951.
115. Dowling, J. T., Freinkel, N., and Ingbar, S. H. *J. Clin. Endocrinol. 16*:280, 1956.
116. Dowling, J. T., Freinkel, N., and Ingbar, S. H. *J. Clin. Invest. 35*:1263, 1956.
117. Dowling, J. T., Freinkel, N., and Ingbar, S. H. *J. Clin. Invest. 39*:1119, 1960.

118. Dumont, J. *Biochim. Biophys. Acta 46*:195, 1961.
119. Dunn, J. T. *J. Biol. Chem. 245*:5954, 1970.
120. Dussault, J., and Fischer, D. A. B. *Program of the Sixth International Thyroid Conference* (Abstracts), Vienna, 1970.
121. Dussault, J., Hobel, S., Calvin, J., De Stefano, J., Erenberg, A., and Fisher, D. A. *Endocrinology 90*:1301, 1972.
122. Dussault, J., Row, V. V., Lickrish, G., and Volpe, R. *J. Clin. Endocrinol. Metabol. 29*: 595, 1969.
123. Dyer, N. C., Brill, A. B., and Glasser, S. R. *Am. J. Obstet. Gynecol. 103*:290, 1969.
124. Dzhalilova, I. K., and Saatov, T. S. *Second All-Union Biochemical Congress. Symposium: Metabolism of Hormones and the Mechanism of Their Action,* Tashkent, 1969, p. 144.
125. Dzhalilova, I. Kh., and Saatov, T. S. in: *Neuro-endocrine Correlation* (in Russian), Obninsk, 1968, p. 98.
126. Easty, G. C., Salter, B. R., and Stanley, P. G. *Biochem. J. 68*:210, 1958.
127. Edelhoch, H. I. *J. Biol. Chem. 237*:2778, 1962.
128. Edelhoch, H. I. *Exp. Ann. Biochim. Méd. 1964*:31.
129. Edelhoch, H. I., and Lippoldt, *J. Biol. Chem. 235*:1335, 1960.
130. Edelhoch, H. I., and Perlman, R. L. *J. Biol. Chem. 243*:2008, 1968.
131. Einhorn, J., and Larson, L. G. *J. Clin. Endocrinol. Metabol. 19*:28, 1959.
132. Einhorn, J., and Wikholm, G. *Acta Endocrinol. 37*:457, 1961.
133. Ekholm, R., and Smeds, S. *J. Ultrastr. Res.* 16:71, 1966.
134. Emrich, D., Muhlen, A. V. zur, Burmeister, G., Zimmermann, H. D., and Beckmann, R. *Acta Endocrinol. 68*:377, 1971.
135. Engstrom, W. W., and Markardt, B. *J. Clin. Endocrinol. 14*:215, 1954.
136. Eskin, I. A. *Fundamentals of the Physiology of the Endocrine Glands* (in Russian), Moscow, 1968.
137. Evans, T. C. *J. Nucl. Med. 8*:157, 1967.
138. Federman, D. D., Robbins, J., and Rall, J. E. *J. Clin. Invest. 37*:1024, 1958.
139. Ferrehi, C. *Pediatrics 37*:460, 1966.
140. Field, J., Dekker, A., Zor, U., and Kaneko, T. *Ann. N. Y. Acad. Sci. 180*:278, 1971.
141. Field, F. P., Fregly, M. J., and Kim, K. J. *Toxicol. Appl. Pharmacol. 21*:556, 1972.
142. Fink, K., and Fink, R. *Science 108*:358, 1948.
143. Fisher, D. A., and Oddie, T. H. *J. Clin. Endocrinol. 23*:811, 1963.
144. Fisher, D. A., and Oddie, T. H. *Am. J. Dis. Child. 107*:574, 1964.
145. Fisher, D. A., et al. *Pediatrics 46*:208, 1970.
146. Fletcher, K. *Biochem. J. 67*:136, 1957.
147. Flock, E. V., and Bollman, J. L. *Biochem. J. 84*:621, 1963.
148. Flock, E. V., Bollman, J. L., Grindlay, J. H., and McKenzie, B. F. *Endocrinology 61*:461, 1957.
149. Flock, E. V., David, C., Stobie, G. H., and Owen, C. A. J. *Endocrinology 73*:422, 1963.
150. Fawcett, D. M., and Kirkwood, S. *J. Biol. Chem. 205*:795, 1953.
151. Foyet, G., and Tixier, R. *Abstracts of Papers FEBS*, 1968, Abstract no. 568.
152. Fraenkel-Conrat, J., and Fraenkel-Conrat, H. *J. Biol. Chem. 135*:199, 1940.
153. Franclin, A. L., Chaikoff, I. L., and Lerner, I. K. *J. Biol. Chem. 153*:161, 1944.
154. Freinkel, N., *Endocrinology, 66*:850, 1960.
155. Freinkel, H., and Ingbar, S. H. *J. Endocrinol. Metabol. 15*:442, 1955.
156. French, F. S., and Wan Wyk, J. J. *J. Pediatr. 64*:589, 1964.
157. Frey, H., and Flock, E. V. *Ann. Endocrinol. 29*:550, 1958.
158. Friis, T., and Sacher, E. *Acta Edocrinol. 18*:428, 1955.
159. Fudzii, S. *Ref. Zh. Biol. Khim. 17C*:267, 1961.
160. Fugo, N. W. *J. Exp. Zool. 85*:271, 1940.
161. Fukuchi, M., Inoue, M., Kumahara, Y. *Folia Endocrinol. (Japan) 45*(10):25, 1970.
162. Furdui, F. I. *A Study of Regulation of Thyroid Functions and the Mechanism of Production of Diffuse Toxic Goiter.* Author's abstract of doctoral dissertation, Kishinev, 1969.
163. Galton, V. A. *Endocrinology 82*:282, 1968.

164. Galton, V. A., and Ingbar, S. H. *Endocrinology 69*:1, 1961.
165. Galton, V. A., and Pitt-Rivers, R. *Biochem. J. 72*:319, 1959.
166. Geloso, J. P. *C. R. Soc. Biol. 150*:2140, 1956.
167. Geloso, J. P. *C. R. Acad. Sci. 246*:168, 1958.
168. Geloso, J. P. *C. R. Soc. Biol. 155*:1239, 1961.
169. Geloso, J. P. *Proceedings of the International Congress of Endocrinology*, London, 1965, part 2, 764.
170. Geloso, J. P. *Ann. Endocrinol. 28 (Suppl.)*:1–79, 1967.
171. Gilman, G. A., and Rall, T. W. *Fed. Proc. 25*:617, 1966.
172. Gilman, G. A., and Rall, T. W. *J. Biol. Chem. 243*:5867, 1968.
173. Gimbette, T. M., and Piffanelli, A. *J. Clin. Pathol. 21*:767, 1968.
174. Gitlin, D., and Biasucci, A. *J. Clin. Endocrinol. 29*:849, 1969.
175. Glynn, B., Elkabir, D. J., Deboarh, D., and Roitt, J. M. *Proc. R. Soc. Med. 61*:1303, 1968.
176. Goldsmith, E. D., Gordon, A. S., and Charipper, H. A. *Am. J. Obstet. Gynecol. 49*:197, 1945.
177. Gorbman, A., Lissitzky, S., Michel, O., et al. *C. R. Soc. Biol. 145*:1642, 1951.
178. Gorbman, A., Lissitzky, S., Michel, O., Michel, R., and Roche, J. *Endocrinology 51*:546, 1952.
179. Gorbman et al. *Endocrinology 60*:565, 1957.
180. Gorbunova, M. P. *Tsitologiya 10*(4):422, 1968.
181. Gorski, J., Toft, D., Stryamala, G., Smith, D., and Notides, A. *Recent Prog. Horm. Res. 24*:45, 1968.
182. Grahame-Smith, D. G., Butcher, R. W., Ney, R. L., and Sutherland, E. W. *J. Biol. Chem. 242*:5535, 1967.
183. Greer, M., and Rockie, C. *Endocrinology 85*:244, 1969.
184. Grégoire, I., Zimozin, N., and Grégoire, I. *C. R. Acad. Sci. 262*:2776, 1966.
185. Grigor'eva, N. F. *Proceedings of a Symposium on Hormonal Factors in Individual Development* (in Russian), Moscow, 1971, p. 63.
186. Gromov, L. I., and Plakutina, G. I. *The Formation of the Endocrine Function in Ontogeny* (in Russian), 1964, p. 137.
187. Gross, J., Ford, D. F., Symchovics, S., and Horton, J. H. *Ciba Found. Colloq. Endocrinol. 10*:182, 1957.
188. Gross, J., and Pitt-Rivers, R. *Lancet 2*:706, 1952.
189. Grumbach, M. M., and Werner, S. C. *J. Clin. Endocrinol. 16*:1392, 1956.
190. Gruenstein, E., and Wynn, G. J. *Theor. Exp. Biol. 26*:343, 1970.
191. Gudernatsch, J. F. *Arch. Entwicklungsmech. Org. 35*(3):457, 1912.
192. Guillemin, R., Dear, W. E., Nichols, B., and Lipsomb, H. *Proc. Soc. Exp. Biol. Med. 101*:107, 1959.
193. Guillemin, R., Yamazaki, E., Jutisz, M., and Sakuz, E. *C. R. Acad. Sci. 255*:1018, 1962.
194. Haddad, H. M., and Rall, T. E. *Endocrinology 67*:413, 1960.
195. Hagemann, U. *Arch. Anat. Path. 327*:71, 1955.
196. Haibach, H. *Endocrinology 88*:918, 1971.
197. Hall, R., Amos, J., Garry, R., and Buxton, R. L. *Br. Med. J. 1970*(5704):274.
198. Hall, P. F., and Myant, N. B. *J. Physiol. 133*:181, 1956.
199. Halmi, N. S., Granner, D. K., Doughmann, D. J., Peters, B. H., and Muller, G. *Endocrinology 67*:70, 1960.
200. Hamada, S., Torizuka, K., Miyake, T. *Gunma Symp. Endocrinol. 3*:153, 1966.
201. Harrington, C. R., and Pitt-Rivers, R. *Nature 144*:205, 1939.
202. Harrington, C. R., Pitt-Rivers, R., Querido, A., Roche, J., and Taurog, A. *Nature 179*: 218, 1957.
203. Harrington, C. R., and Randall, S. S. *Biochem. J. 25*:1032, 1931.
204. Harris, G. W. *Metab. Clin. Exp. 13*(Part 2):117, 1964.
205. Haynes, R. C., Jr. *J. Biol. Chem. 233*:1220, 1958.
206. Haggestad, C. B., and Wells, H. J. *Anat. Rec. 118*:389, 1954.
207. Heidelberger, M., and Pedersen, K. *J. Gen. Physiol. 19*:95, 1935.

208. Heimann, P. *Acta Med. Scand. 187*:323, 1970.
209. Heninger, A. W., Larson, F. C., and Albright, E. C. *J. Clin. Invest. 42*:1761, 1963.
210. Hershman, J. M., Read, D. G., Bailey, A. L., et al. *J. Clin. Endocrinol. 30*:430, 1970.
211. Hillier, A. P. *J. Physiol. 199*:161, 1968.
212. Hillier, A. P. *J. Physiol. 203*:419, 1969.
213. Hillier, A. P. *J. Physiol. 211*:585, 1970.
214. Hillier, A. P. *J. Physiol. 217*:635, 1971.
215. Hillier, A. P. *J. Endocrinol. 50*:181, 1971.
216. Hillmann, G. *Z. Naturforsch. 11b*:424, 1956.
217. Hillmann, G., Keil, B., and Taslimi, P. *Z. Naturforsch. 13b*:820, 1958.
218. Hillmann, G., Keil, B., and Taslimi, P. *Z. Naturforsch. 16b*:28, 1961.
219. Hoch, F. L. *Arch. Biochem. Biophys. 124*:238, 1968.
220. Hodges, R. C., Evans, T. C., and Bradbury, J. T. *J. Clin. Endocrinol. 15*:661, 1955.
221. Hopkins, S., and Thorburn, L. *J. Endocrinol. 1971*(3):549.
222. Horton, E. W. *Physiol. Rev. 49*:122, 1969.
223. Hosoya, T. *Fed. Proc. 24*:605, 1965.
224. Hosoya, T. *Gunma Symp. Endocrinol. 5*:219, 1968.
225. Hosoya, T., Kondo, Y., and Ui, N. *J. Biochem. 52*:180, 1962.
226. Hwang, U. K., and Wells, L. J. *Arch. Anat. Micr. Morphol. Exp. 48*:123, 1959.
227. Igo, R. R., and Mackler, B. *Arch. Biochem. Biophys. 65*:12, 1961.
228. Ingbar, S. H. *J. Clin. Invest. 40*:2053, 1961.
229. Ingbar, S. H., and Freinkel, N. *Recent Prog. Horm. Res. 16*:353, 1960.
230. Inoue, K., Grimm, Y., and Greer, M. A. *Endocrinology 81*:946, 1967.
231. Inoue, K., and Taurog, A. *Endocrinology 83*:816, 1968.
232. Ivanova, E. A., and Levina, S. E. *Dokl. Akad. Nauk SSSR 167*:1423, 1966.
233. Jonckheer, M. H., and Karcher, D. M. *J. Clin. Endocrinol. Metab. 32*:7, 1971.
234. Jörgensen, E. C. *Mayo Clin. Proc. 39*:560, 1964.
235. Jörgensen, E. C., Zenker, N., and Greenberg, C. *J. Biol. Chem. 235*:1732, 1960.
236. Jost, A. *Arch. Anat. Microsc. Morphol., Exp. 42*:168, 1953.
237. Jost, A. *Rev. Suisse Zool. 64*(48):821, 1957.
238. Jost, A. *C. R. Soc. Biol. 153*:1900, 1959.
239. Jost, A. *Proceedings of a Symposium on Hormonal Factors of Individual Development*, Moscow, 1971.
240. Jost, A., Moreau, G., and Fournier, C. *Arch. Anat. Microsc. Morphol. Exp. 49*(4):431, 1960.
241. Jost, A., Morel, F. F., and Marois, M. *C. R. Soc. Biol. 143*:142, 1949.
242. Jost, A., and Vigouroux, E. *Ann. Endocrin. 26*:621, 1965.
243. Kakhana, M. S. *Abstracts of Proceedings of a Conference on the Role of Neuroregulatory and Endocrine Factors in the Activity of the Nervous System in Health and Disease* (in Russian), Leningrad, 1956.
244. Kaneko, T., Zor, U., and Field, J. B. *Metabolism 19*:430, 1970.
245. Karlson, P. *Perspect. Biol. Med. 6*:203, 1963.
246. Kasavina, B. S., Kol'chinskaya, T. A., Bronshtein, M. E., and Ivanova, V. B. *Dokl. Akad. Nauk SSSR 158*:996, 1964.
247. Kayes, J., Maunsbach, A. B., and Ullberg, S. *J. Ultrastr. Res. 7*:339, 1962.
248. Kendall-Taylor, B., and Munro, D. S. *J. Endocrinol. 47*:333, 1970.
249. Khalikov, S. K. *Abstracts of Sectional Proceedings of the Second All-Union Biochemical Congress, Section 5*, Tashkent, 1969, p. 41.
250. Khomasuridze, A. G. *Collected Transactions of the Research Institute of the Physiology and Pathology of Women* (in Russian), Vol. 4, Tbilisi, 1967–1968, p. 409.
251. Khomasuridze, A. G. *The Functional State of the Thyroid Gland in the Offspring of Hypothyroid Rats.* Author's abstract of candidate's dissertation, Moscow, 1969.
252. Kinderen, P. J. der, Houtstrazanz, M., and Schwarz, J. *Clin. Endocrinol. Metabol. 20*:712, 1960.
253. Klainer, L. W., Chi, Y. M., Friedberg, S. L., Rall, T. W., and Sutherland, E. W. *J. Biol. Chem. 237*:1239, 1962.

254. Klopper, A. *Am. J. Obstet. Gynec. 107*:807, 1970.
255. Knopp, J., Stolc, V., and Tong, W. *J. Biol. Chem. 245*:4403, 1970.
256. Kobayashi, I., and Greer, M. *Endocrinology 88*:309, 1971.
257. Kögl, F., and Deenen, L. L. M. van *Acta Endocrinol. 36*:9, 1961.
258. Kolli, E. A. *Byull. Éksp. Biol. Med. 36*:27, 1953.
259. Kolli, E. A. *Abstracts of Proceedings of the Fifth International Biochemical Congress*, Vol. 1, Moscow, 1961, p. 571.
260. Kondo, I., and Ui, N. *Endocrinol. Jpn. 10*:60, 1963.
261. Kondo, I., and Ui, N. *Gunma Symp. Endocrinol. 3*:71, 1966.
262. Kondo, I., De Nayer, P., Labaw, L. W., Robbins, J., and Rall, I. E. *Endocrinology 83*: 1123, 1968.
263. Kozyreff, V., Surks, M. I., and Oppenheimer, J. *Endocrinology 86*:781, 1970.
264. Kuche, F. A., Jr., Humes, J. I., Ivanoff, J., Cirillo, V. J., and Ham, E. A. *Science 169*: 883, 1970.
265. Lassiter, W. C., and Stanbury, J. B. *J. Clin. Endocrinol. Metabol. 18*:903, 1958.
266. Laufberger, V. *Lekarske Rozhledy Časop. Lekaruv Českych*. 1913.
267. Leblond, C. R., and Gross, J. *Endocrinology 43*:306, 1948.
268. Lecocq, R. E., and Dumont, J. E. *J. Biol. Chem. 104*:705, 1967.
269. Lecocq, R. E., Jamy, F., and Dumont, J. *Abstract of Papers, FEBS*, Prague, 1968, Abstract no. 610.
270. Le Lièvre, Ch., and Le Donarin, N. *Ann. Biol. 9*(5–6):285, 1970.
271. Lelong, M., Job, J. C., and Canlorbe, P. *Arch. Fr. Pediat. 22*:333, 1965.
272. Lenart, L. *Riv. Anat. Patol. Oncol. 28*:394, 1965.
273. Levey, G. S., and Pastan, I. *Life Sci. 9*:67, 1970, Part 1.
274. Limanova, E. E. *Probl. Éndokrinol. 1954*(1):70.
275. Limanova, E. E. *Probl. Éndokrinol. 1965*(5):116.
276. Limanova, E. E., and Grodzenskii, D. É. *Probl. Éndokrinol. 1963*(1):23.
277. Lindsey, R. H., and Cohen, P. P. *Endocrinology 76*:734, 1965.
278. Lipman, M. M., Katz, F. H., and Jailey, J. W. *J. Clin. Endocrin. 22*:268, 1962.
279. Lissitzky, S. *Bull. Soc. Chim. Biol. 42*:1187, 1960.
280. Lissitzky, S., Benevent, M. T., Nunez, J., Jacquemin, C., and Roche, J. *Biochim. Biophys. Acta 64*:469, 1962.
281. Lissitzky, S., and Krotemberg, W. *C. R. Acad. Sci. 242*:3002, 1956.
282. Lissitzky, S., Mante, S., Attali, J. C., and Cartouzou, G. *Biochem. Biophys. Res. Commun. 35*:437, 1969.
283. Lissitzky, S., Rolland, M., Reynaud, J., Savary, J., and Lasry, S. *Eur. J. Biochem. 4*: 464, 1968.
284. Lissitzky, S., Roques, M., and Benevent, M. T. *Biochim. Biophys. Acta 41*:252, 1960.
285. Lissitzky, S., Roques, M., Torresani, J., Simon, C., and Bouchillout, S. *Biochim. Biophys. Res. Commun. 16*:249, 1964.
286. Ljungren, J. G. *Acta Chem. Scand. 15*:1772, 1961.
287. Logothetopoulos, J., and Scott, R. F. *J. Physiol. (London) 132*:365, 1956.
288. London, W., Money, W., and Rawson, R. *Endocrinology 73*:205, 1963.
289. Lovenzode, E., and Molea, G. *Biochim. Biophys. Acta 146*:593, 1967.
290. Lowenstein, J. E., and Wollmann, S. H. *Endocrinology 87*:143, 1970.
291. Ludek, J., and Thackery, P. *Biochim. Biophys. Acta 208*:275, 1970.
292. Ludwig, W., and von Mutzenbecher, P., *Z. Physiol. Chem. 159*:195, 1939.
293. Lupulescu, A. *C. R. Soc. Biol. 158*:1450, 1964.
294. Lutherer, L. O., Burns, A. H., Fregby, M. J., and Field, F. P. *Proc. Soc. Exp. Biol. Med. 18*:414, 1971.
295. Lutsin, M. A. *Biokhimiya 33*:306, 1968.
296. Maayan, M. L., and Ingbar, S. H. *Endocrinology 87*:588, 1970.
297. McCann, S. M., and Porter, J. C. *Physiol. Rev. 49*:420, 1969.
298. McCannon, J., Row, V. V., and Volpe, R. *J. Endocrinol. 51*:17, 1971.
299. Macchia, V., and Varrone, S. *FEBS Lett. 13*:342, 1971.
300. MacClendon, J., and Maclennan, C. *Proc. Soc. Exp. Biol. 40*:553, 1939.

301. McGire, E. M., Hutchinson, J. H., Clement, W. E., Kenneky, J. S., and Currie, A. J. *Scott. Med. J.* *5*:189, 1960.
302. McKenzie, J. N. *Recent Prog. Horm. Res.* *23*:1, 1967.
303. Macnaughton, M. C. *Am. J. Obstet. Gynecol.* *97*(7):998, 1967.
304. Man, E. B., Pickering, D. E., Walker, J., and Cooke, R. E. *Pediatrics* *9*:32, 1952.
305. Man, E. B., Mermann, A. C., and Cooke, R. E. *J. Pediatr.* *62*:926, 1963.
306. Mante Bouscayrol, S., Cartouzou, G., Depieds, R., and Lissitzky, S. *Gen. Comp. Endocrinol.* *2*:193, 1962.
307. Maraud, R., and Stoll, R. *Biol. Med.* *50*:313, 1961.
308. Marks, J. F., Hamlin, M., and Zack, P. *J. Pediatr.* *68*:559, 1966.
309. Marks, J. F., Wolfson, J., and Klein, R. J. *Pediatrics* *58*:32, 1961.
310. Matovinovic, J., and Vickery, A. L. *Endocrinology* *64*:149, 1959.
311. Matsuda, K., and Greer, M. A. *Endocrinology* *76*:102, 1965.
312. Matsuura, T., Kon, H., and Cahnmann, J. *J. Org. Chem.* *29*:3058, 1964.
313. Means, J. H., De Groot, L., and Stanbury, J. B., *The Thyroid and Its Diseases,* McGraw-Hill, New York, 1963.
314. Melander, A. *Acta Physiol. Scand.* *83* (Suppl.): 31, 1971.
315. Melander, A., and Sundler, F. *Endocrinology* *90*:188, 1972.
316. Melander, A., Nilsson, E., and Sundler, F. *Endocrinology* *90*:194, 1972.
317. Meltzer, R. I., and Stanaback, R. J. *J. Org. Chem.* *26*:1977, 1961.
318. Merkulov, M. F. *Byull. Éksp. Biol. Med.* *48*(11):65, 1959.
319. Mestman, J. H., Niswonger, J. W., and Anderson, G. V. *Am. J. Obstet. Gynecol.* *103*(3):322, 1969.
320. Michel, R., and Etling, N. *C. R. Soc. Biol.* *151*:36, 1957.
321. Michener, W., Tauxe, W., and Hayles, A. *Pediatrics* *29*:369, 1962.
322. Middlesworth, van L., Jasani, B., and Sinha, K. N. *Proc. Soc. Exp. Biol. Med.* *137*:71, 1971.
323. Mitskevich, M. S. *Dokl. Akad. Nauk SSSR* *58*:693, 1947.
324. Mitskevich, M. S. *Dokl. Akad. Nauk SSSR* *59*:1033, 1948.
325. Mitskevich, M. S. *Dokl. Akad. Nauk SSSR* *69*:277, 1949.
326. Mitskevich, M. S. *Dokl. Akad. Nauk SSSR* *70*:165, 1950.
327. Mitskevich, M. S. *Glands of Internal Secretion in the Embryonic Development of Birds and Mammals* (in Russian) Izd. AN SSSR, Moscow, 1957.
328. Mitskevich, M. S. *Zh. Obshch. Biol.* *22*(1):3, 1962.
329. Mitskevich, M. S. *Proceedings of a Symposium on Hormonal Factors in Individual Development* (in Russian), Moscow, 1971, p. 3.
330. Monroe, R. A., Swanson, E. W., and Wylie, C. E. *J. Dairy Sci.* *34*:507, 1951.
331. Moralis, R., and Goldberg, T. H. *Biochemistry* *6*:2639, 1967.
332. Morton, M. E., and Schwartz, I. R. *Science* *117*:103, 1953.
333. Myant, N. B., *Clin. Sci.* *15*:551, 1956.
334. Myant, N. B. *Clin. Sci.* *17*:75, 1958.
335. Myant, N. B. *Biol. Neonat.* *9*:148, 1966.
336. Nadler, N. J., Sarcar, S. K., and Leblond, C. P. *Endocrinology* *71*:120, 1962.
337. Nagasaka, A., and De Groot, L. J. *Endocrinology* *88*:470, 1971.
338. Nagataki, S., Shizume, K., Matsuda, K., and Ishii, J. *Proc. Soc. Exp. Biol. Med.* *102*:765, 1959.
339. Nagataki, S., Shizume, K., and Okinawa, S. *Endocrinology* *69*:199, 1961.
340. Nair, R. M. G., Barret, J. E., Bowers, C. Y., and Schally, A. V. *Biochemistry* *9*:1103, 1970.
341. Nataf, B., Imbenott, J., Frid, J., and Harel, J. *Proceedings of a Symposium on Hormonal Factors in Individual Development* (in Russian), Moscow, 1971, p. 62.
342. Nataf, B., and Sfez, M. *First International Congress of Endocrinology, Advance Abstracts of Short Communications,* Copenhagen, 1960, p. 607.
343. Nataf, B., and Sfez, M. *C. R. Soc. Biol.* *155*:991, 1961a.
344. Nataf, B., and Sfez, M. *C. R. Soc. Biol.* *155*:1235, 1961b.
345. Nataf, B., Sfez, M., Michel, R., and Roche, J. *C. R. Soc. Biol.* *150*:1088, 1956.

346. Nataf, B., Sfez, M., Michel, R., and Roche, J. *C. R. Soc. Biol. 151*:2089, 1957.
347. Nathanielsz, P. W. *J. Physiol. (London) 211*(11):157, 1970.
348. Nayer, P. de, and Visscher, M. de *Biochim. Biophys. Res. Commun. 36*:639, 1969.
349. Nayer, P. de, and Visscher, M. de *FEBS Lett. 8*:3, 1970.
350. Nicoloff, J. T., Dowling, J. T., and Paton, D. D. *J. Clin. Endocrinol. Metabol. 24*:294, 1964.
351. Nieman, C., and Mead, F. F. *J. Am. Chem. Soc. 63*:2685, 1941.
352. Nigmatov, N. N., and Saipov, T. *Abstracts of Sectional Proceedings of the Second All-Union Biochemical Congress, Section 5,* Tashkent, 1969, p. 36.
353. Nikitovitch, M., and Knobil, E. *J. Clin. Endocrinol. 15*:837, 1955.
354. Nishinaga, A., Cahnmann, H. J., Kon, H., and Matsuura, T. *Biochemistry 7*:388, 1968.
355. Noumura, T. *Jpn. J. Zool. 12*:301, 1959.
356. Novicoff, A. B. *Biol. Bull. 125*:385, 1963.
357. Nunez, J., Mauchamp, J., Macchia, W., Jerusalimi, A., and Roche, J. *Biochem. Biophys. Res. Commun. 20*:71, 1965.
358. Nunez, J., Mauchamp, J., Jerusalimi, A., and Roche, J. *Biochim. Biophys. Acta 145*: 127, 1967.
359. Nunez, J., Mauchamp, J., Macchia, W., and Roche, J. *Biochim. Biophys. Acta 107*:247, 1965.
360. Nunez, J., Mauchamp, J., Pommier, J., Cirkovic, T., and Roche, J. *Biochim. Biophys. Acta 127*:112, 1966.
361. Ogawara Hiroshi, Bilstad, J. M., and Cahnmann, H. J. *Biochim. Biophys. Acta 257*:339, 1972.
362. Olin, P. *Endocrinology 86*(5):1041, 1970.
363. Olin, P., Ekholm, R., and Almeqvist, S. *Endocrinology 87*:1000, 1970.
364. Oppenheimer, J. H., Schwartz, H. L., Shapiro, H., Bernstein, G., Martinez, M., and Surks, M. I. *J. Clin. Invest. 49*:1016, 1970.
365. Oppenheimer, J. H., Surks, M. I., and Schwartz, H. L. *Recent Prog. Horm. Res. 25*:381, 1969.
366. Osorio, C. *Revista Iber. Endocrinol. 15* (Majo):263, 1968.
367. Osorio, C., and Myant, N. *Br. Med. Bull. 16*:159, 1960.
368. Osorio, C., and Myant, N. *Clin. Sci. 23*:277, 1962.
369. Palmer, W. W., Leland, J. P., and Gutman, A. B. *J. Biol. Chem. 125*:615, 1938.
370. Pastan, I. H. in: *Current Topics in Biochemistry,* Academic Press, New York, 1972.
371. Pastan, V., and Katzen, R. *Biochem. Biophys. Res. Commun. 29*:972, 1967.
372. Pastan, I., and Macchia, V. *J. Biol. Chem. 242*:5757, 1968.
373. Pastan, I., and Wollman, S. H. *J. Cell. Biol. 35*:262, 1967.
374. Pavlovic-Hournac, M., Rappoport, L., and Nunez, J. *Exp. Cell. Res. 68*:332, 1971.
375. Peake, R. L., Balasubramaniam, K., and Deiss, W. P. J. *Biochim. Biophys. Acta 148*: 689, 1967.
376. Peake, R. L., Cates, R. I., and Deiss, W. P. *Endocrinology 87*:494, 1970.
377. Pende, N. *Endocrinology. The Pathology and Clinical Features of the Organs of Internal Secretion* (Transl. from Russian), Moscow, 1937.
378. Pérelmutter, L., Delvin, N., and Stepenson, N. R. *Can. J. Biochem. Physiol. 41*:2493, 1963.
379. Perry, R. E., Hodgman, J. E., and Starr, P. *Pediatrics 35*:759, 1965.
380. Peterson, R. R., and Young, W. C. *Endocrinology 50*:218, 1952.
381. Pickering, D. E. *Am. J. Dis. Child. 107*(6):567, 1964.
382. Pickering, D. E., and Kontaxis, N. E. *J. Endocrinol. 23*:267, 1961.
383. Pickering, D. E., Kontaxis, N. E., and Benson, R. C. *Am. J. Dis. Child. 95*:616, 1958.
384. Picon, M. L. O. *C. R. Acad. Sci. 252*:4052, 1961.
385. Pierce, J. G., Rowitch, A. B., Brown, D. M., and Stanley, P. G. *Biochim. Biophys. Acta 111*:247, 1965.
386. Piera, J. G., Carsten, M. E., and Wynston, L. K. *Ann. N. Y. Acad. Sci. 86*:612, 1960.
387. Pincus, G., and Thimann, K. W., eds. *The Hormones,* Vol. 3, Academic Press, New York, 1955.

388. Pind, K. *Acta Endocrinol.* *26*:263, 1957.
389. Pittman, C. A., Chambers, J. B., and Read, V. H. *J. Clin. Invest.* *49*:75a, 1970. (Abstr.)
390. Pitt-Rivers, R., and Rall, I. O. *Endocrinology* *68*:309, 1961.
391. Pitt-Rivers, R., Stanbury, J. B., and Rapp, B. *J. Clin. Endocrinol. Metabol.* *15*:616, 1955.
392. Pitt-Rivers, R., and Tata, J. *The Thyroid Hormones*, Pergamon Press, Oxford, 1959.
393. Pitt-Rivers, R., and Thibault, O. *C. R. Acad. Sci.* *240*:658, 1955.
394. Pitt-Rivers, R., and Trotter, W. R., eds. *The Thyroid Gland,* Butterworths, London, 1964.
395. Plaskett, L. *Biochem. J.* *78*:652, 1961.
396. Ponse, K. *Ann. Endocrinol. (Paris)* *12*:266, 1956.
397. Postel, S. *J. Clin. Endocrinol.* *16*:927, 1956.
398. Postel, S. *Endocrinology* *60*:53, 1957.
399. Primack, M. P., Tapley, D. F., and Buchanan, J. *Biochim. Biophys. Acta* *244*:349, 1971.
400. Primstone, B. I., Hoffenberg, R., and Black, E. *J. Clin. Endocrinol. Metabol.* *23*:336, 1963.
401. Purves, H. D., and Adams, D. D. *Exerpta Med., Int. Congr. Ser.* *26*:25, 1960.
402. Pyzhova, I. K., Turakulov, Ya. Kh., and Ioffe, K. G. *Khim. Prir. Soedin.* *1968* (1): 63.
403. Pyzhova, I. K., Turakulov, Ya. Kh., and Ioffe, K. G. *Biokhimiya* *34*:392, 1969.
404. Rabin, B. S., Kite, I. H., and Rose, N. R. *Proc. Soc. Exp. Biol. Med.* *121*:888, 1966.
405. Rabinowitz, J. L., and Herckera, E. S. *Science* *173*:1242, 1971.
406. Raiti, S. *N. Engl. J. Med.* *277*:456, 1967.
407. Rall, J. E. *Gunma Symp. Endocrinol* *3*:137, 1966.
408. Rall, J. E., Robbins, J., and Lewallen, C. G. in: G. Pincus, K. V. Thinman, and E. B. Astwood, eds. *The Hormones,* Vol. V. Academic Press, New York, 1964, p. 159.
409. Ramwell, P. W., and Shaw, E. in: *Recent Progress in Hormone Research,* Academic Press, New York, 1970.
410. Rather, A., Dhariwal, A., and McCann, S. *Clin. Obstet. Gynecol.* *10*:106, 1967.
411. Reichenberger, J. Deutsch Z. Verdau. Stoffwechselkr. *17*:1939, 1957.
412. Reichlin, S. Neuroendocrinology, in: *Textbook of Endocrinology*, Saunders, Philadelphia, 4th Edition, 1968.
413. Richard, W. H., Larson, F. C., and Albright, E. C. *J. Clin. Invest.* *12*:1761, 1963.
414. Riggs, D. S. *Pharmacol. Rev.* *4*:283, 1952.
415. Riley, J. D., and Sclare, G. *Br. Med. J.* *1*:979, 1957.
416. Robbins, J. *J. Biol. Chem.* *238*:182, 1963.
417. Robbins, J., and Nelson, J. H. *J. Clin. Invest.* *37*:153, 1958.
418. Robbins, J., Wollf, J., and Rall, J. E. *Endocrinology* *64*:37, 1954.
419. Robyn, A. G., Butcher, R. W., and Sutherland, E. W. *Cyclic AMP*, Academic Press, New York, 1972.
420. Roche, J. *Bull. Acad. Nat. Med.* *137*:77 (Febr.), 1953.
421. Roche, J., and Michel, R. *Ann. N. Y. Acad. Sci.* *86*:454, 1960.
422. Roche, J., Michel, R., Etling, N., and Jouan, P. *C. R. Soc. Biol.* *150*:1320, 1956.
423. Roche, J., Michel, R., and Jouan, P. *Biol. Med. (Paris)* *45*:481, 1956.
424. Roche, J., Michel, R., and Lissitzky, S. *C. R. Soc. Biol.* *147*:232, 1959.
425. Roche, J., Michel, R., and Nunez, J. *C. R. Soc. Biol.* *151*:1699, 1957.
426. Roche, J., Michel, R., and Nunez, J. *Acta Endocrinol.* *32*:142, 1959.
427. Roche, J., Michel, R., and Tubiana, M. *Rev. Fr. Etud. Clin. et Biol.* *4*:1051, 1959.
428. Roche, J., Michel, R., and Wulf, W. *C. R. Soc. Biol.* *149*:1604, 1955.
429. Roche, J., Michel, R., Wulf, W., and Nunez, J. *C. R. Acad. Sci.* *240*:921, 1955.
430. Roche, J.. Nunez, J., and Closon, M. *C. R. Soc. Biol.* *154*:2194, 1961.
431. Roche, J., Nunez, J., and Jacquemin, C. *Biochim. Biophys. Acta* *64*:475, 1962.
432. Roche, J., Nunez, J., and Jacquemin, C. *Biochim. Biophys. Acta* *69*:271, 1963.
433. Rodeck, H. *Wochenschr. Kinderheilk.* *106*:87, 1958.
434. Rose, R. G. *Int. J. Appl. Radiat. Isot.* *4*(1–21):50, 1958.
435. Rose, N. R., Kite, J. H., Jr., Doebbler, T. K., and Witebsky, E. in: *Injury, Inflammation and Immunity*, Williams & Wilkins, Baltimore, 1964.

436. Rose, H., Russell, K., and Starr, P. *Am. J. Obstet. Gynec. 86*:767, 1963.
437. Rosenberg, I. N., Ahn, C. S., and Chalfen, M. H. *J. Clin. Endocrinol. Metabol. 21*:554, 1961.
438. Rosenberg, I. N., Athans, J. C., Ahn, C. S., and Behar, A. *Endocrinology 69*:438, 1961.
439. Rosenberg, I. N., Athans, J. C., and Behar, A. *Endocrinology 66*:185, 1960.
440. Ruebner, B., Leeuwen, G., and Korngold, L. *Lancet 1*:1108, 1960.
441. Rumyantseva, O. N., Mitskevich, M. S., and Sergeenkova, G. P. *Proceedings of a Symposium on Hormonal Factors in Individual Development* (in Russian), Moscow, 1971, p. 76.
442. Russell, K. P. *Obstet. Gynecol. Surv. 9*:157, 1954.
443. Russell, K. P., Tanaka, S., Starr, P. *Am. J. Obstet. Gynecol. 79*:718, 1960.
444. Saatov, T. S. *Dokl. Akad. Nauk Uzb. SSR 1965*(2):38.
445. Saatov, T. S, and Dzhalilova, I. *Dokl. Akad. Nauk Uzb. SSR 1972*(2):55.
446. Salakhova, N. S., Kalyaeva, T. A., and Turakulov, Ya. Kh. *Abstracts of Proceedings of the Second All-Union Congress of Endocrinology* (in Russian), Moscow, 1972.
447. Salakhova, N. S., and Turakulov, Ya. Kh. *Seventh Conference of European Comparative Endocrinology*, Abstracts, Budapest, 1973, p. 107.
448. Salvatore, G., Aloj, S., Salvatore, M., and Edelhoch, J. *J. Biol. Chem. 242*:5002, 1967.
449. Sato, S., Szabo, M., Kowalski, K., and Burke, G. *Endocrinology 90*:343, 1972.
450. Scharrer, E., and Gaupp, R. *Z. Gesamte Neurol. Psychiatr. 145*:462, 1933.
451. Schimada, H., and Yasumasu, I. *Gumma Symp. Endocrinol. 3*:47, 1966.
452. Schleusener, H., Murphy, P. V. N., and McKenzie, J. M. *Metabolism 20*:299, 1971.
453. Schulman, S. *Gumma Symp. Endocrinol. 5*:117, 1968.
454. Schussler, G., and Ingbar, S. H. *J. Clin. Invest. 40*:1394, 1961.
455. Schwartz, H. L., Surks, M. T., and Oppenheimer, J. *J. Clin. Invest. 50*:1124, 1971.
456. Sead, R. W., and Goldberg, L. H. *J. Biol. Chem. 240*:764, 1965.
457. Seal, U. S., and Doe, R. P. *Proceedings of the Second International Congress on Endocrinology*, part 1, 1965, p. 325.
458. Seitmuratova, O. Kh., and Khalikov, S. K. *Proceedings of the Second All-Union Biochemical Congress*, Fan, Tashkent, 1969, p. 132.
459. Seitmuratova, O. K., and Khalikov, S. K. *Proceedings of the Second All-Union Biochemical Congress*, Fan, Tashkent, 1969, pp. 132–133.
460. Selin, H. G., and Goldberg, L. H. *J. Biol. Chem. 240*:774, 1965.
461. Seljelid, R. *J. Ultrastr. Res. 17*:195, 1967.
462. Shepard, T. H. *J. Clin. Endocrinol. 27*:945, 1967.
463. Shepard, T. H. *Gen. Comp. Endocrinol.10*:174, 1968.
464. Shiba, T., and Cahnmann, H. J. *J. Org. Chem. 27*:1773, 1962.
465. Shiba, T., Kajiwara, M., Kato, Y., Inoue, K., and Kaneko, T. *Arch. Biochem. Biophys. 140*:90, 1970.
466. Shtange, N. B. *Formation of the Endocrine Function in Ontogeny* (in Russian), Moscow, 1964, p. 119.
467. Simon, C., and Daug, J. *Acta Endocrinol. 68*:(2):367, 1971.
468. Simon, C., Daug, I., Miquelis, R., and Bastiani, P. *Acta Endocrinol. 68*:367, 1971.
469. Simon, C., Roques, F. M., Torresani, J., and Lissitzky, S. *Acta Endocrinol. 53*:271, 1966.
470. Sircar, R. L., and Chaterjee, A. K. *J. Obstet. Gynecol. (India) 20*:38, 1970.
471. Sobel, H. E., Hamburgh, M., and Koblin, R. *First International Congress of Endocrinology, Advance Abstracts of Short Communications*, Copenhagen, 1960, p. 608.
472. Sonnenberg, M., and Money, W. L. *CIBA Found. Colloq. Endocrinol. 11*:38, 1957.
473. Spiro, R. G., and Spiro, M. J. *J. Biol. Chem. 240*:1603, 1965.
474. Spiro, R. G., and Spiro, M. J. *J. Biol. Chem. 241*:1271, 1966.
475. Stanbury, J. B. Familial Goiter, in: *Metabolic Basis of Inherited Disease*, McGraw-Hill, New York, 1966.
476. Stanbury, J. B. *Arg. Reas. Endocrinol. Metabol. 15*(3):145, 1966.
477. Stanbury, J. B., and Morris, M. L. *J. Clin. Endocrinol. Metabol. 17*:1324, 1957.
478. Stanley, P. *Biochem. J. 63*:581, 1951.
479. Stein, O., and Gross, J. *Endocrinology 75*:787, 1964.

480. Sterling, K. in: *Recent Progress in Hormone Research*, Academic Press, New York, 1970.
481. Sterling, R., Brenner, M. A., and Newman, E. S. *Science 169*:1099, 1970.
482. Sunshine, P. *Pediatrics 36*:986, 1965.
483. Surks, M. I., Weinbach, S., and Volport, E. *Endocrinology 82*:1156, 1968.
484. Sutherland, E. W., and Rall, T. W. *J. Biol. Chem. 232*:1077, 1958.
485. Sutherland, E. W., Oye, I., and Butcher, R. W. *Recent Prog. Horm. Res. 21*:623, 1965.
486. Sutherland, E. W., and Rall, T. W. *Advance Abstract Symposium Lectures of the First International Congress of Endocrinology*, Copenhagen, 1960, p. 171.
487. Suzuki, M. *Gunma Symp. Endocrinol. 3*:81, 1966.
488. Suzuki, M., Nagashima, M., and Yamomoto, K. *Gen. Comp. Endocrinol. 1*:103, 1961.
489. Talanti, S., and Hopsu, V. I. *Acta Endocrinol. 35*:841, 1960.
490. Tata, J. R. *Proc. Soc. Exp. Biol. Med.* 95, 1957.
491. Tata, J. R. *Biochim. Biophys. Acta 28*:91, 1958.
492. Tata, J. R. *Bull. Soc. Chim. Biol. 42*:1171, 1960.
493. Tata, J. R. *Nature 187*:1025, 1960.
494. Tata, J. R. in: *Biological Action of Thyroid Hormones at the Cellular and Molecular Levels*, 1964.
495. Tata, J. R. *Seventh International Congress of Biochemistry*, Tokyo, 1967, p. 281.
496. Tata, J. R., Ernster, L., and Suranyl, E. M. *Biochim. Biophys. Acta 60*:480, 1962.
497. Tata, J. R., Widnell, C. C., and Gratzer, W. B. *Clin. Chim. Acta 6*:819, 1961.
498. Taurog, A. *Second Mid-West Conference on the Thyroid*, University of Missouri, Columbia, 1967, p. 87.
499. Taurog, A. *Gunma Symp. Endocrinol. 5*:219, 1968.
500. Taurog, A. in: *Recent Progress in Hormone Research*, Academic Press, New York, 1970.
501. Taurog, A., Briggs, F., and Chaikoff, I. L. *J. Biol. Chem. 194*:655, 1952.
502. Taurog, A., Potter, G. D., and Chaikoff, J. L. *J. Biol. Chem. 213*:119, 1955.
503. Taurog, A., Potter, J. C., and Thio, D. T. *Endocrinology 74*:901, 1964.
504. Taurog, A., Potter, G. D., Tong, W., and Chaikoff, I. L. *Endocrinology 58*:132, 1956.
505. Taurog, A., Tong, W., and Chaikoff, I. L. *J. Biol. Chem. 184*:83, 1950.
506. Taurog, A., Tong, W., and Chaikoff, I. L. *Endocrinology 62*:664, 1958.
507. Terjung, R., and Tipton, C. M. *Am. J. Physiol. 220*:1840, 1971.
508. Tervilla, L. *Ann. Chir. Gynaecol. Fenn. 55*:298, 1966.
509. Thalhammer, O., *Pränatale Erkrankungen des Menschen*, Thieme Verlag, Stuttgart, 1967.
510. Thibault, O. *C. R. Soc. Biol. 149*:877, 1955.
511. Thibault, O. *C. R. Soc. Biol. 151*:475, 1957.
512. Thibault, O., and Lachaze, A. *C. R. Soc. Biol. 145*:797, 1951.
513. Thomson, J. A., and Goldberg, J. *Endocrinology 32*:805, 1968.
514. Tomita, K., Young, J. W., and Lardy, H. A. *Gumma Symp. Endocrinol. 5*:85, 1968.
515. Tomita, K., Lardy, H. A., Larson, F. C., and Albright, E. C. *J. Biol. Chem. 224*:387, 1957.
516. Tong, W. *Endocrinology 76*:163, 1965.
517. Tong, W. *Gunma Symp. Endocrinol. 3*:61, 1966.
518. Tong, W. *Endocrinology 80*:1101, 1967.
519. Tong, W. in: *Progress in Endocrinology, Excerpta Med. Found.*, 1969, p. 669.
520. Tong, W., Kerkof, P., and Chaikoff, I. L. *Biochim. Biophys. Acta 60*:1, 1962.
521. Torresani, J., Roques, M., and Lissitzky, S. *Bull. Soc. Chim. Biol. 52*:775, 1970.
522. Trendelenburg, P. *Hormones* (Transl. from Russian), Moscow, 1936.
523. Trikojus, V. M. *Gunma Symp. Endocrinol. 5*:247, 1967.
524. Trunnel, J. B., and Wade, M. A. *J. Clin. Endocrinol. Metabol. 15*:197, 1955.
525. Tsarikovskaya, N. G., and Miloslavskii, M. Ya. *Safeguarding the Health of the Mother and Newborn Infant* (in Russian), Kiev, 1964, p. 206.
526. Turakulov, Ya. Kh. *Iodine Metabolism and Thyroid Hormones* (in Russian), Izd. Akad. Nauk Uzb. SSR, Tashkent, 1959.
527. Turakulov, Ya. Kh. *Biochemistry of the Thyroid Hormones Under Normal Conditions and in Thyroid Pathology* (in Russian), Izd. Akad. Nauk Uzb. SSR, Tashkent, 1962.

528. Turakulov, Ya. Kh. *The Biochemistry and Pathochemistry of the Thyroid Gland* (in Russian), Tashkent, 1963.
529. Turakulov, Ya. Kh., Khalikov, S. K., and Seitmuratova, O. Kh. *Uzb. Biol. Zh. 1971* (6):3.
530. Turakulov, Ya. Kh., Khusainova, F., and Mirakhmedov, A. K. *Dokl. Akad. Nauk. SSSR 195*(3):740, 1970.
531. Turakulov, Ya. Kh., L'vovich, N. A., Gagel'gans, A. I., and Mirakhmedov, A. K. *Uzb. Biol. Zh 1972*(1):3.
532. Turakulov, Ya. Kh., Mirakhmedov, A. K., L'vovich, N. A., and Rakhmatullaeva, F. *Probl. Éndokrinol. 17*(6):105, 1972.
533. Turakulov, Ya. Kh., Mirakhmedov, M. M., and Yangunaev, R. A. *Byull. Éksp. Biol. Med. 74*(12):41, 1972.
534. Turakulov, Ya. Kh., Saatov, T., Khamidov, D. Kh., Khalikov, S. K., and Mirakhmedov, A. K. *Probl. Éndokrinol. 18*(1):55, 1972.
535. Turakulov, Ya. Kh., Seitmuratova, O. Kh., and Khalikov, S. K. *Uzb. Biol. Zh. 1971* (4):69.
536. Ui, N. *Gunma Symp. Endocrinol. 6*:171, 1969.
537. Valenta, L., and Béraud, T. *J. Endocrinol. 31*:422, 1970.
538. Van der Laan, J. E., and Van der Laan, W. P. *Endocrinology 40*:403, 1947.
539. Van Heyningen, H. E. *Endocrinology 69*:720, 1961.
540. Van Zyl, A., and Edelhoch, H. *J. Biol. Chem. 242*:2423, 1967.
541. Verain, A., Verain-Pinoy, A. *C. R. Acad. Sci. 251*:3079, 1960.
542. Vind, H. P., Kharasch, K., and Stowell, E. C. *J. Biol. Chem. 223*:108, 1956.
543. Voitkevich, A. A. *Probl. Éndokrinol. Gormonoter. 5*:(1):31, 1959.
544. Voitkevich, A. A. *Probl. Éndokrinol. 10*(6):82, 1964.
545. Voitkevich, A. A. *Neurosecretion* (in Russina), Meditsina, Leningrad, 1967.
546. Voitkevich, A. A., and Tkachev, A. V. *Probl. Éndokrinol. Gormonoter. 12*(1):111, 1966.
547. Vunder, T. A. *Probl. Endokrinol. Gormonoter. 1*(2):15, 1955.
548. Waterman, A. J., and Gorbman, A. *J. Exp. Zool. 132*:509, 1956.
549. Weiss, B. *J. Biol. Chem. 201*:31, 1953.
550. Wells, L. Y. Univ. Minn. Med. Bull. *31*:(6):186, 1960.
551. Werner, S. C., Block, R. J., and Mandl, R. H. *J. Clin. Endocrinol. Metabol. 20*:205, 1960.
552. Wetzil, B. K., Spicer, S. S., and Wollman, S. H. *J. Cell. Biol. 25*:593, 1965.
553. Williams, J. A., Berens, S. C., and Wolff, J. *Endocrinology 88*:1385, 1971.
554. Williams, J., and Wolff, J. *Proc. Nat. Acad. Sci.* (*Washington*) *67*:1901, 1970.
555. Wilson, B., Raghupathy, E., Tonoue, T., and Tong, W. *Endocrinology 83*:877, 1968.
556. Wolf, J., Chaikoff, I. L., and Nichols, C. N. *Endocrinology 44*:510, 1949.
557. Wollman, S. H., Spicer, S. S., and Burstone, M. S. *J. Cell. Biol. 21*:191, 1964.
558. Wollman, S. H., and Wodinsky, J. *Endocrinology 56*:9, 1955.
559. Wynn, J., and Gibbs, R. *J. Biol. Chem. 237*:3499, 1962.
560. Wynston, L. K., Free, C. A., and Pierce, J. G. *J. Biol. Chem. 235*:85, 1960.
561. Yamada, T., Iino, S., and Greer, M. A. *Endocrinology 69*:1, 1961.
562. Yamamoto, K. *Jpn. J. Physiol. 9*:394, 1959.
563. Yamasaki, E., Noguchi, A., Slingerland, D. N. *J. Clin. Endocrinol. Metabol. 19*:1437, 1959.
564. Yamashita, K. H., and Field, J. B. *J. Clin. Invest. 51*:463, 1972.
565. Zondek, H. *Acta Med. Scand. 103*:251, 1940.

PART II

Physiological Effects of the Thyroid Hormones

The thyroid gland has a powerful influence over the activities of the whole body. If the function of the gland is for any reason lost, serious disturbances of chemical and morphological structure arise and are manifested as physical and mental disorders. The diversity of the action of thyroid hormones on physiological functions, on the metabolic rate, and on the activity of various enzyme systems both in the body as a whole and in tissue preparations has been known for a long time. Our knowledge of the role of thyroid hormones is based on experiments in which a particular thyroid hormone has been given to healthy and athyrotic animals and on extensive clinical observations on patients with hyperthyroid and hypothyroid states.

The effect of thyroid hormones *in vivo* is expressed as reactions of whole organs and of individual physiological functions and morphological structures. The internal secretions of the thyroid gland modify growth and metamorphosis, the utilization of oxygen by the body as a whole or by tissue preparations *in vitro*, various aspects of metabolism, and the activity of particular enzyme systems.

The extreme diversity of the effects observed after injection of thyroid hormone may reflect the primary action of this agent on a single link fundamental to the mechanism of biochemical processes in the cell or on a single morphological structure responsible for the proper integration of processes at the cell level. These problems will be examined fully later. Here I shall merely state that when the action of a thyroid hormone is discussed, the term is used not only with respect to the thyroxine and triiodothyronine produced in the thyroid gland, but also to several of their derivatives and analogs. However, we know that all compounds with the biological activity of thyroid hormones belong chemically to the thyronine group, the aromatic rings of which contain iodine atoms.

Two opposite views are held on the action of thyroid hormones in the intact organism. Some workers assert that the mechanism of the effect of thyroid hormones is nervous and that the hormone affects the state of neurons of the central nervous system either through a reflex or directly, and that it exhibits its peripheral action through the activity of these CNS cells. Another group of workers insists that hormones reach the body tissues by the humoral route and exert their effect directly at the cell level. This problem has been examined in detail by Genes [198] in his survey.

There is, of course, no doubt about the action of thyroid hormones on the cells of the central nervous system, especially on the diencephalon and also on the posterior and anterior lobes of the pituitary. This is clear from many investigations in which thyroxine and triiodothyronine accumulated in the brain in relatively high concentrations after injection of hormones labeled with radioactive iodine. Presumably thyroid hormones modify metabolism in the nerve tissue and thus could exert their action through the CNS.

Meanwhile, evidence of the direct action of thyroxine and other active forms of thyroid hormone on oxygen utilization by tissue slices and homogenates, on the uncoupling of oxidative phosphorylation by the action of thyroxine on mitochondria, and on its effect on enzyme activity and on metabolic processes in isolated tissues, and so on has accumulated in the literature.

It is difficult to support the view that the thyroid hormone has no other peripheral effect than that exerted through the central nervous system. The action of thyroxine on the nerve cells of the brain is manifestly also an expression of its peripheral effect: By modifying the metabolism of nerve cells thyroxine can exert its action through the CNS. I therefore consider that these two possible modes of action of thyroid hormones—humoral, directly on the tissues and organs, and nervous, through the CNS—are not necessarily opposed to each other. They are both based on changes in cell metabolism resulting from the direct action of thyroxine. Logically the nervous and humoral mechanisms of action of the thyroid hormones of the peripheral tissues and organs are complementary.

The physiological effects of the thyroid hormones are reflected in practically all manifestations of bodily activity, and their investigation can provide valuable information on the approach to be used to study the mechanism of action of the hormones at the cellular, subcellular, and molecular levels.

However, the very diversity of these effects is itself a serious obstacle to the analysis of the mechanism of action of the thyroid hormones.

Another difficulty in examining the physiological role of thyroid hormones is the impossibility of assessing it in the intact organism. The data from pathological physiology and the clinical picture of diseases of the thyroid gland, accompanied by a deficient or excessive supply of thyroxine and triiodothyronine to the blood stream, are essential for this purpose. Under such conditions it is by no means certain that many of the pathological manifestations are the direct result of changes in activity of the thyroid gland and indeed may reflect pharmacological rather than physiological effects of its hormones.

Now is evidently the time to attempt a systematic analysis of the available data, in the knowledge that such an attempt must at present be restricted to some of the most clearly defined effects of these hormones. In this section I shall first examine the most general effects of the thyroid hormones (their effect on growth and differentiation of the tissues, on the basal metabolism and various aspects of intermediate metabolism), and I shall then examine changes in the functions of the most important organs and systems of the body in the presence of a deficiency or excess of thyroid hormones. This examination must naturally be limited to certain of the most vital processes and systems or to those to whose experimental investigation the authors of this book have contributed directly.

Tissue Growth and Differentiation

Thyroxine was for a long time thought to be a true growth hormone. This view was based on the short stature of cretins and the delayed growth of thyroidectomized animals. However, the effects of loss of thyroid function or of a deficiency of thyroid hormones in the body differ depending on the animal's age. The younger the animal, the more severe the effect of thyroid deficiency on its general condition. Thyroidectomy in the tadpole, for instance, prevents metamorphosis. A similar arrest of metamorphosis is also observed in the salamander after removal of its thyroid gland.

The effect of thyroid hormones on metamorphosis in amphibians is usually regarded as the clearest manifestation of the action of these hormones on differentiation of the body tissues. Metamorphosis, under the control of thyroid hormones, is not limited to changes in the external appearance of the animal but also includes various biochemical changes and, in particular, modification of the system for the detoxication of ammonia (the formation of the urea cycle), changes in the structure of the hemoglobin, the appearance of new digestive enzymes, and the quickening of respiration. It is not yet clear which of these effects is primary. All that can be said is that the direct cause commencing the synthesis of urea is evidently the appearance of a new enzyme—carbamyl phosphate synthetase—in the tadpole [463]. Meanwhile the synthesis of other enzymes, especially of the succinate oxidase complex, in the mitochondria is reduced during metamorphosis and RNA synthesis is increased [190].

Some interesting results were obtained in 1959 by Wilt [651]. His observations showed that thyroxine induces resorption of the tadpole tail even *in vitro*. The possibility therefore cannot be ruled out that the formation of new proteins during metamorphosis is brought about by the catabolic action of thyroid hormones, for an increase in the concentration of free amino acids in the blood can stimulate protein synthesis in the tissues. Paik and Cohen [463] in fact showed that amputation of 60% of the total mass of the tail in tadpoles prevents the characteristic increase in carbamyl phosphate synthetase in the liver observed during metamorphosis.

In other classes (birds, mammals) thyroidectomy retards growth and differentiation; the earlier the thyroid gland is removed, the greater the effect. This rule stands out particularly clearly in mammals. Kids, calves, piglets, foals, and donkeys thyroidectomized at an early age cease to grow. The development of their gonads is stopped and their metabolic rate falls sharply. Removal of the thyroid gland from young rabbits produces marked changes: delayed growth of the skeleton, hypothermia, deposition of fat, etc. Finally, the results of thyroidectomy of young monkeys are highly demonstrative. These animals are greatly retarded in growth, they become extremely lethargic, and they are abnormally fat. Earlier investigators emphasized that thyroidectomy of these animals in the adult state does not produce such marked disturbances.

In clinical practice a state of hypothyroidism can occur as the result of the removal of thyroid tissue at operation and the destruction of thyroid tissue through an overdosage of radioactive iodine or X-rays, in acute suppurative thyroiditis, in the final stage of chronic thyroiditis, or in metastatic carcinoma, tuberculosis, and other diseases of the thyroid gland.

Thyroid insufficiency, i.e., inability of the thyroid gland to produce its hormone in the amount required to satisfy the normal functions of the body and to maintain the normal level of thyroid hormones in the blood stream, can also develop spontaneously. Spontaneous thyroid insufficiency is found most frequently in man. In some cases the degree of hypothyroidism may be slight, but in others total aplasia or agenesis of the thyroid gland is observed. Just as under experimental conditions the result depends on the age at thyroidectomy, so the patient's condition is largely determined by the age of onset of the disease. The severest form is the syndrome of total functional insufficiency of the thyroid gland in the newborn, otherwise known as cretinism, based on congenital aplasia of the gland.

Congenital cretinism is the result of an embryonic developmental defect of the thyroid gland. The study of the uptake of radioactive iodine in this condition reveals complete absence of thyroid tissue capable of accumulating iodine or the presence of only a very small quantity of thyroid tissue. Some workers consider that inherited factors may be the cause of congenital cretinism. Most investigators, however, ascribe an important role to various harmful factors affecting the mother during pregnancy. These factors include an unsatisfactory diet, the action of toxins, severe infections, and so on.

Failure of the processes of differentiation of all the tissues and, in particular, of the CNS leads to many serious disturbances of mental activity. Such subjects are totally without any manifestation of intellectual activity, and they may even lack the instinctive functions of self-preservation and cleanliness. They are left only with a demand for food, usually expressed as a harsh and inarticulate cry, but they are unable to satisfy their need themselves. Severe disturbances affecting all parts of the central and peripheral nervous system are the features which distinguish congenital cretinism most clearly from other forms of hypothyroidism, and they may often not respond readily to treatment with thyroid preparations.

Thyroid insufficiency in childhood or adolescence (the acquired form) is usually called *juvenile hypothyroidism* or childhood or juvenile myxedema. Inflammatory or degenerative changes in the thyroid gland arising as a result of infectious diseases of childhood are regarded as the main causes of these forms of hypothyroidism.

The sequelae of thyroid insufficiency, occurring after thyroidectomy, are best studied experimentally in young animals. After removal of their thyroid gland they develop various disorders, more especially disturbances of growth and trophic and metabolic disturbances. All symptoms arising as a result of thyroid insufficiency are essentially linked with these fundamental disturbances.

Disturbances of growth are manifested chiefly in the skeleton. Growth of the whole body ceases prematurely in the young animals and growth of the long bones is particularly retarded. As a result the thyroidectomized animal acquires the characteristic appearance of a dwarf: The body is spherical and the limbs and tail short. Not only is ossification disturbed in such animals but specific degeneration of the epiphyseal cartilages is also observed: normal cell proliferation is limited, the ground substance swells and spaces appear in it, the cavities in the cartilage enlarge into vesicles, and the cells atrophy or some may disappear altogether.

Ossification begins from numerous irregular foci scattered through the zone of altered cartilage. These foci ultimately enlarge and join to form centers of irregular shape, often porous or lacking a distinct outline. If the hypothyroidism develops later in life, centers already ossified are usually not affected, although sometimes changes are found in the cartilaginous tissue of the epiphyseal line of the femur, leading to a reduction in size of the epiphyses. The presence of this form of epiphyseal dysgenesis is one of the most characteristic features of early hypothyroidism. In other forms of growth retardation, this type of epiphyseal dysgenesis is not found. The discovery of dysgenesis in certain centers, moreover, often points to the date of origin of the thyroid deficiency. Some enzyme systems in the cartilage tissue concerned with growth and ossification are considered to be dependent on thyroid hormones. Development of the teeth is also delayed parallel to the delay in endochondrial ossification.

Thyroidectomy in adult animals in which the skeleton is already formed gives rise to local disorders of growth. For a long time the view was widely held that thyroid hormones directly affect growth of the skeleton and that the disturbances of growth in thyroid insufficiency are due to the absence of thyroid hormones. However, this view was questioned as a result of work showing that inhibition of growth in thyroidectomized rats can be caused by a deficiency of pituitary somatotropic hormone [35]. Injection of thyroxine into hypophysectomized animals stimulated their growth only very slightly, whereas pituitary somatotropic hormone stimulated growth of thyroidectomized rats strongly. On the other hand, the combined action of growth hormone and thyroid hormone led to more rapid growth of the bones, internal organs, and skeletal muscles than each of the hormones separately. However, in the presence of large doses of thyroxine the growth effect of somatotropic hormone may be weakened. The effect of thyroxine differs from that of somatotropic hormone by the fact that it does not change the protein content in bone tissue.

The effect of a deficiency and excess of thyroid hormones on growth and development of the skeletal system has been studied in detail by M. and R. Silberberg [548]. These workers showed that thyroid hormones act primarily on the ossification of cartilage, stimulating its proliferation, and they also act on the final development and closing of the epiphyses. The time of appearance of the centers of ossification also depends on thyroid function [450]. The healing of fractures is particularly slow in thyroidectomized animals.

In thyrotoxicosis, however, evidence of resorption of bone can be observed. Excess of thyroxine inhibits regeneration of the surface layer of the cornea after burns and delays cell division during epithelization [562]. Prolonged administration of thyroxine or TSH to guinea pigs considerably inhibits the drawing together of the surface during healing of skin wounds whereas thyroidectomy does not affect this process [427]. It was shown in Gol'ber's laboratory that the increase in the concentration and synthesis of nucleic acids and protein in the liver after partial hepatectomy is reduced in rabbits with thyrotoxicosis [464]. These facts show that an excess of thyroid hormones inhibits regeneration.

Severe hypothyroidism in man leads to the development of myxedema, based on trophic changes in the skin and its appendages, chiefly through albuminous and mucoid infiltration. The accumulation of mucoid material gives the skin its characteristic appearance of edema. In more severe cases the subcutaneous cellular tissue becomes thickened (a marked increase in the concentration of mucoproteins) and the skin becomes coarse, fixed, and dry, and scaling of the skin is frequently observed. These skin disturbances are linked with particular histological changes, including hyperkeratosis and degenerative changes in the epidermal cells with occlusion of the mouths of the follicles. The connective-tissue layer of the skin in this condition is edematous and the collagen and elastic fibers are displaced by large accumulation of mucinous material consisting chiefly of mucopolysaccharides, hyaluronic acid, and chondroitinsulfuric acid. Nielson et al. [445] consider that in thyroid insufficiency hyaluronic acid accumulates in large quantities and contributes to the swelling of the connective tissue of the skin.

Nitrogen retained because of inhibition of endogenous protein metabolism plays a role in the increased formation of mucoproteins in the fluid of the myxedematous tissue. Water and salts also accumulate in the tissues. The edema may also spread to the mucous membranes. Subcutaneous or submucous mucoprotein infiltration causes thickening of the lips and a marked increase in their size; the tongue consequently protudes, and as a result the mouth is permanently open. Sometimes the vocal cords are thickened, leading to hoarseness and disturbances of speech. The speech becomes slow and indistinct.

Trophic changes in the hair and nails are highly characteristic of myxedema. Growth of the hair is considerably slowed, and it becomes dry, brittle, and fragile. Often the hair falls out in large quantities, causing diffuse or localized baldness. This applies in particular to the axillary and pubic hair and to the hair in the lateral third of the eyebrows (the Hertog-Levy sign). The effect of thyroid insufficiency on the beard or on hair growth in other parts of the trunk is negligible. The nails become thin, ridged transversely and longitudinally, and brittle. Often defective lunules and white spots in the matrix are observed.

Various types of pigmentation of the skin can be seen in thyrotoxicosis. Sometimes there is darkening of the skin of the eyelids (Jellinek's sign), the face, neck, linea alba of the abdomen, the loin, the extensor surfaces of the limbs, and elsewhere. These signs are supposedly connected with a deficiency of the adrenal cortex which usually develops in advanced thyrotoxicosis. However, pigmentation of the mucous membranes, highly characteristic of Addison's disease, is usually not observed in thyrotoxicosis. In some cases of thyrotoxicosis areas of depigmentation appear on the skin. These observations suggest local disturbances of pigment metabolism. The exact mechanism of these disturbances is not clear.

Metabolism

The most constant and characteristic feature of thyroid insufficiency is the slowing of all metabolic processes and, in particular, a sharp decrease in the basal metabolic rate, which in thyroidectomized animals may be reduced by 30–45%. As a result of the lowered basal metabolism, animals of this type become relatively insensitive to temporary oxygen deprivation. For instance, whereas a normal rabbit utilizes 1.82 liters oxygen per kilogram body weight per hour, the thyroidectomized rabbit utilizes only 0.887 liter. Tissue respiration and the curve of oxygen dissociation in the blood are considerably lowered. However, anaerobic catabolism is inhibited to the same degree as the oxidative phase of metabolism. Inhibition of the hydrolysis and oxidation of metabolites leads to the limitation of catabolism in all stages of metabolism.

The resultant effect of this general slowing of all forms of energy metabolism in hypothyroidism is a marked decrease in heat production. In thyroidectomized animals, just as in animals in which the thyroid gland is blocked by antithyroid agents, both the external and internal body temperatures are lowered. The hypothermia observed is the result chiefly of a marked decrease in heat production.

Hyperthyroidism, whether spontaneous or due to administration of large doses of extrinsic thyroid hormones, is characterized by a constant increase in the intensity of dissimilatory processes, especially oxidation. An important effect is an increase in heat metabolism. After administration of thyroid hormones, the body temperature rises. Feeding thyroid extract or injecting thyroid hormones may increase heat production by 170% in dogs and by 300% in rabbits. Heat production is also stimulated by thyroid hormones in rats, mice, and pigeons. Heat production in patients with thyrotoxicosis is increased by 200% or more.

The calorigenic action of thyroid hormones is also manifested as a sharp increase in the oxygen consumption. This occurs under basal metabolic conditions (increased BMR), but it is particularly marked during work, when the oxygen consumption rises in proportion to the increase in muscular activity. Since about 1900 many investigations into various aspects of this effect, in both clinical and experimental forms of hyperthyroidism, have been published. Work in this direction has been summarized by Boyd [86]. Until it became possible to determine iodine chemically in the blood and to use radioactive iodine for diagnostic purposes, the investigation of basal metabolism was essentially the only criterion that could be used to assess the state of thyroid gland function. The wide range of usefulness of this parameter is evidence that increased oxygen consumption under the influence of thyroid hormones reflects one of their fundamental properties and comes close to the primary disturbance of cell metabolism arising through their action. This hypothesis is supported by the quantitative relationship between the increase in metabolism and the dose of the hormone [479, 579].

It is very important to note that increased oxygen consumption is observed not only in experiments *in vivo* but also after the addition of thyroid hormones *in vitro* to organs and to tissue slices, homogenates, and subcellular fractions. The heart taken from an animal with thyrotoxicosis consumes more oxygen per unit time than the isolated heart of the healthy animal. Slices of such a heart, and also of the liver, kidneys, spinal cord, and other organs, in turn utilize more oxygen and oxidize added substrates more rapidly than under normal conditions [12]. Mitochondria or even submitochondrial particles isolated from the tissues of animals with thyrotoxicosis or the tissues of healthy animals, if treated *in vitro* with thyroid hormones, also utilize more oxygen [254, 364, 366, 379, 408]. Consequently, the calorigenic effect of thyroid hormones is manifested not only at the cellular level, but also at the subcellular and even at the molecular level. The calorigenic effect is thus a convenient criterion for comparing changes induced by thyroxine at all these levels with its effects on the intact animal.

Protein Metabolism. Data on the role of thyroid hormones in the growth, development, and differentiation of tissues and in reparative phenomena are evidence of their effect on protein metabolism. In 1951, Skow [558] forcibly fed rats equally and found a much smaller deposition of protein in thyroidectomized than in intact animals. Salganik [517] showed that in rats kept on a low-protein diet thyroid extract increases but methylthiouracil (a thyrostatic agent), on the contrary, reduces the nitrogen concentration in the liver tissue. These observations indicate an anabolic effect of thyroid hormones with respect to nitrogen metabolism. Yet the clinical records of patients with hyperthyroidism abound with descriptions of the manifestations of the catabolic action of these hormones.

In many of these reports a sharp rise in the rate of dissimilatory processes, including increased excretion of nitrogen, on the borderline of cachexia, is described as one of the clearest features of thyrotoxicosis [30, 157, 519]. Injection of thyroxine into rats lowers the creatine content in skeletal and heart muscle]80]. The excretion of creatine in the urine is simultaneously increased. This increase is evidently based on inhibition of the phosphorylation of creatine as a result both of a deficiency of ATP]195, 221, 531] and of inhibition of creatine phosphokinase activity [367, 371]. Increased breakdown of tissue proteins in the presence of an excess of thyroid hormones in the body is manifested as the more rapid disappearance of labeled amino acid from the organ proteins determined at measured times after its injection into the blood stream [308]. Activity of proteolytic enzymes in the tissues is considerably increased [212, 380, 605, 639]. These factors all contribute to a sharp increase in nonprotein nitrogen in the blood and tissues.

According to Gol'ber [212] and Smyk and Fishchenko [566] hyperthyroidism disturbs urea formation in the liver. Arslanov [30] showed that despite the acceleration of urea formation, the sharp activation of dissimilatory processes leads to their relative insufficiency, so that the ammonia concentration in the tissues may rise [592]. If ammonium salts are administered to hyperthyroid animals, less of them are excreted as urea than in control animals [205, 566]. The serum albumin concentration is usually low in thyrotoxicosis, whereas the concentration of the globulin fractions may rise [30]. Meanwhile, Kekki [325], using chromatography and electrophoresis, observed an increase in the synthesis of the albumin and α-globulin fractions of the plasma proteins in hyperthyroidism and a decrease in the synthesis of γ-globulin. Thyroid deficiency was accompanied by the opposite changes.

Hypothyroidism leads to retention of nitrogeneous products in the body. Creatine accumulates in the heart [665] and skeletal [605] muscles and the creatine phosphate concentration increases; the blood glutathione level rises [543]. The excretion of creatine and urea in the urine is reduced [428]. Tissue slices of thyroidectomized rats excrete amino acids and proteins more slowly into the incubation medium [332]. The total protein concentration rises slightly in the serum and cerebrospinal fluid, chiefly on account of an increase in the globulin fractions. However, these changes are all connected with the inhibition of protein catabolism rather than with the activation of protein synthesis. On the contrary, the intensity of protein synthesis is lowered [305, 569, 665], as is the concentration of nucleic acids in the tissues [75].

There is much experimental evidence to show that low doses of thyroxine and triiodothyronine stimulate protein synthesis, whereas high concentrations of thyroid hormones inhibit this process. Actually, even the same dose of thyroxine differs in its effects, depending on the level of thyroid function. Crispell et al. [129] showed that triiodothyronine, if administered to euthyroid persons, reduces the rate of protein synthesis as reflected in the retention of ^{15}N-glycine; however, the same dose of hormone increased the lowered level of protein synthesis in patients with myxedema to normal. Stein and Gross [580] found that triiodothyronine stimulates protein biosynthesis in liver homogenates of thyroidectomized but not of intact rats. Some investigators [318, 511] found that daily administration of 5–10 μg thyroxine to thyroidectomized rats increased the rate of protein synthesis, but administration of doses of the hormone 10 times larger to thyroidectomized or intact animals either reduced or completely prevented the formation of new protein molecules in the tissues. Dutoit [151] reported in 1951 that liver slices of rats to which thyroxine had been given incorporated labeled alanine into protein more rapidly. Conversely, thyroidectomy retarded this process. It was difficult to interpret the data indicating stimulation of protein synthesis by thyroid hormones in the light of the well-known and obvious catabolic effect of these hormones under clinical conditions. They were therefore disregarded for a long time.

In the late 1950s and early 1960s, however, the problem of the anabolic effect of thyroid hormones came under close scrutiny in connection with the analysis of the molecular mechanisms of their action. Sokoloff et al. [568, 569, 570] showed that in rats receiving small doses of thyroid hormones various tissues (excluding those whose oxygen consumption is not increased by thyroxine) incorporate labeled amino acids into protein faster than in control animals. A low level of synthesis of serum antibodies was found in thyroidectomized rabbits, and administration of thyroxine let to an increase in this level (sometimes above normal) and in the rate of the reaction to antigen. The concentration of parenchymatous protein was low in liver biopsy material from patients with thyrotoxicosis [447]. Meanwhile, the protein content in the liver was increased in rats fed with thyroid preparations [399]. After subcutaneous injection of a single large dose of thyroxine (400 μg) into rats, the protein content in the liver was initially increased, but it soon fell below the initial level [584]. Panachin and Kandror [464] found that the initial stages of thyrotoxicosis produced in rabbits by administration of thyroid extract are accompanied by an increase in the concentration and synthesis of protein in the liver (as reflected in the incorporation of ^{14}C-glycine), but the degree of this increase was progressively reduced as the administration of thyroid extract continued. In the hearts of these animals Kandror et al. [314, 315] found an initial acceleration of incorporation of labeled methionine and glycine into protein (including into actomyosin), followed by inhibition of this process (in severe toxicosis). The concentration of free amino acids in the blood, liver, and skeletal [127, 189] and heart [84, 306] muscles in animals with experimental thyrotoxicosis is increased, further evidence of the inhibition of peptide synthesis. In rats with thyrotoxicosis the synthesis of amino acids in the liver is also reduced, to judge from the smaller amount of alanine formed from pyruvate and ammonium bicarbonate [106].

The conflicting data on the effect of thyroxine on protein synthesis can evidently be explained by the fact that the effect of the hormone depends on its dose. Intraperitoneal injection of 100 μg thyroxine into rats daily for 6–16 days or incubation of liver homogenates with 1×10^{-5}–1×10^{-4} M thyroxine increased the rate of incorporation of amino acids into protein. Higher doses of the hormone inhibited protein synthesis both *in vivo* and *in vitro*. Similarly, bone marrow slices from young rabbits, when incubated with 1×10^{-7} M thyroxine or triiodothyronine incorporated histidine more rapidly into protein, but higher concentrations of the hormone slowed protein synthesis [438]. Nevertheless, thyroid hormones are essential for a normal level of protein synthesis, for these processes are inhibited in thyroidectomized animals.

Thyroxine injections increase the total RNA content in the rat liver, which Reid [497] attributes to acceleration of the synthesis of soluble RNA by the supernatant fraction of the cells. Panachin [464] also observed an increase in the total RNA concentration in the liver of rabbits with relatively mild thyroid overdosage. The uptake of label into RNA was accelerated. Kandror and Svyatkina [589] also found an increase in the RNA content in the heart muscle of these animals. In the early stages of thyrotoxicosis incorporation of inorganic phosphate into RNA of the nuclei and ribosomes was increased, but in severe toxicosis (with a loss of weight of more than 30%) the renewal of RNA of these subcellular fractions was distinctly inhibited. Unlike Reid's observations [497], in these experiments no change was found in RNA synthesis in the supernatant fraction. Sorokin and Turakulov [571] found diverse changes in the rate of RNA synthesis in different tissues of rats under the influence of thyroid hormones.

This short survey could be considerably extended by the addition of data on the character and sequence of the changes in nucleic acid and protein metabolism of the cell as a whole and of its various subcellular fractions and also on the correlation of these changes with other manifestations of the action of thyroid hormones. These data will be examined in Part III, in which modern views on the molecular mechanism of action of thyroid hormones are considered.

Lipid Metabolism. Small doses of thyroid hormones increase the assimilation of fat from the intestine. Large doses of the hormone stimulate peristalsis so that the food passes more quickly through the intestine and the fat cannot be absorbed. As a result, steatorrhea develops. There are conflicting reports in the literature on the effect of thyroid hormones on lipid synthesis, and these contradictions can by no means always be explained by differences in the dose of hormones used. Many investigations have demonstrated the acceleration of lipid synthesis by the action of thyroxine or triiodothyronine. The rate of synthesis of cholesterol is increased in man and in rats receiving thyroid hormones [347, 459], making the hypocholesteremia observed in thyrotoxicosis difficult to explain. However, simultaneous stimulation of the conversion of cholesterol into bile acids [158] and the elimination of cholesterol from the body [505] provide an explanation for this observation. Thyroxine increases the deposition of fat in the brown adipose tissue of rats, acting in this respect synergistically with cortisone [361]. However, it is not yet proved whether lipid synthesis is increased under these conditions. To judge from the incorporation of labeled precursors, thyroid hormones stimulate the rate of synthesis of cholesterol and fatty acids in rats and also in tissue slices of these animals [103, 133, 176, 318, 404, 409, 575]. Meanwhile, the rate of cholesterol synthesis [520] was found to be reduced in liver homogenates from thyrotoxic rats, and its concentration in the whole tissue also was reduced [255]. The total lipid reserves in the body are reduced in patients with thyrotoxicosis [641]. However, information on the lipid content in the liver in thyrotoxicosis is contradictory. Clinicians who have investigatged the liver of patients with thyrotoxicosis by punch biopsy have usually observed fatty infiltration of the organ. However, in experimental animals, although some workers [4, 5, 641] have found that the content of total lipids in the liver is reduced, according to others [467] it is unchanged, but most investigators have found [211, 461, 526] that it is increased.

The contradictory nature of results obtained by different workers for the fat content in the liver can probably be explained by the fact that they carried out only single tests in different stages of thyrotoxicosis and used different doses of thyroid hormones. The results of experiments by Gol'ber and Negovskaya [441] showed that the lipid content in the liver is considerably increased in rats fed with thyroid extract. Similar results were obtained by histochemical investigation of lipids in the liver [91]. Rachev [490] cites experiments which showed that hyperlipemia develops in thyrotoxicosis. However, Negovskaya [441] found that the total serum lipid level in these animals is low.

Gol'ber and Negovskaya found lowered lipolytic activity of the liver in rats with toxicosis due to thyroid extract; this observation could shed important light on the pathogenesis of the lipid accumulation in the liver. Travina also considers that lipid accumulation of the liver is connected with a decrease in the lipase activity in the organ in thyrotoxicosis. Gol'ber and Negovskaya found a decrease in the β-lipoprotein content in the liver of experimental animals fed with thyroid extract. The β-lipoprotein level in the blood serum falls as thyrotoxicosis increases in severity, as other workers have also observed [2, 87, 150, 244, 456, 505, 560, 576].

The phospholipic content in the liver is unchanged in animals fed with thyroid extract, but at the same time the serum phospholipid concentration falls sharply. This shows that the liberation of fatty acids from the liver as components of phospholipids is obstructed. A decrease in the plasma phospholipid concentration is also found in patients with thyrotoxicosis [2, 145, 516]. As a result of their analysis, Gol'ber and Negovskaya identify the following factors as responsible for the accumulation of fat in the liver in thyrotoxicosis: (a) a decrease in the liver glycogen, (b) stimulation of lipid mobilization, (c) disturbance of the formation of β-lipoproteins as the result of a disturbance of the protein-synthesizing function of the liver, (d) inadequate elimination of triglycerides in the form of β-lipoproteins and of fatty acids in the form of phospholipids, (e) a decrease in the hydrolysis of triglycerides.

Thyroidectomy, like myxedema, is accompanied by reduced synthesis of cholesterol [86, 176, 239]. Replacement therapy with thyroid hormones returns the rate of synthesis of cholesterol and fatty acids in patients with myxedema to normal [390].

The experiments of Fletcher and Myant [177] clearly demonstrated how the effect of thyroxine depends on its dose. For example, administration of 20 μg thyroxine to rats accelerated cholesterol synthesis from acetate in cell-free preparations of the liver, but administration of 30–50 μg thyroxine slowed this process. These workers observed the inhibition of fatty acid synthesis by all doses of the hormone used, and they attributed it to ATP deficiency because of exhaustion of the glycogen reserves.

In connection with the effect of thyroid hormones on lipid metabolism some interesting results were obtained by Fraenkel-Conrat and Greenberg [183], Gershberg and Kuhl [201], and by Hung [288], who found a decrease in the concentration of coenzyme A in the liver of patients and animals with thyrotoxicosis. On the other hand, thyroxine is essential for the synthesis of this compound, for the conversion of pantothenic acid into coenzyme A does not take place in the absence of the hormone [591, 610].

Thyroid hormones evidently participate in regulation of the lipid level not only in the tissues, but also in the blood. There is experimental [226, 441, 559] and clinical [152, 500] evidence that if an excess of thyroid hormones is present in the body, the concentration of free fatty acids rises in the arterial and venous blood. Experiments conducted in Gol'ber's laboratory showed that the concentration of NEFA (nonesterified fatty acids) is increased also in the cerebrospinal fluid of rabbits with experimental thyrotoxicosis.

The change in the rate of lipid synthesis under the influence of thyroid hormones is not the only mechanism regulating the lipid level in the tissues and blood. Thyroid hormones can also change the rate of mobilization of fat from the depots and its oxidation. In the course of its influence on the mobilization of fat from the depots, thyroxine engages in complex interactions with other lipid-mobilizing factors [298]. It is, therefore, very difficult to distinguish the isolated effect of thyroid hormones on the tissue lipid reserves. According to Negovskaya [441], prolonged administration of thyroid extract to rats increases the lipolytic activity of adipose tissue. Schwartz and Debons [524] observed the faster liberation of free fatty acids from the adipose tissue of dogs receiving thyroid hormones. The rate of disappearance of NEFA from the blood increased at the same time. An increase in the rate of circulation of the plasma NEFA in thyrotoxicosis also was observed by Eaton et al. [152] and Gold et al. [226]. The opposite changes were observed in hypothyroid animals.

A decrease in the blood NEFA level and in NEFA absorption by the tissues in hypothyroidism were also reported by Scott et al. [525] and Hamburger et al. [253]. Bressler and Wittels [89] found that administration of thyroxine to guinea pigs increases the oxidation of fatty acids by heart homogenates at the expense of other substrates. These workers attribute this result to an increase in the concentration of free carnitine and acylcarnitine in the tissues. In the experiments of Skuratovskaya [559] on hyperthyroid cats with catheterization of the coronary sinus, an increase in the contribution of free fatty acids to the oxidative metabolism of the heart muscle was also observed (as shown by the ratio between the assimilation of NEFA and oxygen by the myocardium). The respiratory quotient of the heart is reduced in thyrotoxicosis.

It is interesting to note that, according to White and Engel [646], triiodothyronine itself does not accelerate the liberation of NEFA from adipose tissue *in vitro*. Admittedly, it was also shown later that triiodothyronine activates lipolysis in adipose tissue *in vitro* [110, 628], which some investigators attribute to activation of adenyl cyclase and inhibition of phosphodiesterase. As a result, cyclic AMP, a lipase activator, accumulates in the tissues. However, the work of Levey et al. [386] and of Laraia and Ready [364] showed that adenyl cyclase activity in the tissues (the myocardium, for example) of hyperthyroidized animals is not increased or may actually be reduced.

Despite the fact that the lipolytic activity of the heart muscle is considerably increased in animals receiving thyroid preparations [20, 83, 559], after the addition of triiodothyronine it is unchanged in myocardial tissue *in vitro* [525, 559]. The possibility cannot be ruled out that the increased mobilization of fatty acids from the depots (which Challoner [110] observed in experiments *in vitro* as reflected in an increase in the glycerol level in the absence of other oxidation substrates) may therefore reflect the usual shift in equilibrium of the reaction in response to the more rapid disappearance of its product. The rate of oxidation of fatty acids in homogenates and mitochondria of the tissues (heart, liver) of rats receiving thyroxine in fact rises sharply [136, 274]. The respiratory quotient falls to 0.7 in patients with thyrotoxicosis [152, 458] and in animals receiving thyroid hormones [148], indicating preferential oxidation of fat. Since the initial stages of oxidation of fatty acids require ATP, the acceleration of these processes may be connected with the effect of thyroxine on the formation of high-energy compounds. On the other hand, this action of thyroid hormones must be allowed for when their influence on energy metabolism is studied.

In severe cases of diffuse toxic goiter in man and also in experimental thyrotoxicosis in animals produced by feeding with thyroid extract, hyperketonemia may be observed [212, 380]. In mild cases of hyperthyroidism, ketonemia is absent. In prolonged thyrotoxicosis with utilization of the greater part of the reserve, the risks connected with a metabolism in which lipids do not participate must arise. This state of affairs leads to increased utilization of proteins and to a profound disturbance of the metabolism of the body.

In conclusion, some workers [66, 149, 271, 378] are inclined to regard the decrease in the serum cholesterol concentration as an independent effect of *thioactive* compounds unconnected with the general effect of thyroid hormones on metabolism.

Carbohydrate Metabolism. Thyroid hormones participate in the regulation of the blood sugar, although their role in this respect is subsidiary. These hormones evidently influence glucose formation, by stimulating gluconeogenesis from amino acids, and also its utilization in the tissues. Glucose catabolism by the anaerobic route is considerably accelerated by thyroxine [57, 574]. The mechanism of this acceleration is not yet clear. In particular, it is not known whether it takes place through an increase in the synthesis of enzymes catalyzing the rate-limiting stages of glycolysis or on account of some effect of thyroxine on phosphorus metabolism, as a result of which the content of inorganic phosphate in the cell rises and the "brake" on glycolysis is thereby released (the Pasteur effect).

Increased assimilation or oxidation of glucose (or both together) was observed in the muscles of hyperthyroid rabbits [426], the liver of hyperthyroid rats [99], and also after the addition of thyroid hormones to cultures of chick embryonic fibroblasts [249] and ascites carcinoma cells [58, 107, 264]. A single intraperitoneal injection of 50–100 μg thyroxine into rats is sufficient to accelerate the utilization of intravenously injected glucose [117]. To judge from the rate of lactic acid formation, the tissues of the diaphragm and salivary glands of rats receiving thyroid preparations convert glucose more rapidly by the glycolytic route. It is curious to note that the addition of 1×10^{-3} M azide to these tissues, although not affecting glycolysis in control animals, inhibits it in hyperthyroid rats. These findings may indicate that the acceleration of glycolysis is not a direct effect of the thyroid hormones but a reflection of disturbance of a metabolic pathway common to the enzyme systems of glycolysis and respiration [230]. As Hoch [273] points out, phosphorus metabolism could be the pathway in question. On the other hand, reports have been published that physiologically inactive analogs of thyroxine (which do not increase the oxygen consumption of the body) also accelerate glycolysis [262]. At the same time, thyroid hormones are known to stimulate glycolysis, not by the direct activation of the enzymes of the glycolytic cycle, but by another mechanism. According to Bargoni et al. [57] the activity of only two glycolytic enzymes—enolase and lactate dehydrogenase—is increased in the liver of rats with experimental thyrotoxicosis; the activity of the other enzymes is unchanged, except that the phosphoglucomutase activity falls. Thyroxine *in vitro* inhibits purified glyceraldehyde-3-phosphate dehydrogenase [655]. As

Hoch [273] rightly points out, enolase or lactate dehydrogenase is unlikely to catalyze the rate-limiting stages of glycolysis, and for that reason the stimulant effect of the thyroid hormones on the anaerobic conversions of glucose must evidently be regarded as indirect.

Besides glycolysis, the thyroid hormones also activate another pathway of glucose metabolism, the hexose monophosphate shunt. This is a system of enzymes and coenzymes oxidizing glucose to CO_2. This system of enzymes is well represented, in particular, in mature erythrocytes. Necheles and Beutler [439] showed that incubation of erythrocytes with triiodothyronine increases the rate of oxygen utilization and that this is the result of stimulation of the hexose monophosphate shunt. The degree of increase of the oxygen utilization varied in direct proportions to the concentration of the hormone. A similar effect, although weaker, was observed in response to the action of thyroxine. The fact that a similar, or even greater, increase in oxygen utilization took place under the influence of triiodothyronine in hemolyzed erythrocytes indicates that this effect is not the result of the action of the hormone on membrane permeability.

Thyroid hormones have been shown to affect activity of the enzymes of the hexose monophosphate shunt. High glucose-6-phosphate dehydrogenase activity was found in 11 of 12 patients with thyrotoxicosis; in two cases the determinations were repeated after the patients had recovered and the enzyme activity was then back to normal. Other workers confirmed a sharp increase in the activity of this enzyme in most cases of hyperthyroidism [51, 77, 638]. Pearson and Dzuyan found normal glucose-6-phosphate dehydrogenase activity in the erythrocytes in patients with hypothyroidism, but Root [504] described a decrease in its activity in the erythrocytes of hypothyroid children. After treatment the activity of this enzyme rose considerably. Dried thyroid gland or triiodothyronine, administered to a healthy person, caused a marked increase in the enzyme activity in the erythrocytes, which later returned to normal. Glock and McLean [210] described increased glucose-6-phosphate dehydrogenase activity in the liver of rats receiving thyroxine earlier still. Activation of the hexose monophosphate shunt by thyroid hormones has also been described in heart tissue. Besides glucose-6-phosphate dehydrogenase, thyroxine also increases the activity of another enzyme belonging to this pathway of glucose conversion: 6-phosphogluconate dehydrogenase [57, 395]. However, in contrast to the constant and clear effect obtained *in vivo*, incubation of erythrocytes with triiodothyronine *in vitro* did not increase enzyme activity. According to Wolff and Wolff [655] high concentrations of thyroxine *in vitro* actually inhibit glucose-6-phosphate dehydrogenase isolated from yeast.

In contrast to the observation that thyroxine stimulates activity of the hexose monophosphate shunt, some results pointing in the opposite direction have been published. Dow and Allen [146] found that the total oxidation of glucose by the glycolytic pathway is increased in hyperthyroid rats, whereas the hexose monophosphate shunt is completely inhibited. Redding and Johnson [496] studied the erythrocytes of patients with thyrotoxicosis and also found increased glycolysis and inhibition of the hexose monophosphate shunt. This problem requires further investigation.

According to most observations an excess of thyroid hormones in the body leads to a decrease in the content of glycogen (especially its metabolically active forms) in the liver and muscles [30, 116, 120, 211, 242, 335, 397, 426, 441]. If the thyroid function is deficient or if the gland is inhibited by thyrostatic preparations, an increase in the glycogen content in the liver and muscles is frequently observed. The decrease in the glycogen content in the organs in thyrotoxicosis is accompanied by a sharp decrease in their ATP content [68, 112]. In the experiments of Gol'ber, Kandror, et al. [211, 219, 220] the glycogen content in the liver and myocardium was sharply reduced in rabbits after prolonged feeding with large doses of thyroid extract and also in hyperthyroidized cats and rats. In some cases it was completely impossible to detect any glycogen in the liver. Histochemical investigations confirmed the results of the biochemical tests [91]. Meanwhile the concentration of high-energy phosphates (ATP and creatine phosphate) in the tissues fell considerably. The content of ATP and creatine phosphate also fell sharply in the heart muscle of rats and guinea pigs receiving thyroid preparations [68, 412]. The fact that some investigators [476] did not observe this phenomenon in hyperthyroidized dogs can evidently be explained by the very high resistance of these animals to thyroid hormones [1]. Meanwhile, in other animals, administration of these hormones does not always lead to a decrease in the ATP concentration in the tissues [116]. Buccino et al. [96], in experiments in which thyroxine was given to cats, actually found a small increase in the ATP reserves in the myocardium. Hypothyroidism was accompanied by the opposite changes.

An increase in the glycogen level under the influence of thyroid preparations was observed in a series of investigations. For instance, after a single injection of thyroxine into rats, the glycogen content rose in the liver [584] and skeletal muscles [382, 383]. The opposite action of this hormone on the glycogen content in the tissues is evidently explained by differences in its dose. Wertheimer and Benter [643, 644] showed in fact that low doses of thyroxine increased glycogen synthesis *in vivo* and *in vitro*, whereas high doses inhibit this process.

Administration of large doses of sugar by mouth to thyroidectomized animals often does not lead to an increase in the blood glucose level or to glucosuria. However, intravenous injection of glucose into such animals is usually followed by hyperglycemia. These observations indicate a slowing of the absorption of glucose from the alimentary tract in hypothyroidism.

Intravenous injection of galactose or glucose in the presence of a raised level of thyroid hormones in the body does not give a constant picture. Some workers [22] describe a normal type of blood sugar curve whereas others [648] observed a *delayed* type of curve characteristic of diabetes. It is difficult to reconcile these facts with the more rapid utilization of glucose by the tissues mentioned above. Sugar loading in thyrotoxicosis also gives a *diabetic* curve, possibly because of increased absorption of hexoses from the gastrointestinal tract [21, 385]. On this account, administration of thyroid hormones to some species of animals (dogs) aggravates diabetes produced, for example, by removal of the pancreas. However, the course of diabetes in pancreatectomized rats is unaffected by thyroxine. *Thyrogenic* diabetes is evidently associated with exhaustion of the β-cells of the pancreas arising in prolonged thyrotoxicosis [53]. Like the action of thyroid hormones on other types of metabolism, their effect on carbohydrate metabolism is also closely linked with the effects of other hormones, especially insulin and adrenalin.

Water and Electrolyte Metabolism. Disturbances of water and electrolyte metabolism in thyroid dysfunction are among the clearest manifestations of thyroid pathology. Although most workers state that the mechanism of these changes is extrarenal, nevertheless, considering the metabolic changes produced by thyroid hormones in the renal parenchyma, it must be assumed that the influence of these hormones on the activity of the kidneys must play an important role in the genesis of the changes in the water and electrolyte balance caused by an excess or deficiency of thyroid hormones.

After administering large doses of thyroid extract experimentally to rabbits for a long time, Kandror et al. [313] found phasic changes in diuresis in the animals. In severe and prolonged thyrotoxicosis the volume of urine excreted daily by the experimental animals was much less than in the controls. The classical function tests did not give a definite answer to the question of whether kidney function was disturbed in thyrotoxicosis. However, the use of more delicate methods, enabling the various kidney functions to be tested separately, showed a frequent decrease in glomerular filtration in patients with thyrotoxicosis [469], especially in severe forms of the disease. A decrease in the tubular reabsorption of water [513] and in the concentrating power of the kidneys has also been described under the influence of thyroid hormones. The tubular secretion is more often increased. Thyroidectomy in dogs is accompanied by some decrease in the clearance of diodrast and in its maximal tubular secretion [266]. The reabsorption of glucose also is increased [155]. According to Genes and Lesnoi [199], water loading (through a gastric fistula) in dogs leads to increased diuresis in animals receiving thyroid tissue with their food and to reduced diuresis in thyroidectomized animals. The investigations of Pashkov [465] on patients with thyrotoxicosis differing in severity and duration showed a disturbance of kidney functions. The polyuria observed in relatively mild stages of the disease is replaced by oliguria as the thyrotoxicosis becomes more severe. Function tests revealed retention of water in the body in severe thyrotoxicosis.

In connection with these clinical observations it is interesting to mention the experimental data of Gol'ber and Kandror [217], who found an increase in the content of water in the tissues (myocardium) in rabbits with severe thyrotoxicosis produced by feeding with thyroid extract. The loss of extracellular fluid and sodium ions arising under the influence of small doses of thyroid hormone evidently leads to an *extracellular dehydration* of the body. This is largely responsible for the sharp loss of weight with an increase in the dosage of the hormones and in the duration of their administration. Hypotonic extracellular fluid can be displaced inside the cells, which not only restores osmotic equilibrium, but also causes the cells to swell. In other words, after the first phase of extracellular dehydration there follows a phase of cellular hyperhydration. Another contributory factor is the increased catabolism in thyrotoxicosis, with the increased formation of endogenous water.

The changes in the content and distribution of water and electrolytes in the tissues observed in the presence of a deficiency or excess of thyroid hormones in the body may also be linked with a disturbance of the activity of the many systems controlling water and electrolyte metabolism and kidney function. However, thyroid hormones can themselves, evidently, affect the permeability of biological membranes to water and ions. In some experiments, for instance, even low concentrations of thyroxine (1×10^{-6} M) *in vitro* changed the permeability of the toad urinary bladder and skin to water and certain electrolytes.

Since electrolytes are often direct regulators of the intensity of biochemical reactions in the cell, it is important to analyze in rather more detail the interaction of some of them with thyroid hormones. There is conflicting evidence on the effects of thyroid hormones on potassium and sodium metabolism in the body. Some workers [36, 493, 494] found no changes in the metabolism of these cations in thyrotoxicosis, whereas others observed either hyperkaliemia and hyperkaliurea [81, 103] or a decrease in the level of exchangeable potassium *in vivo* [434, 641]. Despite the absence of sharp changes in the total potassium content in the erythrocytes in patients with thyrotoxicosis, the uptake of ^{43}K by these cells was reduced. Similar results were obtained by administering triiodothyronine to healthy human subjects [43]. If tissue preparations are incubated with thyroxine, they often lose potassium ions, and the ratio between their intracellular and extracellular potassium is reduced [596].

The change in permeability of the intracellular organelles to K^+ taking place under the influence of thyroid hormones [432] leads to swelling of the mitochondria and also to the onset of muscular paralysis [273]. Kandror and Kryukova [312] showed that the sodium concentration in the blood plasma of rabbits receiving large doses of thyroid extract for long periods of time falls, whereas its concentration in the erythrocytes and heart muscle tissue rises. So far as potassium is concerned, in such thyrotoxic rabbits there was no accompanying decrease in its concentration in whole blood, although it fell in the erythrocytes and rose in the plasma. The potassium concentration in the myocardium of the left ventricle, which has only a very small content of extracellular fluid, was less than in the control. These workers interpreted their results as showing potassium deprivation of the cells and their corresponding enrichment with sodium in severe thyrotoxicosis.

Interaction between thyroid hormones and magnesium ions is particularly interesting because these ions participate in many enzymic reactions connected with the metabolism of high-energy phosphate. According to one view, thyroxine and triiodothyronine form chelated complexes with magnesium and thus prevent its participation in enzymic reactions [196, 365, 490]; this effect plays an important role in the mechanism of action of thyroid hormones. However, this hypothesis has still to be proved, for it cannot explain why some enzyme systems activated by magnesium (muscle creatine phosphokinase, for example) are inhibited in thyrotoxicosis, whereas others (mitochondrial ATPase, muscle hexokinase, for example), on the contrary, increase their activity [565]. Meanwhile changes in thyroid function are reflected in the magnesium metabolism. In patients with myxedema, for instance, triiodothyronine treatment rapidly increased the magnesium excretion with the urine [594]. Some workers [484, 567] described a decrease in the concentration of protein-bound magnesium in the blood serum in thyrotoxicosis, although others [108, 125, 549] did not observe this effect. The total magnesium concentration in the blood serum is reduced in experimental thyrotoxicosis [632], but the requirement of this cation is increased. Kandror and Kryukova [312] observed no considerable changes in the plasma magnesium concentration in rabbits receiving thyroid extract, whereas its concentration in the erythrocytes and myocardium fell. By injecting magnesium into such animals (by iontophoresis), Gol'ber and co-workers were able to reverse some of the metabolic changes in the myocardium considerably. When an analogous procedure was carried out on patients with thyrotoxicosis, their body weight increased, their tachycardia was reduced or disappeared completely, and their basal metabolic rate and blood pressure fell [25]. Rachev [490] found that incubation of the mitochondria from various tissues of hyperthyroidized rabbits with an optimal concentration of magnesium ions considerably reduces the severity of the changes in oxidative phosphorylation. Rachev accordingly injected magnesium chloride into the experimental animals and obtained a marked improvement in the clinical picture of the disease and a decrease in the mitochondrial changes.

The similarity between the *molecular* effects of the thyroid hormones and the action of calcium ions determines the interest shown in relations between these factors in the body. Both synergistic [164, 577] and antagonistic [366] relations between calcium and thyroxine can be found in the literature. Staehelin [577] also considers that thyroxine acts through changes in the concentration of free calcium ions in the body. It has been shown, for example, that in experimental calcium deficiency thyroxine does not increase the oxygen consumption of animals.

Sometimes equally severe disturbances of the calcium balance occur in thyrotoxicosis as in hyperparathyroidism. The principal changes are recorded in the bones, but other tissues also are affected. Biopsy of bone tissue [180] and fluoroscopy [40] reveal marked osteoporosis in thyrotoxicosis. The bones and muscles of rats with experimental thyrotoxicosis accumulate less ^{45}Ca than normal, but the radioactivity of the liver and uterus is increased under these circumstances [656]. Administration of thyroid extract to rabbits leads to phasic changes in the plasma calcium concentration: At first it rises a little, but as the pathological changes progress it decreases. The calcium concentration in the heart muscle falls a little, but in the erythrocytes it rises [312]. Investigation of the excretion of calcium in the urine and feces in thyrotoxicosis or hypothyroidism does not always reveal a disturbance of calcium metabolism. It is stated that calcium ions inhibit the synthesis of thyroid hormones or increase the renal iodine clearance [595].

In the analysis of relations between thyroid function and calcium metabolism it must be remembered that the changes which arise are not necessarily the result of direct interaction between these factors. The calcium balance may be disturbed as a result of changes in phosphorus metabolism, because of complex interaction between the thyroid and parathyroid glands, and, finally, because of changes in the secretion of the special thyroid hormone, thyrocalcitonin.

Thyroid Hormones and Vitamins. Some of the physiological manifestations of a deficiency or excess of thyroid hormones in the body resemble the effects of a disturbance of vitamin metabolism produced by changes in the bodily requirements of these compounds, changes in their absorption or utilization. This aspect of the action of thyroxine and triiodothyronine has assumed particular importance in the light of the connection postulated by Utevskii [618] between hormones, vitamins, and enzymes.

However, the evidence regarding the ability to prevent particular features of thyroid pathology by means of particular vitamins is conflicting [147, 494]. Ershoff [160] showed in 1947 that feeding whole liver preparations to growing rats receiving thyroid hormones prevents the loss of weight of the animals that otherwise takes place regularly under those conditions. However, this effect could not be attributed to the action of any of the proteins present in the liver or to any vitamins yet known. It is difficult to see the manifestation of any concrete avitaminosis in the clinical picture of hypothyroidism, even if severe. In most cases all that can be said is that there may be certain features of hypovitaminoses. Human requirements of thiamine have been shown to be increased in thyrotoxicosis [494], while the concentration of free thiamine and of diphosphothiamine in the blood is reduced [648]. The total thiamine content is also reduced in the liver, but not in the spleen (which does not respond to thyroid hormones by an increase in respiration). These changes are due not only to the more rapid utilization of vitamin B_1, but also to its increased elimination from the body in the urine, feces, and sweat [147, 648]. Judging by the increase in the blood diphosphothiamine level after administration of vitamin B_1, the phosphorylation of thiamine is undisturbed in thyrotoxicosis in man [648]. Feeding rats with thyroid preparations or administration of thyroxine to them is followed by a decrease in the tissue cocarboxylase concentration. Injections of thiamine into control and experimental animals increase the tissue cocarboxylase level, but in hyperthyroidized rats this level falls quicker than in the control rats. Peters and Rossiter [473] ascribe this to the more rapid destruction of the coenzyme in the tissues and not to a disturbance of thiamine phosphorylation. Rachev [490] cites evidence that the addition of vitamin B_1 to the food of hyperthyroidized animals often lowers the basal metabolic rate, reduces the tachycardia, and causes an increase in the body weight. Meanwhile, Bhagat and Lockett [72] showed in 1961 that administration of thyroxine to animals with severe avitaminosis-B_1 does not increase their oxygen consumption. This contradiction remains unexplained.

An excess of thyroid hormones in the body is not accompanied by any visible manifestations of vitamin B_6 deficiency. However, the supply of pyridoxine to the tissues is limited [39, 654]. The concentration of pyridoxal-5-phosphate in the liver and heart muscle of rats receiving thyroxine was considerably reduced because of a disturbance of the phosphorylation of pyridoxine and not because of a decrease in its content [360, 410]. Thyroidectomy leads to an increase in the concentration of pyridoxal-5-phosphate in the liver. In rats receiving thyroxine in a dose of 10 μg daily for 15 days the cysteine desulfhydrase activity disappears and the activity of serine and threonine dehydrogenases and of alanine-glutamate transaminase falls sharply in the liver. Addition of pyridoxal-5-phosphate to the animal's diet or the addition of this coenzyme to the incubation medium of liver slices restores the activity of all these enzymes. Similar results have been obtained with respect to the effect of thyroxine *in vitro* [283].

Meanwhile a decrease in the activity of various pyridoxal enzymes observed in the liver of animals receiving large doses of thyroxine or triiodothyronine (cysteine and dihydroxyphenylalanine decarboxylases, for example) is only partly prevented by pyridoxal-5-phosphate *in vitro* [105, 360, 645]. These results indicate that small doses of thyroid hormones disturb the phosphorylation of pyridoxine, whereas large doses may inhibit the synthesis of the apoenzyme also [273].

With a change in thyroid function the metabolism of vitamin B_{12} is also disturbed. Its content in the tissues and blood of rats receiving thyroid preparations falls considerably [13, 202, 319]. Similar changes take place in hypothyroidism in man and experimental animals. In the case of thyroid deficiency, the main cause of the decrease in the vitamin B_{12} content in the body is a disturbance in its absorption due to the atrophic gastritis which often develops in this condition [603]. However, there is evidence that a deficiency of the secretion of the gastric intrinsic factor in hypothyroidism is not the only cause of the disturbance of vitamin B_{12} absorption [73, 381, 455]. Hellegers et al. [268] consider that the low serum concentration of vitamin B_{12} in children is a sign of cretinism.

There is evidence that the effect of thyroid hormones on intracellular metabolism is closely bound with the utilization of vitamin B_{12}. In healthy persons and also in patients with thyrotoxicosis and myxedema, Ziffer et al. [666] determined the excretion of vitamin B_{12} in the urine and its serum concentration after intramuscular injection of 50 μg of this vitamin. In hyperthyroidism the serum vitamin B_{12} level and its excretion in the urine was lower than in healthy subjects, whereas the converse was the case of hypothyroidism. Vitamin B_{12} counteracts the delay in growth observed when thyroid gland tissue is fed to young animals [70, 156]. Even a small dose of crystalline cyanocobalamin completely prevented the lethal effect of 200 μg thyroxine in rats with avitaminosis-B_{12} [587]. Whereas injections of thyroxine in control animals reduced the DNA content in the liver, in rats with avitaminosis-B_{12} thyroxine increased the DNA content in the liver [355]. These results may point to interaction between the hormone and vitamin in the regulation of nucleic acid synthesis. Spontaneous vitamin B_{12} deficiency is rare in animals, and one way of producing this state is by feeding with thyroid preparations. The vitamin B_{12} level in the tissues falls in thyrotoxicosis parallel to the decrease in the glutathione level in the liver and blood and the decrease in incorporation of cysteine into the glutathione of the liver. Gershoff et al. [202] found that the reduced tissue vitamin B_{12} concentration in thyrotoxicosis can be restored to normal by increasing the magnesium content in the diet. Administration of vitamin B_{12} prevents the various metabolic disturbances arising in rats receiving thyroid preparations [160, 172, 202, 319, 581]. Fatterpaker et al. [172] even accept that an intracellular deficiency of vitamin B_{12} is the primary manifestation of thyrotoxicosis. Vitamin B_{12} is undoubtedly necessary for certain fundamental metabolic processes in the cell, and one of the effects of thyroid hormones is probably accompanied by the more rapid utilization of the vitamin in the course of these processes. The more rapid metabolism occurring in the presence of an excess of thyroid hormones is also responsible for the greater consumption of vitamin C. Its content in the blood and tissues falls in this condition, its excretion rises, and the bodily requirement also rises [147, 544]. At the same time there is no definite connection between thyroid activity and ascorbic acid metabolism [494]. Berg [68] showed as long ago as 1937 that the administration of vitamin C to animals with experimental thyrotoxicosis improves the contractile function of the heart muscle. The creatinuria decreases under these conditions. According to Byshevskii [104], avitaminosis-C increases the excretion of iodine from the body.

The change in thyroid activity is also reflected in the fate of the lipid-soluble vitamins, especially vitamin A. In hypothyroidism, for instance, the serum vitamin A concentration falls. This evidently takes place because of blocking of the conversion of carotene into vitamin A, for hypothyroidism is accompanied by hypercarotenemia. Administration of thyroxine under these conditions restores the rate of synthesis of the vitamin [300]. When the young rats which began to receive thyroid preparations with their food as soon as they stopped receiving their mothers' milk were given carotene, the quantity of vitamin A which accumulated was greater than in control animals [482]. The rate of conversion of carotene into vitamin A is also increased by thyroid hormones in rabbits and guinea pigs. However, prolonged oversaturation with thyroid preparations is accompanied by severe manifestations of avitaminosis-A [482]. In guinea pigs receiving thyroxine the vitamin A content in the liver rises at first but then falls [483]. These observations show that the effect of thyroid hormones on vitamin A synthesis, like their effect on the synthesis of other organic compounds in the body, is biphasic. Furthermore, the possibility cannot be ruled out that the reduced vitamin A content in the body in severe thyrotoxicosis is connected with the sharp loss of fat and, consequently, with loss of the ability to store carotene and vitamin A in the tissues. A disturbance of the absorption of carotene also plays an important role.

Thyroxine promotes not only the formation of vitamin A but also its conversion into retinine, for this hormone (like, 2,4-dinitrophenol) improves dark adaptation of the eyes in man [468]. These observations have been confirmed in experiments on the tadpole retina [651]. Vignais [631] also found that thyroxine and vitamin A produce opposite changes in liver transhydrogenase activity in rats with avitaminosis-A. However, the role of these effects in the explanation of the mechanism of action of the hormone is not yet clear. Sheets and Struck [539] found a decrease in the oxygen utilization in hyperthyroidized animals after receiving large doses of vitamin A. On the other hand, Oliverau and Serfaty [457] in histophysiological investigations demonstrated a decrease in thyroid gland activity and a decrease in the number of β-cells in the pituitary in vitamin A deficiency.

Excessive quantities of thyroid hormones presumably can give rise to symptoms of vitamin D deficiency *in vivo*, although information on the tissue levels of this vitamin in thyrotoxicosis is apparently not available. Thyrotoxicosis is in fact accompanied by increased calcium excretion, and administration of vitamin D under these conditions restores the normal calcium metabolism [147]. In hypothyroidism, however, it is impossible to restore the calcium and phosphorus metabolism to normal by vitamin D alone. Under these conditions thyroid hormones must be given at the same time.

There is very little information in the literature on changes in the remaining vitamins during disturbances of thyroid function. For example, it has been stated that avitaminosis-E, like thyrotoxicosis, is accompanied by increased utilization of oxygen by the surviving tissues. A deficiency of pantothenic acid gives rise to manifestations similar to those of hyperthyroidism, and the severity of particular features of thyrotoxicosis can be reduced by its administration. This may well be connected with the role of coenzyme A in metabolism, for pantothenic acid is a component of this coenzyme. An excess of thyroid hormones also leads to increased excretion of riboflavin derivatives from the body [4].

In the light of the facts concerning interaction between thyroid hormones and vitamins described above, it can be concluded that many of the changes in metabolism which were mentioned are connected with a disturbance of the activity of enzymes concerned with protein, lipid, and carbohydrate metabolism. Meanwhile the vitally important question of priority among the disturbances of enzyme reactions under the influence of thyroid hormones remains unanswered.

Action on the Nervous System

Much clinical and experimental material concerning the effect of thyroid hormones on the activity of the nervous system has now been gathered. Although under the controlling influence of direct or humorally mediated nervous impulses, the thyroid gland itself can exert a powerful influence on processes taking place at different levels of the central and autonomic nervous systems.

Action on the Central Nervous System

In thyrotoxicosis various nervous and mental disorders are almost constantly observed. Botkin [85], many years ago, in his clinical lecture on Basedow's or Graves' disease, emphasized that the most constant and characteristic symptoms of this disease are mental changes. Emotional disturbances in patients with thyrotoxicosis, as well as their increased excitability and a proneness to rapid fatigue, have been noted by other authors. Meanwhile, as the severity of the toxicosis increases, opposite phenomena in the central nervous system begin to dominate the picture: The patients are apparently apathetic and lethargic.

The peripheral neurological symptoms of thyrotoxicosis are very clear and extremely varied. One of the most interesting and complex problems in the study of the effect of thyroid hormone on the nervous system is the pathogenesis of the motor disturbances. Much clinical material has been gathered on this question. The commonest symptoms of the motor disturbances are those of hyperkinesia (tremor, choreiform spasms). Besides muscular weakness, atrophy of the muscles is often observed in patients with thyrotoxicosis and may be particularly marked in the late stages of the disease. The motor disorders in thyrotoxicosis are often accompanied by diencephalic symptoms. This fact has led some investigators to suggest that the function of the basal ganglia, concerned with the regulation of muscle tone, is disturbed in thyrotoxicosis [241, 512].

The existence of gross destructive changes in the nervous system in patients dying from thyrotoxicosis was mentioned in papers published at the end of the nineteenth century. In more recent publications, especially in the last decade, the importance of changes in the permeability of the vascular wall, leading to degenerative changes in nerve tissue, has been emphasized.

Histological study of specimens obtained at autopsy from 15 patients dying from thyrotoxicosis of increasing severity and morphological studies of the nervous systems of animals with experimental thyrotoxicosis demonstrated edema, congestion, and gross changes of a destructive and degenerative nature in the cerebral cortex, basal ganglia, and spinal cord [186, 187].

On the basis of extensive clinical and morphological material and also of a histological study of changes in the central nervous system of animals with experimental thyrotoxicosis, Aizenshtein [14, 15] concluded that there is a close connection between the clinical manifestations of thyrotoxicosis and the morphological changes in the nervous system. These include mainly a disturbance of vascular permeability and severe edema of the brain tissue, with marked degenerative changes among its cells. Because of the motor manifestations in the clinical picture of thyrotoxicosis, Aizenshtein paid great attention in his work to the histological study of the state of the spinal cord. He found that the severity of damage to the spinal motoneurons is about the same as in the cells of the cerebral hemispheres, and sometimes it was actually more severe.

Experimental investigations of disturbances of higher nervous activity have greatly broadened our ideas of the state of the nervous system in thyrotoxicosis. Ponirovskii [481], in 1924, and Rozanov [509], in 1925, for instance, showed that thyroid extract produces excitation of cortical functions in dogs. In their investigation into the effects of different doses of thyroid hormones on conditioned-reflex activity in dogs fed for long periods with thyroid hormones, Zavadovskii and Zak [663] found that these disturbances developed in phases. In the first phase they found weakening of positive conditioned-reflex reactions and the abolition of differentiation; in the second phase excitability was increased and the duration of both conditioned and unconditioned salivatory reflexes was shortened.

Changes in higher nervous activity of animals also were found to depend on the dose if only a single dose of thyroid hormones was given. Pribytkova [486], for example, showed that administration of 0.5–1 mg thyroxine leads to inhibition of conditioned reflexes during the first 24 h, whereas a dose of 0.125–0.5 mg causes a marked decrease in the reflex but only on the third day after administration of the preparation. Kuz'menko [358] also found a decrease in the excitability of the brain under the influence of large doses and an increase after administration of small doses of thyroxine. Higher nervous activity in the presence of an excess or deficiency of thyroid hormones also was investigated in Pavlov's laboratory, in particular by Petrova [475], who found a disturbance of cortical activity in dogs after prolonged feeding with thyroid extract, with predominance of stimulation and with manifestations of motor excitation. Exhaustion of cortical activity occurred sooner in animals with a weak type of higher nervous activity. Similar results were obtained by Samoilova [518], Konge [339], and Pugachev [487]. According to Baranov, Speranskaya, and Tendler [56], higher nervous activity is disturbed even after doses of thyroid hormones which do not affect the basal metabolic rate. After feeding thyroid extract to dogs for a long time, these workers found a decrease in the aggregated value of the positive conditioned reflexes despite no change in the basal metabolic rate.

The functional state of the central nervous system also shows considerable changes in the presence of a deficiency of thyroid hormones. In monkeys thyroidectomized soon after birth, growth and normal development of the brain cease, and development of the central nervous system is disturbed. If the deficiency of thyroid function appears in a later period, after complete maturation of the brain, neither pathology of development nor true degenerative changes are observed, but ability to form conditioned reflexes is retarded. For example, as long ago as in 1924, Pavlov's collaborator Val'kov [621] showed that thyroidectomy in animals is followed by considerable disturbances in conditioned-reflex activity. Food reflexes nine months after the operation were formed with difficulty, and they never reached their usual stability. To maintain the reflexes at the necessary level, they had to be reinforced daily. Val'kov concluded from his experiments that a deficiency of thyroid function leads to weakening of both excitatory and inhibitory cortical reflexes.

Genes [197] states that after removal of the thyroid gland, unconditioned as well as conditioned reflexes are weakened. In young rabbits 8–9 weeks after the operation, for instance, the reflex of contraction of the dorsal skin in response to tactile stimulation disappears. Thyroidectomy in sheep leads to a marked decrease in the food reflex, diminution of motor activity, and depression of defensive reflexes.

The impossibility of producing guarding and passive–defensive reflexes in thyroidectomized animals and their inability to carry out complex forms of analysis and synthesis were described by Val'kov [621], Azimov [45], Zavadovskii [662], and Morrison and Cunningham [431]. Thyroidectomy in young rooks also delays the formation of new types of behavioral reflexes, and sometimes involution may actually be seen: Reflexes characteristic of the earlier stages of postnatal development appear [627].

Clinical observations also provide evidence of the weakening of excitability in the central nervous system in hypothyroidism. Krasnogorskii [345] investigated the state of the higher nervous activity in patients with athyroid cretinism and found that conditioned-reflex formation was extremely retarded. Even after many combinations, the conditioned connections were unstable and weak and their latent period was long. If not reinforced, they quickly disappeared and were restored slowly.

Changes in excitability of the central nervous system under the influence of thyroid hormones have also been demonstrated during investigations of the course of electrically induced convulsions in animals [146, 466, 596].

Clinical observations indicating the relatively high sensitivity of the central nervous system to an excess or deficiency of thyroid hormones have been confirmed by numerous experimental investigations. In both cases the fundamental nervous processes of excitation and inhibition are evidently affected, being more so for inhibition.

The central effects of thyroid hormones have also been studied by electroencephalography, which permits an evaluation of the characteristics of cortical electrical activity and the character of corticosubcortical relations. Numerous investigations showed that if the content of thyroid hormones in the body is low, the electrical activity of the brain is reduced [135, 282, 322, 334, 346]. In patients with myxedema a decrease in the amplitude and frequency of the α-waves occurred. In severe cases, there was a total absence of α-waves which were replaced by β- and Δ-rhythms. A characteristic feature was the uniformity of the electrical activity in different parts of the brain and weakening or total absence of the response to photic stimulation. Nieman [446] described patients with myxedema whose EEG in all leads consisted of an almost uniform tracing with waves at a frequency of 4–5 per sec and with a maximal amplitude of 10 μV. Administration of thyroid preparations to these patients restored the electrical activity of the brain and thus demonstrated that the pathological changes in the EEG are connected with a deficiency of thyroid hormones. Depression of electrical activity of the brain in hypothyroidism after thyroidectomy has also been obtained experimentally [16, 59, 88].

Ross and Shwab [507] studied the EEG changes associated with increased thyroid function and observed an increase in brain activity in patients with thyrotoxicosis, manifested as an increase in frequency of the α-rhythm. Many investigators [123, 204, 421] later confirmed these observations. Deineka and Serkov [135] studied the EEG in patients with Basedow's disease and found that the changes in the EEG were dependent on the severity of the disease. An increase in the amplitude of the EEG waves was recorded only in patients with a mild form of thyrotoxicosis. They showed an increase in the amplitude of the α-waves and spreading of a regular α-rhythm to all parts of the brain. In patients with severe thyrotoxicosis, the amplitude of the EEG rhythms was lowered, and the rhythm binding response to photic stimulation was considerably weakened. A connection between the severity of the disease and changes in the EEG of patients with thyrotoxicosis also was observed by Kovalev [343]. He stated that the normal EEG was restored in most patients after subtotal thyroidectomy and disappearance of the clinical manifestations of the disease. On the whole, thyrotoxicosis is characterized by increased electrical activity and by manifestations of desynchronization and an increase in the frequency of the α-rhythms against the background of a decrease in the general amplitude of the EEG, together with the appearance of volleys of slow, high-amplitude discharges [119, 174, 302, 422, 443].

Changes in the electrical activity of the brain in response to an increase in the content of thyroid hormones in the body has frequently been reproduced under experimental conditions [16, 292, 303, 405, 600, 634]. Akishina, Lutsenko, and Markova [16] found phasic changes in the EEG of animals after administration of thyroid extract. In the initial period of administration of thyroid hormone to the animals, low-amplitude fast waves appeared on the spontaneous EEG. As further thyroid hormone was given, the electrical activity changed, with a decrease in the frequency and amplitude of the waves. The response to photic stimulation at the beginning of the observations revealed precise rhythm binding at all frequencies used, but at the end it was found only at low frequencies. The change in the character of rhythm binding, in these workers' opinion, is explained by a change in the physiological lability of the brain cells. The observations of Akishina et al. agree with the clinical observations of Krump [348] on patients with thyrotoxicosis of varied severity.

In the last decade research into the study of the central effects of thyroid hormones and, in particular, on their interaction with the nonspecific systems of the brain has developed intensively. For example, Benetato et al. [65] studied the effect of thyroid hormones on the central nervous system of the dog under *encéphale isolé* conditions and concluded that these hormones exert their central action on the reticulohypothalamic formation. It was concluded that many changes in the central nervous system in thyrotoxicosis are determined by the particularly high sensitivity of the reticular formation to thyroid hormones.

Marits [405, 406, 407] studied the dependence of electrical activity in the rostral part of the reticular formation and cortex on the state of thyroid gland function. He showed that electrical activity of the mesencephalic reticular formation and cerebral cortex is considerably depressed in thyroidectomized dogs. Meanwhile the sensitivity of the reticular formation to the activating action of adrenalin was considerably reduced in these animals. Administration of thyroxine to the animals restored the electrical activity of the reticular formation and also its sensitivity to adrenalin. Normal cortical activity was restored only after recovery of the rhythms in reticular structures. Marits concluded that the decrease in cortical electrical activity after thyroidectomy is due to a diminution of ascending activating influences from the nonspecific brain structures whose normal function evidently depends largely on the functional state of the thyroid gland. The same conclusion was reached by Kakhana [303], who showed that electrical activity of the brain-stem reticular formation and also of the visual cortex is increased in dogs 4 h after feeding with thyroid extract.

The intermediary role of the nonspecific brain systems in the action of thyroid hormones is confirmed by the observations of Vartapetov et al. [626]. These workers showed that the action of thyroid extract in dogs is exhibited slowly and weakly if chlorpromazine, which blocks adrenergic structures of the reticular formation, is administered at the same time.

Wilson et al. [650] studied the nature of the ascending activating effects of the brain-stem reticular system and observed a decrease in the duration of the activation reaction of the EEG in response to photic stimulation three days after oral administration of triiodothyronine to healthy human subjects. Further evidence of the lowered level of activity of the reticular structures was given by the decrease in amplitude of secondary responses in the reticular structures of the brain to peripheral stimulation. These observations show that the effects of thyroid hormones are mediated through the nonspecific systems of the brain. However, differences between the effects arising are evidently determined by the doses of the hormones and the methods of their administration.

Information obtained by the experimental study of the effects of thyroid hormones on the function of the spinal centers is very limited. Nevertheless, this problem deserves the most serious attention from both the theoretical and the practical points of view, for the segmental apparatus of the spinal cord is closely associated with the cortical, diencephalic, and brain-stem structures in the regulation of motor activity. Attempts to reveal the participation of the spinal cord in the pathogenesis of motor disturbances in patients with thyrotoxicosis have been carried out as part of the investigation of the character of the tendon reflexes in this disease. Some workers have shown that the latent period and duration of the reflex response are considerably shortened [375, 471, 561].

Electromyographic tests have also been carried out on patients with thyroid hyperfunction. The most detailed study of patients with thyrotoxicosis by the electromyographic method was undertaken by Fol'b [179]. He investigated 72 patients with thyrotoxicosis of varying severity. Decreased electrical activity corresponding to the maximal strength of contraction was observed in all patients, even in those with mild thyrotoxicosis. Pathological rhythms were found in 18 patients, in 3 of them even in the resting state. Similar changes were observed by Ogorodova [454]. These findings indicate that spinal motoneurons are definitely concerned in the mechanism of this pathological state.

Gol'ber, Gaidina, and Ignatkov [214, 215, 216] analyzed the effect of thyroid hormones on the function of the segmental apparatus of the spinal cord experimentally. In cats with experimental thyrotoxicosis produced by feeding with thyroid extract, they found shortening of the latent period and duration of the monosynaptic reflex responses indicating facilitation of the conduction of excitation along the monosynaptic reflex arc. To analyze the character of the changes in inhibition in the spinal segmental system of animals with thyrotoxicosis, these workers studied the various types of central inhibition by the method of monosynaptic testing. They found a disturbance of all types of inhibition, most clearly demonstrable in the late, prolonged (presynaptic) inhibition. Special experiments showed that the weakening of this type of inhibition was connected with a decrease in presynaptic depolarization of the thick, fast-conducting afferent fibers. A decrease in amplitude of the dorsal root potentials also was observed in animals with thyrotoxicosis; this is indirect evidence of a decrease in the depolarization of the primary afferents.

Results obtained in Gol'ber's laboratory revealed weakening of both inhibitory and facilitatory influences of the medullary reticular formation on reflex activity of the spinal centers in animals with experimental thyrotoxicosis [19]. Under these circumstances, evidently not only the activity of the spinal mechanisms, but also certain other forms of higher control, are disturbed.

These observations shed some light on the pathogenesis of the motor disturbances in thyrotoxicosis. Leaving aside those aspects of the origin of the muscular disturbances that are connected with metabolic changes in the muscles (changes in the contractile properties of protein complexes and their relations with high-energy phosphorus compounds), it can be postulated that important roles in the mechanism of origin of the motor disorders in thyrotoxicosis may be played, first, by descending influences from higher structures of the central nervous system and, second, by the direct action of an excess of thyroid hormones on the spinal reflex arc. This hypothesis is confirmed by the observations of Ford and Rhines [182], who found selective accumulation of ^{131}I-labeled triiodothyronine in the ventral horns of the spinal cord of experimental rats.

Changes in excitability in the presence of an excess or deficiency of thyroid hormones raise the question of the mechanisms producing changes in the functional state of the central nervous system. It is claimed that changes in the excitability of the brain are connected with the effect of thyroid hormones on various aspects of metabolism and, in particular, with an increased basal metabolic rate. Ross and Shwab [507], Lindsley and Rubinstein [389], and Rohmer et al. [503] consider that changes in the electrical activity of the brain are the results of an increased basal metabolic rate in hyperthyroidism. However, Rubin et al. [510] and Hoagland et al. [272] showed that the increase in electrical activity of the brain after administration of thyroxine occurs even without any change in the basal metabolic rate. Moreover, Timiras and Woodbury [596], by analysis of the central action of thyroxine, found that DNP which, like thyroxine, stimulates the basal metabolism, does not change the excitability of the brain.

The sensitivity of the central nervous system to anoxia is greatly increased in hyperthyroidism [328], and it has been suggested that the thyroid hormones increase the oxygen demand of the brain. Results have been obtained to show a decrease in the oxygen demand, the oxidation of glucose, and the velocity of the cerebral blood flow in hypothyroid states [451, 522]. It is therefore not surprising that attempts have been made to link the disturbances of electrical activity in thyrotoxicosis with changes in the general cell metabolism and, in particular, in carbohydrate metabolism [552] or with the anoxia produced by the metabolic disorders.

Travina [598], Yasenchak [660], and Nevstrueva, Dolina, and Sokolova [444] found changes in protein metabolism in hyperthyroidism, while Timiras and Woodbury [596] found changes in potassium and sodium metabolism. Zhukova [665] performed a histochemical study of protein metabolism in the spinal cord of albino rats after a single injection of L-thyroxine. Quantitative cytophotometric analysis showed stimulation of metabolism 2 h after the injection. The changes in dehydrogenase activity studied in these experiments revealed disturbances of both aerobic and anaerobic oxidation.

From the standpoint of modern physiology, the functions of the central nervous system are largely determined by the state of the synapses responsible for the fundamental manifestations of nervous activity—excitation and inhibition—and also by the sensitivity of the nervous system to humoral and chemical agents. This raises the question whether functional changes in the central nervous system can be attributed to the effects of thyroid hormones on synaptic transmission. The important role of synapses in the production of the effects of thyroid hormones is emphasized by Vogralik and Mironova [634]. These workers explain the mechanism of development of changes in brain electrical activity in thyrotoxicosis by hyperactivity of the synapses in the central nervous system, resulting in improved conduction of nervous impulses through the synapses because of the increased formation or the slower destruction of acetylcholine in them. At the time when the EEG rhythms are quickened in patients with thyrotoxicosis or after administration of thyroid extract to healthy persons, the blood acetylcholine level rises considerably. The content of adrenalin and cholinesterase remains almost unchanged. Vogralik and Mironova conclude that the increased conduction of nervous impulses in cholinergic synapses causes profound functional disturbances in the nervous system as well as the state of synaptic hyperactivity described above. Thus, there are not only changes in the EEG rhythms, but hyperkinesia, tremor, and muscular weakness.

There is in fact considerable evidence, although much of it is conflicting, to show that thyroid hormones do affect acetylcholine metabolism *in vivo*. Kassil' and Plotitsina [321], Glants [208], and Koudelkova and Vik [341] observed a raised blood acetylcholine level in hyperthyroidism. However, according to Georgieva and Kuz'mina [200], an increase in the acetylcholine concentration may also occur in hypothyroidism. The information concerning the effect of thyroid hormones on cholinesterase activity is no less contradictory. An increase in serum cholinesterase activity in hyperthyroidism was observed by Antopol et al. [28], Faber [168], and Uono [616]. An increase in cholesterase activity in the liver under the influence of thyroxine was found by Quandramagna et al. [488]. Meanwhile, Hoffman [276] and Hawkins et al. [262] found a decrease in the serum cholinesterase activity in hyperthyroidism. The same effect was found after a single dose of thyroxine. The ability of the blood serum to hydrolyze acetylcholine is connected with pseudocholinesterase activity. By contrast with pseudocholinesterase, the true cholinesterase activity of the blood is unchanged in thyroid dysfunction [262].

The influence of thyroid hormones on acetylcholine metabolism in the central nervous system has been demonstrated experimentally. Kakushkina and Tatarko [304] found a decrease in the acetylcholine content in the brain tissue of dogs after thyroidectomy. On the other hand, if the level of thyroid hormones in dogs was raised, the acetylcholine concentration in their brain was unchanged and the cholinesterase became less active.

Tucek and Diepold [602] found no changes in the acetylcholine concentration in the cortex and subcortical formations of the brain in rats receiving thyroid extract but found an increase in the content of substances participating in acetylcholine synthesis. The cholinesterase activity in the cortex was indistinguishable from the control, and, although it was increased in the medulla and basal ganglia, the increase was not significant. A definite increase in the cholinesterase activity of the brain in rats with hyperthyroidism was observed by Hamburgh and Flexner [252].

Research showing that thyroid hormones may modify the reactivity of the tissues to acetylcholine is of considerable interest. It has been shown, for instance, that the miotic action of pilocarpine is weakened in thyroidectomized animals [599] and the reaction to atropine is intensified. Conversely, administration of small doses of thyroxine to healthy animals increases the sensitivity of the intestinal receptors to acetylcholine [506], but a study of the effects of acetylcholine and neostigmine on the heart showed that thyroxine increases their negative chronotropic and dromotropic action [635]. Glants [208] showed that hyperthyroidism is accompanied by an increase, and hypothyroidism by a decrease in the intensity of the spastic response to eserine. The changes in the motor response to eserine were evidently connected with a disturbance of cholinergic transmission in the central nervous system. This is also shown by the experiments of Ugol'nikov [615], who found weakening of arecoline and nicotine convulsions in rats with hypothyroidism. Babichev [46] studied the behavior of synaptic conduction in the sympathetic ganglion and found that the excitability of the ganglion is increased by thyroxine but reduced if the thyroid gland is blocked by methylthiouracil.

In the study of the effect of thyroid hormones on reactivity of central adrenergic and cholinergic structures of the central nervous system, Gol'ber et al. [214] found increased reactivity of both cholinergic and adrenergic structures in thyrotoxicosis. Other evidence of changes in the function of central adrenergic structures was given by the work of Benetato et al. [65], Marits [407], Kakhana [303], and others already mentioned above.

In the writers' view, changes in the reactivity of the cholinergic structures of the nervous system are not evidence of an excess of acetylcholine in the synapses. Furthermore, Gaidina, Gol'ber, and Kryzhanovskii [192] gave thyroid extract to rats and observed a disturbance of neuromuscular synaptic function (the latent period of the response of the muscles to indirect stimulation was lengthened, the durations of the absolute and relative refractory phases were increased, Vvedenskii inhibition began to occur at lower frequencies, and a complete block of transmission began to appear at higher frequencies of stimulation than in control experiments). These parameters began to return toward their control values, i.e., the normal function of the synapse began to be restored, after administration of neostigmine. These observations point to a deficiency of the mediator in skeletal muscle synapses. A decrease in the acetylcholine content in the neuromuscular synapse was observed by Pickens and Lockett [477].

The mechanism of action of thyroid hormones of the nervous system is thus very complex and includes components such as changes in tissue metabolism and in the functions of peripheral organs and tissues. However, besides the broad nonspecific spectrum of action of the thyroid hormones they can also evidently exert a specific action on nervous structures particularly sensitive to them.

The Autonomic Nervous System

The effect of thyroid hormones on the state of the autonomic innervation of organs and tissues has been studied much less than their effects on somatic nerves. This problem is closely bound up with the question of intermediate stages in the action of thyroid hormones on the cell, for many investigators regard changes in the functions of the autonomic nervous system as the primary cause of the ultimate effects of thyroxine and triiodothyronine.

Many changes in the rhythm of the cardiac contractions characteristic of thyrotoxicosis (atrial fibrillation and flutter, sinus arrhythmia, ventricular extrasystoles, sinoatrial and intra-atrial block, lengthening of the P–Q interval of the ECG, etc.) are generally attributed to the influence of the vagus nerve [114, 178, 363, 491]. Many workers [188, 401, 485, 557], therefore, consider that these manifestations of thyrotoxicosis are the result of an increase in the influence of the vagus nerves on the heart in this disease. The view that a *vagus factor* is concerned in the genesis of cardiac arrhythmias in thyrotoxicosis was first expressed by Nahum and Hoff [435], Wise and Hoff [652], and Altschule [23]. These workers showed that atrial fibrillation does not arise after electric shock alone but does develop if acetylcholine is injected simultaneously. They studied the frequency of development of atrial fibrillation by injecting acetyl-β-methylcholine into four patients with Basedow's disease. All the patients developed atrial fibrillation, preceded by sinoatrial block. Injection of the same dose of acetylcholine into healthy subjects did not give rise to such severe arrhythmias.

They concluded that spontaneous atrial fibrillation in patients with thyrotoxicosis is observed if depressor effects of the vagus nerves or the sensitivity of the patients to vagus effects is increased in the course of the disease. In this way the marked prominence of *parasympathetic* symptoms such as perspiration, hyperemia of the skin, and hyperactivity of the gastrointestinal tract in patients with thyrotoxicosis was emphasized, and the possibility of a reflex increase in tone of the vagus nerve in response to tachycardia or to elevation of the blood pressure was noted.

In an attempt to link the increased sensitivity of the heart to acetylcholine with the view that thyrotoxicosis is a state of *sympathetic hyperactivity*, Hoffman et al. [277] expressed a different opinion. On the basis of McDowall's [393] observation that the heart contains reserves of adrenergic substances reactive to acetylcholine, these workers postulated that the action of acetylcholine in the thyrotoxic heart is accompanied by the liberation of these substances. "We must therefore speak, not of an increase in the sensitivity of the thyrotoxic heart to acetylcholine, but of an increase in its sensitivity to adrenalin" [393].

McDowall's theory was not supported by other workers [324, 330, 613], and the views of Hoffman et al. [277] were criticized even by supporters of the concept that the effects of thyroid hormones were induced by a "catecholamine genesis." Raab [489] postulates that there is an increase in the liberation of active acetylcholine under the influence of thyroxine and that in thyrotoxicosis "activitiy of both the adrenergic and the cholinergic systems is increased."

To assess the state of the parasympathetic innervation of the heart, Shakhnarovich and Kandror [534] investigated the spontaneous electrical activity of the vagus nerves. Their experiment showed that the frequency of efferent impulses conducted along the vagus nerve increases progressively in rabbits fed with thyroid extract. The frequency of efferent impulses along the vagus nerve was increased two weeks after the beginning of thyroid feeding, but thereafter it remained unchanged. The mean amplitude of each spike leaving the centers of the vagus nerves fell progressively during the development of thyrotoxicosis.

As regards electrophysiological indices of the state of the vagus nerve, these workers found a marked decrease in the action potential response and threshold of excitation and also in the duration of the action potential in rabbits with thyrotoxicosis caused by thyroid feeding. The refractory period of the nerve was shortened. The response of the heart to stimulation of the vagus nerve was less in hyperthyroid than in the control animals. In most experimental rabbits it was impossible, in general, to reproduce the bradycardia usually observed during stimulation of the vagus nerve; a paradoxical effect in the form of an increased heart rate and elevation of the blood pressure was observed in some animals.

The experiments of Kryukova [351] indicate that stimulation of hypothalamic structures presumed to be connected with the centers of the vagus nerves in thyroid extract treated rabbits induces initially a stronger inhibition of the pacemaker activity of the sinus node than in the control (as shown by the possibility of obtaining bradycardia in response to stimulation by a subliminal current). Later, stimulation of hypothalamic structures (by *liminal* and *supraliminal* strengths of current) was accompanied by a progressive decrease in the effect. Furthermore, starting from the 14th day of experimental thyrotoxicosis in rabbits, stimulation of the peripheral ends of the divided vagus nerves leads to a progressively weaker inhibition of pacemaker activity of the sinus node than in the control. Under these conditions the sinus node *escapes* from the influence of the vagus nerves sooner than in the control (Fig. 5). Repetitive stimulation of the peripheral ends of the vagus nerves in the control animals constantly proved effective, whereas in the experimental rabbits (even when supraliminal strengths of stimulating current were used) they were ineffective.

These results suggest that the initial increase and subsequent sharp decrease in the effects of parasympathetic impulses on pacemaker activity of the sinus node are connected with a disturbance of mechanisms at the level of the heart itself or a disturbance of the transmission of influences from the nerve to the heart. While they reflect difficulties in the mechanism whereby parasympathetic influences act on the heart in the presence of an excess of thyroid hormones in the body, these observations at the same time help to explain why in thyrotoxicosis the effects of the vagus nerve, which ought to counteract the increased heart rate, are absent.

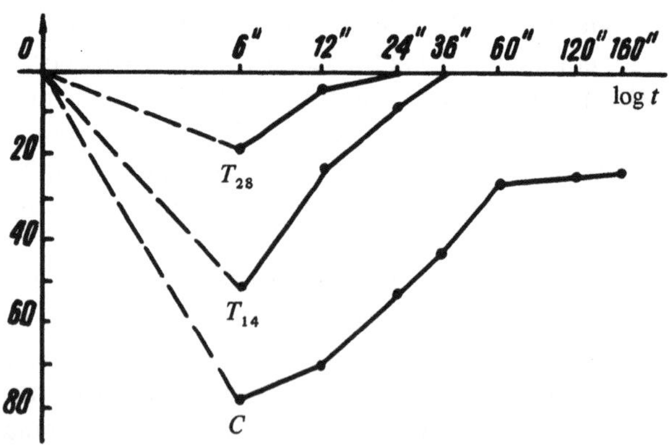

Fig. 5. Degree and duration of bradycardia during stimulation of vagus nerve in control (C) and experimental rabbits: T_{14}–thyrotoxicosis for 2 weeks; T_{28}–thyrotoxicosis for 4 weeks (decrease in heart rate, according to Kryukova, 128% of initial value).

To explain the causes of the changes in the effectiveness of parasympathetic influences observed in thyrotoxicosis, the humoral mechanisms of neuromuscular transmission have been studied. The data in the literature on the state of the acetylcholine–cholinesterase system in thyrotoxicosis are mainly concerned with the concentrations of these substances in the blood and nervous system. An early and persistent increase in the acetylcholine concentration in the blood in thyrotoxicosis was found experimentally and clinically by Glants [208] and Vogralik [634]. Salei and Stepanova [516] obtained less clear results, which could have been due to the different model of thyrotoxicosis used: They fed dogs with small doses of thyroid extract for two months.

According to Golovach [231], the blood acetylcholine concentration in patients with thyrotoxicosis was much lower than in healthy persons, and the lowest values were obtained in severe forms of the disease. A small increase in the concentration of acetylcholine-like substances in the cerebrospinal fluid after injection of thyroid hormones into the blood stream was found by Kassil' and Plotitsina [321]. On the basis of the increased concentration of acetylcholine in the cortex, medulla, and basal ganglia [602, 623] in experimental thyrotoxicosis, an increase in the rate of acetylcholine synthesis in nervous tissue was postulated, for the activity of true cholinesterase in this condition was unchanged [602]. In other experiments [46, 555], however, thyrotoxicosis was accompanied by a decrease in cholinesterase activity in different parts of the nervous system. Moreover, it cannot be concluded that the increase in the acetylcholine concentration in thyrotoxicosis is due to its more rapid synthesis, since the increase could be equally well explained by inhibition of the breakdown of the mediator. Information on cholinesterase activity in the blood is contradictory. In the opinion of most investigators the cholinesterase activity in thyrotoxicosis is increased [24, 27, 46, 153, 207, 231, 276], but according to others it is reduced [208, 634].

Although the data for the state of the acetylcholine–cholinesterase system in the blood and nervous system in experimental thyrotoxicosis have led many investigators to postulate strengthening of cholinergic responses in this pathological state [208, 634], they do not explain the ineffectiveness of vagus influences on the heart, and they actually make this fact even more difficult to understand. With an increase in the severity of the toxicosis in rabbits, the acetylcholine content in the right atrium falls, although cholinesterase activity is unchanged. This could indicate inhibition of the synthesis of the mediator. An increase in the acetylcholine concentration was found, however, in the blood of hyperthyroid rabbits. These observations indicate that the concentration of mediator in the blood does not evidently reflect the amount actually in the region of contact between nerve and organ.

The decrease in the acetylcholine content in the region of contact between the vagus nerves and the heart muscle is evidently the reason for ineffectiveness of the stimulation of these nerves in thyrotoxicosis, for administration of neostigmine, preventing the breakdown of acetylcholine by cholinesterase, completely restored the inhibitory action of the vagus nerves of the heart. There is a more extensive (and more contradictory) literature on the state of the *sympathetic* portion of the autonomic nervous system during changes in the secretory activity of the thyroid gland.

The experiments of Shakhnarovich [533] on rabbits receiving thyroid extract for two and four weeks showed that the frequency of spontaneous activity along the preganglionic trunk during the development of thyrotoxicosis is virtually unchanged, although some tendency for the frequency to decrease may be detected in the late stages of the disease. The voltage of the activity is decreased at these times chiefly on account of a decrease in the mean amplitude of each spike. The frequency of activity in the postganglionic trunk remained at the control level during the first two weeks of thyrotoxicosis but then fell considerably. Similar changes were found in the voltage of the activity, as a result of a decrease both in the firing rate and in the mean amplitude of each spike.

Sheveleva [542] perfused the sympathetic ganglion of the cat with thyroxine and obtained results indicating increased activity in postganglionic fibers (stimulation of contraction of the nictitating membrane). After the intra-arterial injection of large doses of L-thyroxine (over 500 μg) into cats, Babichev [46, 47] found, however, that spontaneous activity of the pre- and postganglionic fibers of the superior cervical and inferior mesenteric sympathetic ganglia was considerably reduced. With an increase in the severity of thyrotoxicosis in rabbits, Shakhnarovich [533] found that the excitability of cells of the superior cervical sympathetic ganglion increased. This was manifested as a marked decrease in the threshold of their stimulation.

In animals receiving thyroid extract for two weeks, the amplitude of the recorded action potential was slightly reduced. This decrease became statistically significant in the later stage of experimental thyrotoxicosis. With a progressive increase in the severity of thyrotoxicosis in the rabbits, the reproducibility of postexcitation potentiation in the sympathetic ganglion in rabbits increased. However, the degree of postexcitation potentiation in the experimental animals was less than in the control (when it could be reproduced). In a relatively early stage of experimental thyrotoxicosis the lability of the ganglion increased a little, but in severe toxicosis it was below the control level.

Confirmation of the more rapid exhaustion of the sympathetic ganglion in thyrotoxicosis was obtained in experiments in which functional resistance was measured. In animals with experimental thyrotoxicosis the time during which the ganglion could reproduce a standard frequency of stimulation without reduction of amplitude was considerably shortened. Babichev [46] injected various doses of L-thyroxine into cats for 5 days and then observed a decrease in the threshold and refractoriness of the superior cervical sympathetic ganglion. With an increase in the dosage of the hormone injected, functional resistance and lability of the ganglion and the degree of post-tetanic potentiation also were reduced.

Shakhnarovich [533] investigated the conduction of impulses along the postganglionic sympathetic trunk in animals with thyrotoxicosis and also found a decrease in the threshold of stimulation, a decrease in amplitude of the action potential, and shortening of its duration and of the refractory period of the nerve trunk. Many workers [142, 184, 233, 278, 281, 470] have observed a decrease in the catecholamine concentration in the adrenals of hyperthyroidized animals. Lhotka et al. [388] found atrophic and degenerative changes in the adrenal medulla of rats receiving large doses of thyroid preparations. In 1951, Hökfelt [278] reported that the initial adrenalin concentration in the adrenals was lower in hypothyroid rats than in the control, and that injection of insulin into the animals led to a smaller decrease in its concentration than in the controls. Harrison [257] found that insulin hypoglycemia in patients with thyrotoxicosis leads to a smaller increase in the noradrenalin excretion than in healthy persons.

In a recent careful experimental study of this problem, Johnson [299] found a marked decrease in the ability of the adrenal medulla of animals with thyrotoxicosis to respond with a liberation of catecholamines to reflex stimulation of the gland. A sharp decrease in the total content of catecholamines in the myocardium was observed by Abelin and Ryser [6]. In the experiments of Utevskii and But, McMillan and Rand [398], and Beaven et al. [63], the catecholamine concentration in the tissues of hyperthyroid animals was normal or reduced. According to Osinskaya [460], small doses of thyroid extract cause virtually no change in the noradrenalin content in the rabbit heart whereas larger doses of the preparation, given over long periods of time, cause a sharp decrease in the contents not only of catecholamines, but also of substances with the properties of their quinoid oxidation products.

Zhangelova [664] investigated the catecholamine content in the adrenal, myocardium, brain, and liver of rabbits with experimental thyrotoxicosis. She found that in mild and moderately severe thyrotoxicosis, the adrenalin content in all the organs studied was the same as in the control. In animals with prolonged and severe thyrotoxicosis, the adrenalin concentration in the adrenals was reduced by almost 70%, and the noradrenalin concentration in the heart by 60% and in the brain and liver by 50%. The adrenalin concentration in the liver also was reduced by more than 30%. The content of substances with the properties of oxidation products of the pyrocatecholamines in the tissues was virtually unchanged. Characteristically, the content of free and bound forms of the catecholamines fell sharply in the organs of the hyperthyroidized animals.

Kardashev et al. [317] showed that the adrenalin concentration in the adrenals, heart, and several other organs rises during thyroid hypofunction. According to the observations of Wurtman et al. [659], the ability of the heart muscle of hyperthyroidized animals to inactivate catecholamines by binding with them is reduced. However, Johnson [299] showed that, after stimulation of catecholamine secretion by the adrenals, the level of these compounds rises in the heart of hyperthyroidized rats actually by a somewhat greater degree than in the heart of control animals, although the adrenal of the former produces less of the catecholamines (judging from their excretion in the urine). Harrison [257] analyzed the corresponding data in the literature and concluded that there is no evidence of elevation of the blood catecholamines in thyrotoxicosis.

In most clinical observations [356, 376, 653] normal excretion of adrenalin and noradrenalin was found in the urine. Ugoleva [614], however, reported a decrease in the daily excretion of adrenalin and a less marked increase in the excretion of noradrenalin by patients with thyrotoxicosis. Like Bülbring [97], Ugoleva regards her findings as evidence of a reduced rate of methylation of noradrenalin in the body because of ATP deficiency. Meanwhile, Baru [61] observed a sharp decrease in the 24-hourly excretion of noradrenalin in a similar group of patients, and this was later confirmed by Golovach [231]. Meanwhile, the excretion of adrenalin was more frequently increased. Negoescu et al. [440] found that the adrenalin excretion in the urine is not increased in all cases of thyrotoxicosis, whereas the excretion of noradrenalin is more frequently reduced. Wiswell et al. [653] state that the 24-hourly excretion of noradrenalin rises in hypothyroidism but not in hyperthyroidism.

Kandror et al. [313] determined the catecholamine content in various organs of rabbits receiving high doses of thyroid extract for one month. They found that the content of adrenalin in the adrenals, of noradrenalin in the myocardium, and of both adrenalin and noradrenalin in the 24-hourly urine of the animals was reduced. These workers at the same time noted a sharp increase in the DOPA content in the tissues of the hyperthyroid rabbits. On the basis of this, they postulated inhibition of catecholamine synthesis at the DOPA-decarboxylase stage. Kandror et al. [313] also found that the excretion of vanillin-mandelic and homovanillic acids in the urine is slightly reduced in rabbits with thyrotoxicosis. These results make it imperative to estimate the activity of enzymes decomposing catecholamines.

From the reports of Harrison [257], it would be hard to imagine a more contradictory series of reports than those which have been published on the effect of hyperthyroidism on monoamine oxidase activity. In the earlier communications [280, 645], an increase in the activity of the enzyme was described in the liver of hyperthyroid animals (rabbits, guinea pigs, rats). Later, however, inhibition of liver monoamine oxidase was more frequently observed in response to an excess of thyroid hormones *in vivo* [98, 143, 573, 599, 619]. These observations were also confirmed in patients with thyrotoxicosis in whom the enzyme activity was reduced in the tissues of the jejunum obtained by biopsy [387]. Meanwhile, Kuschke et al. [357] found increased liver monoamine oxidase activity in patients with thyrotoxicosis. These workers reached this conclusion on the grounds that after administration of equal doses of serotonin to patients with thyrotoxicosis and to healthy subjects the former excreted more 5-hydroxyindoleacetic acid (5-HIAA). These findings agree with the results obtained by Kandror and Shapiro [316] in rabbits with thyrotoxicosis. Stoilov et al. [585] also described an increase in the 5-HIAA excretion in patients with hyperactivity of the thyroid gland.

Gorkin [236] concluded that mitochondrial monoamine oxidase embraces a series of different enzymes, differing in both their physicochemical properties and their substrate specificity. In the experiments of Gorkin et al. [237], monoamine oxidase activity in the myocardium and liver of rabbits receiving thyroid extract was, therefore, measured with respect to several substrates. They found that oxidative deamination of serotonin, benzylamine, and dopamine in the heart of the experimental animals was reduced, whereas deamination of tyramine was virtually unchanged. Deamination of serotonin in the liver increased, while that of the other monoamine oxidase substrates was unchanged. Consequently, the inhibition of monoamine oxidase by thyroid hormones does not lead to an increase in the active concentrations of adrenalin and noradrenalin. Thus, in the presence of an excess of thyroid hormones in the body, the active concentration of catecholamines is not increased. What process can then be considered which may cause the observed increases: the synthesis and secretion of catecholamines or delay in their inactivation?

Both spontaneous hyperthyroidism and artificial saturation of the body with thyroid preparations are accompanied by an increase in the glycogenolytic action of adrenalin. This phenomenon is less marked with respect to the glycogen of voluntary and cardiac muscle and is not manifested at all unless thyrotoxicosis produces the almost total exhaustion of the glycogen reserves in the organs [1]. Harrison [257] points out that an increase in the calorigenic effect of adrenalin in thyrotoxicosis has been demonstrated too often for it to be questioned.

The results of investigations in which the sensitivity of hyperthyroid animals to catecholamines was measured by other tests have given even more contradictory results. The experiments of Kandror and Éster [165, 311] showed that the response of the arterial pressure to a standard dose of adrenalin develops later and more slowly in hyperthyroid rabbits and reaches a lower level than in control animals. These observations evidently conflict with the view that the sensitivity of organs and systems to catecholamines is increased in thyrotoxicosis.

Despite the contradictory nature of the data, the information given in this section indicates a decrease in the intensity of effects of the autonomic nervous system on the organs and tissues of animals receiving thyroid preparations.

Action on the Cardiovascular System

The action of thyroid hormones on the cardiovascular system is clearly manifested by the severe disturbances of the heart in Basedow's disease. The view has been expressed that the thyroid hormones have a specific cardiotoxic action independent of their metabolic effect. Other workers consider that the heart becomes insensitive to vagal impulses in thyrotoxicosis. Furthermore, an additional load on the heart is created by the acceleration of metabolism in the body as a whole observed in hyperthyroidism. By contrast, if there is a deficiency of thyroid hormones in the body, i.e., in hypothyroidism, the oxygen consumption falls, with accompanying changes in the quantitative parameters of the circulation: The minute and stroke volume of the heart are reduced and the arteriovenous difference of oxygen concentration is considerably increased. There is no doubt that these functional changes in the heart muscle in hypothyroidism are based on a disturbance of its metabolism.

Disturbances of metabolism in the heart muscle in hypothyroidism and athyroidism affect primarily the rate of oxygen consumption by the myocardium. The uptake of oxygen by the heart is lowered in patients with hypothyroidism, just as it is in thyroidectomized animals. Respiration is considerably depressed in heart slices of thyroidectomized animals. Substantial changes are also observed in the carbohydrate–phosphorus metabolism of the heart muscle in hypothyroidism. According to Dagaeva [132], the content of ATP and creatine phosphate (CP) is increased in the heart muscle of rats in which the thyroid gland has been blocked by 6-methylthiouracil.

Changes in structural metabolism are of considerable importance. The study of this problem is particularly interesting for it can shed some light on the cause of the enlargement of the heart in hypothyroidism. Zhukova [665] investigated the content of total and nonprotein nitrogen, the concentrations of amino acids (as amino nitrogen), urea, creatine, and creatinine in the myocardium, and the renewal of the heart muscle proteins by studying the degree of incorporation of labeled amino acids at various times after injection. These investigations showed that there was no increase in the content of either total nitrogen or protein nitrogen in the myocardium. Indeed, the nonprotein nitrogen content was actually increased considerably. The coefficient of proteolysis was raised accordingly. Meanwhile, the urea nitrogen content fell considerably, but the amino acid nitrogen was almost unchanged. The increase in the nonprotein nitrogen took place on account of an increase in the creatine and creatinine nitrogen in the heart muscle. Further, Zhukova's study of the rate of incorporation of methionine-^{35}S into heart muscle proteins showed that the rate of protein synthesis is actually slightly reduced in hypothyroidism. These results make it doubtful that hypertrophy of the heart muscle is the cause of the enlargement of the heart in hypothyroidism. Depression of thyroid gland function also gives rise to a relatively specific electrocardiographic syndrome. Low-amplitude waves are a characteristic feature of the ECG in hypothyroidism.

Taken as a whole, the data on the state of the cardiovascular system in hypothyroidism indicate that the changes taking place are secondary. Presumably, changes affecting the heart reflect disturbances of the intensity of its tissue metabolism. In prolonged hypothyroidism or athyroidism, however, degenerative changes, acquiring a pathological importance of their own, may develop in the heart muscle.

Very distinct changes arise in the state of the circulatory system as a result of an excess of thyroid hormones in the body. Changes in the heart give rise to the earliest and clearest symptoms of thyrotoxicosis, and in most cases they determine the severity and prognosis of the disease. That is why these changes were and are still the subject of continued research.

Among the many different manifestations of cardiovascular pathology in thyrotoxicosis two in particular can be distinguished: disturbances of the cardiac rhythm and hemodynamic disturbances leading to the very rapid onset of circulatory failure. Disturbances of the cardiac rhythm constitute an invariable component of the clinical picture of thyrotoxicosis. Some, such as sinus tachycardia, are constant features, whereas others are found more rarely.

The fact that spontaneous arhythmias develop more rarely under experimental conditions, when the number of operative factors is more limited than under clinical conditions, as well as the paroxysmal character of this sign have led some workers to consider the view that the thyrotoxic heart has a tendency toward the development of arhythmias rather than to regard the disturbances of the cardiac rhythm as a characteristic feature of thyrotoxicosis [435, 472, 572].

The experiments of Kryukova et al. [351, 352] on rabbits showed that administration of thyroid extract to animals regularly leads to tachycardia. On the 5th day of the experiments, the heart rate was increased by 12% and on the 14th day by over 30%. However, in rabbits receiving thyroid extract for one month, the heart rate was almost the same as that recorded in animals receiving thyroid for two weeks. Characteristic results were obtained in experiments in which the thyrotoxic heart was exposed to additional factors. Focal or diffuse ischemia of the myocardium or the imposition of an artificial rhythm of the heart in thyrotoxicosis led to arrhythmias of various types much more often than in control animals. Thus the thyrotoxic heart has a much greater tendency to respond to factors disturbing the rhythm, irrespective of the actual mechanism of operation of these additional factors. These results emphasize the importance of accidental factors, not easily controlled or monitored, in the genesis of the cardiac arrhythmias in thyrotoxicosis.

Kryukova [351] showed that there was at first a small increase in the acetylcholine content in the right atrium, followed by a sharp decrease in rabbits with experimental thyrotoxicosis. This differs from control animals wherein the distribution of acetylcholine in the heart corresponds to the gradient of automatic activity (highest in the right atrium, lowest in the left ventricle). In the other parts of the heart the acetylcholine content was practically unchanged. These findings suggest that exhaustion of the sinus automatism in thyrotoxicosis is possible.

An investigation of the excitability of the left ventricle of the heart in hyperthyroid rabbits in Gol'ber's laboratory demonstrated lowering of the threshold in both phases of the repolarization period when the myocardium is excitable under normal conditions. In addition, the study revealed a progressive shortening of the refractory period of the heart muscle. In other words, these experiments showed a marked increase in the excitability of the thyrotoxic heart.

After their analysis of the mechanism of onset of flutter and fibrillation of the heart in patients with thyrotoxicosis, Nahum and Hoff [435] postulated in 1935 that the only common factor in the mechanisms of action of thyroxine and acetylcholine is their ability to increase the excitability of the myocardium. The shortening of the refractory period of the heart as a whole may be the result of the premature ending of the action potential in certain groups of muscle fibers, and it may, therefore, imply an increase in the degree of electrical heterogeneity of the myocardium.

In addition, the experimental data now available can also be regarded as indicating shortening of the action potential itself in some of the heart muscle cells, for it cannot begin before the impulse from the sinus node reaches the ventricles, and it ends sooner than in the rest of the myocardium. Consequently, experiments in which the excitability of the heart was determined in its various phases provide evidence of shortening of the action potential in some fibers of the left ventricular myocardium. Reuter [499] observed a more rapid course of the various phases of repolarization in the atrial muscle under the influence of thyroid hormones.

It is interesting to note that with an increase in dose of the thyroid hormones all phases of repolarization of the muscle fiber proceed more rapidly, so that the action potential in them is shortened. As has been stated already, no shortening of the action potential for the ventricular myocardium under the influence of thyroid hormones was demonstrated in these experiments.

Kryukova's observations [351] show that the situation recorded by Reuter in the atrial muscle can also occur in the muscle of the left ventricle if the animal receives high doses of thyroid hormones for a long period. The question accordingly arises of the mechanisms by which the action potential is shortened in the fibers of the thyrotoxic heart.

There is conflicting information in the literature about the potassium and sodium concentration in the fluid media of the body in thyrotoxicosis. Boekelman [81], for instance, observed an increase in potassium in the erythrocytes of patients with thyrotoxicosis. However, later observations [43, 337] obtained using isotopes not only did not confirm this finding but revealed directly opposite changes. Matyushin et al. [413] found an increase in the potassium content in the heart of hyperthyroid rats. Admittedly, in animals receiving thyroid extract the change in weight was extremely small, so that it is questionable whether thyrotoxicosis was in fact present in this case.

In the experiments of Shepotin and Mil'ko [540] with radioactive potassium, the left ventricle and right atrium of hyperthyroid rabbits incorporated less of the isotope than in the control. This could be evidence of reduced ability of the cell to accumulate potassium against the concentration gradient. The work of Kandror et al. [224, 310] showed that in hyperthyroid rabbits the potassium ion concentration is reduced and the sodium ion concentration increased in the heart muscle. Judging from changes in the concentrations of these ions in the plasma and erythrocytes, thyrotoxicosis lowers the potassium level within the myocardial fibers.

These changes found in the concentration of monovalent cations shed light on the causes of the increased excitability of the myocardial fibers. The decrease in the intracellular potassium concentration and increase in the sodium concentration signify some initial *depolarization* of the membrane, i.e., approximation of the resting potential to the level of the threshold po-

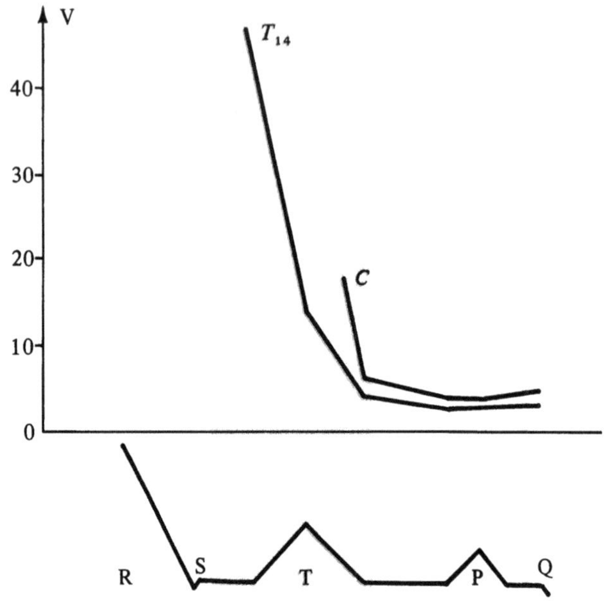

Fig. 6. Thresholds of stimulation (testing pulse) in various phases of the cardiac cycle in control (C) and hyperthyroid (T_{14} –treated 14 days) rabbits.

tential (in the direction toward zero potential). Under these conditions the threshold value of the testing pulse should be reduced, and this is in fact what happens (Figure 6). Moreover, the myocardial cell under these conditions is evidently able to contract in response to an impulse of lower amplitude arising from the pacemaker cells. A decrease in the resting potential produced by different methods has been shown to shorten the action potential. The shift of resting potential and the consequent shortening of the action potential in the cells of the sinus node may be responsible for the tachycardia observed in thyrotoxicosis [307, 310].

The second group of changes characteristically affecting the cardiovascular system in hyperthyroidism includes those responsible for the rapid development of circulatory failure. These include changes in the hemodynamics and function of the myocardium as well as biochemical and structural changes in the heart muscle itself. In Basedow's disease, cell and tissue respiration is increased to a particularly marked degree. It is perfectly evident, therefore, that thyrotoxicosis must be accompanied by considerable changes in the circulatory system, the system concerned with the transport of nutrients and oxygen.

Elevation of the arterial pressure under the influence of thyroid hormones is found regularly in animals of different species: dogs, rabbits, rats, etc. These findings are in agreement with clinical observations.

Kogan-Yasnyi [336], Shurygin [547], Malyugin [400], Klyachko [333], and others have observed a parallel between the severity of thyrotoxicosis and the degree of elevation of the systolic blood pressure. In 1958 Rajmon [492] found after examining 200 patients with diffuse toxic goiter that their systolic pressure was between 180 and 190 mm Hg. Removal of the goiter restored the pressure to normal. Similar results were obtained by Günter [245]. These workers' observations were made on patients with a severe degree of thyrotoxicosis not responding to conservative treatment. Such a considerable increase in the systolic blood pressure could have been due to the severity of the disease. According to Kennedy [327] and Naumova [437], toxic goiter is accompanied by elevation of the blood pressure even in children, in whom it is hard to expect the existence of an initial hypertension and vascular changes.

In the experiments of Kandror and Éster [311], the arterial pressure was measured by means of an electromanometer by direct puncture of the carotid artery in rabbits receiving thyroid extract for one month. They showed that thyrotoxicosis is accompanied by a progressive rise of both the systolic and the diastolic blood pressure. The diastolic pressure rose less than the systolic, so that the pulse pressure was increased.

Measurement of the venous pressure by the direct method in the left jugular vein showed that it is reduced very slightly in rabbits receiving thyroid extract for two weeks but raised somewhat in animals receiving the same treatment for one month. This evidently means that with the progressive development of thyrotoxicosis from administration of thyroid extract, there is a tendency for the venous pressure to rise.

It is evidently firmly established that the velocity of the blood flow rises in thyrotoxicosis. However, the quickened blood flow in this disease continues only as long as the heart can cope with the load. When cardiovascular failure arises, the blood flow is slowed [62, 67, 178, 414]. Since the velocity of the blood flow rises initially, the discovery even of normal values of this parameter in thyrotoxicosis may indicate decompensation of the circulation. Bachmann and Griese [48] found a faster blood flow than normal in patients with thyrotoxicosis even in the stage of decompensation of the circulation. The arterial blood flow in the limbs was particularly high.

The view that thyrotoxicosis is accompanied by an increase in the blood volume in the body became firmly established in 1920–30. In 1933 Jonas and Horejsi [301] described correlation between the blood volume and the basal metabolism. Bussel' [100] also observed correlation between the blood volume, the severity of thyrotoxicosis, and the minute volume of the heart. Regarding the increase in the circulating blood volume in thyrotoxicosis as a result of contraction of the spleen and the liberation of the blood stored in it, Bussel' described experiments in which thyroidectomy prevented the increase in the circulating blood volume in rabbits during physical exertion. However, the administration of thyroid hormones to the animals restored the ability of the spleen to contract in response to physical exertion.

On the other hand, Hegglin et al. [264] described only a very moderate increase in the blood volume, expressed per square meter of the body surface in patients with thyrotoxicosis. According to Mori [430], the increase in the blood volume in thyrotoxicosis is apparent because of the considerable wasting of the patients. Observations made by Kandror and Éster [311] on rabbits with experimental thyrotoxicosis showed a small decrease in the circulating blood volume. However, when expressed per unit of body weight, the blood volume was increased in animals with thyrotoxicosis.

The minute volume of the heart may be connected with the intensity of metabolism in the tissues, i.e., with their oxygen consumption and, in addition, evidently with the ability of the myocardium to satisfy this demand. Besides increasing the minute volume, the body can also utilize additional mechanisms in order to satisfy the oxygen requirements of the tissues. Among these mechanisms, an important place is occupied by the more complete extraction of oxygen from the arterial blood, leading to an increase in the arteriovenous difference. In thyrotoxicosis the oxygen requirements of the tissues are increased, as is reflected in the increased basal metabolism, a cardinal feature of the disease. Investigations have shown that the arteriovenous oxygen difference is not increased in thyrotoxicosis and, for that reason, there must be an increase in the minute volume of the heart. In fact, starting with the investigations of Plesch [480], many workers have found an increase in the minute volume in thyrotoxicosis. A similar increase in minute volume has also been observed in experimental thyrotoxicosis. In experiments on rats receiving thyroxine, for instance, Beznak [71] found that the increase in minute volume is a linear function of the dose of the hormone. This increase reached a maximum by the 5th week of the experiment when a tendency appeared for the arteriovenous oxygen difference to increase. Meanwhile the mortality among the experimental animals rose sharply.

Experiments on rabbits [222] have clearly shown that, in order to satisfy the increasing oxygen requirements of the tissues in thyrotoxicosis, several different mechanisms are activated in succession. Initially only the minute volume of the heart is increased, and it may do so to such an extent that the utilization of oxygen from the blood may actually be reduced. Later, however, when for some reason the minute volume begins to fall, the second mechanism is mobilized and the arteriovenous oxygen difference increases.

The view that in thyrotoxicosis the tissues cannot utilize oxygen from the blood has not been confirmed experimentally. This problem may amount to nothing more than explaining the causes by which in the early stages of the pathological changes the mechanism of an increase in minute volume of the heart is utilized rather than extraction of more oxygen from each volume of blood.

The results of determination of the individual parameters defining the contractile function of the myocardium in hyperthyroidized rabbits receiving thyroid extract for 2 and 4 weeks are given in Table XI. Since the general direction of the changes in all parameters is the same, there are solid grounds for speaking of an increase in the contractile function of the heart in thyrotoxicosis. Two sets of circumstances demand attention. First, whatever parameter is used to judge the contractile function of the heart, there was an increase in function for two weeks after the beginning of thyroid feeding. Subsequently these functions did not increase despite the administration of larger doses of thyroid associated with the higher demands presented to the circulation by the body. Second, the degree of increase of the contractile function in thyrotoxicosis differs depending on which parameter of this function is used. For example, the TTI (tension time index) increased less than did the $(dp/dt)_{max}$ and the mean rate of expulsion of blood from the ventricle during the systole. These differences evidently reflect differences in the degree of correlation between the parameters given and the

Table XI. Parameters of the Contractile Function of the Heart in Rabbits with Experimental Thyrotoxicosis (after Kandror and Salakhova [315])

	I Control $n = 7$*	II Thyrotoxicosis 14 days $n = 11$		III Thyrotoxicosis 28 days $n = 10$		
Parameter	M ± m	M ± m	$P_{I\text{-}II}$	M ± m	$P_{I\text{-}III}$	$P_{II\text{-}III}$
Maximal pressure in left ventricle, mm Hg	110.4 ± 10.4	165.2 ± 10.8	0.05	173.3 ± 12	0.01	0.5
Maximal rate of increase of pressure in left ventricle, $(dp/dt)_{max}$ mm Hg/sec	3488 ± 597	6504 ± 724	0.01	6760 ± 980	0.05	0.5
Tension time index mm Hg · sec/min	2148 ± 318	3375 ± 308	0.05	3404 ± 225	0.01	1
Index of cardiac effort, mm Hg · beat/ min · 10^{-3}	26.4± 3.7	59.6 ± 6.3	0.001	69.5 ± 5.2	0.001	0.2

*n denotes number of experiments.

intensity of expenditure of energy by the myocardium during its contraction.

There is little information in the literature on the contractile function of the myocardium in thyrotoxicosis. By catheterization of the aorta and determination of the minute volume and heart rate in 8 patients with thyrotoxicosis, Howitt et al. [285] studied TTI, $(dp/dt)_{max}$ (from the pressure in the aorta), and various other parameters. They showed, in particular, that the period of expulsion of blood during ventricular systole is shortened, and the stroke work of the heart, the stroke force of the left ventricle, the mean velocity of systolic expulsion, and the TTI and $(dp/dt)_{max}$ are increased. The results of these investigations thus fully supported the results obtained by the present writers on rabbits.

The parameters described above reflect the contractile function of the heart as a whole to some degree, but they do not allow the intensity of function of each unit mass of the myocardium to be assessed. The investigations of Meerson [415] have shown that these two parameters do not necessarily agree. To assess the intensity of function of the structures (IFS) of an organ, Meerson suggested using an index reflecting the quantity of function performed by one gram of tissue of that organ. It is the IFS and not the function of the organ as a whole which is the decisive factor causing hypertrophy of the overfunctioning organ. To calculate IFS, the values of the various parameters of the contractile function of the heart were divided by the weight of the left ventricle. The quotients characterize the intensity of function of each gram of myocardial tissue of the left ventricle (Table XII). These facts indicate that in the late stages of experimental thyrotoxicosis, despite increased demands made on the heart by the periphery, its contractile function is not increased. The dynamics of the contractile function of the heart in hyperthyroidized rabbits corresponds to the dynamics of the IFS of that organ.

In this connection it is interesting to estimate the functional reserve of the heart in hyperthyroid animals. This parameter of the state of the myocardium was determined by Salakhova [514] from the ratio between the contractile function of the heart before and after complete, temporary occlusion of the aorta. The corresponding determination showed that, in rabbits receiving thyroid extract for 2 and 4 weeks, the increase in actual contractile function of the heart was not accompanied by the same increase in its maximal attainable function. As a result of this, the functional reserve, regardless of the parameter used to define the contractile function of the heart, was much lower in thyrotoxicosis than under normal conditions.

Characteristically, Graettinger et al. [240], investigating patients with Basedow's disease in a resting state, found that their minute volume was high, although after physical or other exertion it did not increase further (as

Table XII. Contractile Function of Each Gram of Myocardium of the Left Ventricle (IFS) Calculated from Various Parameters in Experimental Animals (M ± m)

Parameter	Control	Thyrotoxicosis 2 weeks	Thyrotoxicosis 4 weeks
Work, kg·m/min/g	0.24 ± 0.02	0.35 ± 0.03 $P < 0.05$	0.30 ± 0.02 $P < 0.05$ $P_1 = 0.2$
Maximal pressure in left ventricle, mm Hg/g	18.1 ± 1.04	22.4 ± 1.26 $P < 0.009$	21.8 ± 0.87 $P < 0.009$ $P_1 = 0.6$
Tension time index, mm Hg·sec/g	451 ± 52	665 ± 57 $P < 0.05$	756 ± 54 $P < 0.01$ $P_1 = 0.3$
$(dp/dt)_{max}$, mm Hg/sec/g	717 ± 93.4	1300 ± 149 $P < 0.01$	1531 ± 272 $P < 0.05$ $P_1 > 0.4$
Index of cardiac effort, mm Hg·beats/min·10^{-3}	5.6	12	18
Mean rate of expulsion, ml/sec/g	3.88	5.33	4.3

it does in healthy persons). It can be concluded, therefore, that in thyrotoxicosis the myocardium performs intensive hyperfunction. The level of its true function increases so much that the functional reserve of the heart falls, regardless of the maximal attainable function (whether reduced, maintained at the control level, or even slightly increased).

Fresh evidence of the impossibility of a further increase in the contractile function of the myocardium in thyrotoxicosis was obtained in experiments in which an additional functional load was placed on the heart, by increasing the resistance to the cardiac output. These experiments were carried out by Salakhova [514, 515] on rabbits in which aortic stenosis was produced before or during feeding with thyroid extract by the application of a metal ring. The experiments showed that exhaustion of the functional reserves of the heart in thyrotoxicosis prevented the development of myocardial hyperfunction in the emergency stage of compensatory hyperfunction of the heart (CHH). Despite the great increase in contractile activity of the heart muscle compared with intact animals, the rabbits of this experimental group developed cardiovascular failure (hyperemia of the lungs, congestive enlargement of the liver, ascites, pleural effusion). Similar results were obtained in the series of experiments in which thyrotoxicosis was produced in a later stage of CHH. The excess of thyroid hormones evidently prevented the development of adaptation of the myocardium to the increased load, and the myocardium reverted into the emergency stage of CHH.

Although the contractile function of the heart is greater than normal, this does not, therefore, mean that cardiovascular failure cannot exist at the same time. The explanation lies in the inability of the myocardial function to match the needs of the body. In thyrotoxicosis, the myocardium is evidently working at the limit of its functional powers; in severe disease, because of exhaustion of the functional reserves, signs of a decrease in the actual activity of the heart appear.

The experiments of Gol'ber, Kandror, and Salakhova [225] on hyperthyroid rabbits demonstrated phasic changes in myocardial contractility. In the relatively early stages of the toxicosis it increased, but at the end of the experiment (one month after the beginning of administration of thyroid extract) it fell to normal or below normal values. These observations show that the rapid onset of cardiac failure in thyrotoxicosis is based on exhaustion of the functional reserves of the myocardium. According to the literature, the most important mechanism maintaining the functional reserves during increased activity of the heart is hypertrophy of the organ, leading to distribution of the greater function over a greater mass [415]. To understand the pathogenesis of heart failure in thyrotoxicosis, we must therefore analyze the supply of structural materials for the thyrotoxic heart. A detailed study of this problem has been made [310, 638] on rabbits receiving increasing doses of thyroid extract for a long time. These experiments showed that intensive hyperfunction of the heart in thyrotoxicosis develops against the background of only a very small increase in the mass of the heart muscle. Calculation of the relative weight of the left ventricle (compared with the initial body weight of the animals of the various experimental groups) showed that it was only 18% higher than the control value in animals fed with thyroid extract for two weeks. Continuation of the thyroid feeding did not bring about any further increase in the mass of the ventricle. In rabbits receiving thyroid extract for four weeks the relative weight of the left ventricle was not increased further, but was actually slightly reduced. It was now only 13% higher than the control. Special determination of the water content in the heart muscle showed that this difference is due to hydration of the thyrotoxic heart; the dry weight of the left ventricle was indistinguishable from the control.

These findings raised doubts about the reality of the hypertrophy of the heart in animals after the prolonged administration of large doses of thyroid hormones. They acted as the starting point for research into the nucleic acid and protein metabolism of the myocardium in experimental animals. The results showed that prolonged administration of large doses of thyroid extract to rabbits led to a definite decrease in the protein concentration in the myocardium of the left ventricle. This occurred despite a marked increase in the concentration of nonprotein nitrogen and, in particular, of free amino acids nitrogen. Evidence was thus obtained that protein breakdown in the thyrotoxic heart predominates over protein synthesis.

In experiments in which methionine-^{35}S was injected intravenously into animals and the radioactivity liberated from the myocardial protein at various times after injection of the amino acid was measured, it was observed that the protein from the left ventricle of the experimental animals was freed from the previously incorporated amino acid much more rapidly than in control rabbits. In agreement with these observations the proteolytic activity of the myocardium increased during the progressive development of thyrotoxicosis in rabbits receiving thyroid extract. All these results point to a marked increase in the intensity of protein catabolism in the myocardium in thyrotoxicosis, and they show that protein synthesis lags behind its breakdown.

To investigate protein synthesis in the myocardium of hyperthyroidized animals in more detail, methionine-^{35}S and glycine-^{14}C were injected intravenously and the rate of incorporation of these amino acids into myocardial proteins of the left ventricle was then estimated. These experiments showed that feeding for one week with thyroid extract leads to an increase in the incorporation of the label into protein of the mitochondrial fraction of the muscle of the left ventricle. By the 14th day of the experiment greater radioactivity than in the control was recorded both in the total protein and in the actomyosin of the thyrotoxic heart, although the radioactivity of the mitochondrial protein was now less than in the control. One month after the beginning of thyroid administration, the incorporation of glycine-^{14}C into the myocardial protein was distinctly lower than in the control animals. Experiments in which methionine-^{35}S was given yielded similar results.

An increase in the contractile function of the heart, accompanied by intensified breakdown of functioning protein structures, in thyrotoxicosis this leads to intensification of the synthesis of these structures only in the early stages. As the disease progresses, increased myocardial function is not accompanied by further activation of protein synthesis. On the contrary, this process is clearly inhibited.

In view of the close link between the intensity of protein synthesis and nucleic acid synthesis in the organ, the rate of incorporation of radioactive phosphate (^{32}P) into RNA of the heart muscle was also investigated. These experiments showed that until the 14th day of thyroid administration, the total RNA of the myocardium of the left ventricle incorporated more label than in the control animals. Similar changes were osberved with respect to the RNA of nuclei and ribosomes isolated by differential centrifugation from heart muscle tissue homogenates. However, by the 28th day after beginning the thyroid administration, the incorporation of ^{32}P into total cell

RNA and also into RNA of the nuclei and ribosomes from the tissues of the left ventricle in experimental animals was appreciably decreased, comparable to the incorporation of labeled amino acids into the various myocardial proteins. With respect to RNA of the hyaloplasm, no significant changes in the rate of renewal could be observed. The disturbance of the normal correlation between the level of physiological function of the myocardium and the level of synthesis of functioning structures within the muscle evidently lies at the basis of exhaustion of the functional reserves of the thyrotoxic heart and the rapid onset of cardiac decompensation.

In the analysis of this problem, the question inevitably arises of the causes of the disturbance of these mechanisms maintaining the functional reserves of the heart in thyrotoxicosis. The considerable increase in protein breakdown in the heart of the experimental animals, which evidently serves as the source of *wear and tear metabolites*, the means by which information is usually sent from the cytoplasm of the cell into the nucleus, provides evidence that in thyrotoxicosis certain factors prevent this information from being utilized by the genetic apparatus of the myocardial cells. In my opinion, changes arising under the influence of thyroid hormones in the structural and biochemical organization of the mitochondria of the myocardial cells play the principal role among these factors. Investigations in Gol'ber's laboratory have revealed sharp deformation of the mitochondria in the heart muscle of the left ventricle and profound depletion of the energy resources (ATP, CP, glycogen) in rabbits with experimental thyrotoxicosis, in agreement with other workers. A study of the effect of different doses of thyroxine on the structure and function of the mitochondria of cardiac and skeletal muscles of rats [607] showed that small doses of the hormone cause an increase in the number and density of cristae in the mitochondria, i.e., the growth and formation of new *units* of respiration and phosphorylation, whereas toxic doses lead to complete destruction with swelling of the mitochondria, clarification of the matrix, and a decrease in the number of cristae.

Very probably it is the deficiency of biologically utilizable energy that lies at the basis of the disturbance between the levels of function of the heart and its structural metabolism, i.e., disturbance of the mechanisms maintaining the functional reserve of the myocardium. Evidently the deficiency of the supply of energy for the contractile function of the heart may play a very important role in the depression of this function in the late stages of thyrotoxicosis. However, the decrease in the functional reserve of the myocardium when its actual function is still considerably increased can evidently be explained also by the inadequate supply of energy for the mechanisms of biosynthesis of the functioning structures. When energy formation is deficient, the utilization of more energy for the needs of the specific activity of the heart creates a strikingly demonstrative model of the competitive relationships between the needs for physiological function of an organ and the needs for the processes of its structural metabolism. Experiments in which an additional functional load was applied to the thyrotoxic heart [314] confirmed this conclusion. Under these conditions the inhibition of protein synthesis in the myocardium began sooner, and it was more marked in degree than in *pure* thyrotoxicosis. The causes of the changes arising in the heart in the presence of a deficiency or excess of thyroid hormones in the body must evidently be sought in changes at the cellular and subcellular levels of the organ.

Action on Other Organs and Tissues

Thyroid Hormones and the Blood System

Disturbances of thyroid function as a rule are accompanied by changes in the blood system [54, 218, 547, 620]. These changes largely depend on the character of the disturbances, i.e., on whether hypo- or hyperfunction of the gland is present.

The main effect of the thyroid gland on hematopoiesis is its action on the red blood cells. Thyroid hormones influence erythropoiesis and the total volume of red blood cells in the circulating blood. This fact has been confirmed repeatedly by clinical and experimental investigations. However, the mechanism by which thyroid function is linked with the red blood cells is still the subject of differences of opinion despite much research.

The most regular changes in the blood were observed when thyroid function was depressed. Thyroidectomy in man has often been shown to cause the development of anemia of various types. It has also been observed in spontaneous myxedema [31, 44, 101], although anemia was found in only 50–60% of cases and it was mainly mild, hypochromic, and macrocytic in type.

Nevertheless, despite a wealth of clinical observations, no definite conclusions have yet been drawn regarding the effect of thyroid deficiency on erythropoiesis. An important contribution to the study of the role of the thyroid gland in erythropoiesis was made by experiments in which the thyroid gland was removed from animals. The anemia developing after thyroidectomy in cats, dogs, monkeys, and rabbits was described more than 60 years ago [331]. Usually the anemia develops in the course of 20 or 30 days after thyroidectomy, and both the hemoglobin concentration and the number of circulating red cells are reduced. The number of reticulocytes varies and the uptake of ^{59}Fe is reduced [620]. Later experiments repeatedly confirmed the association between thyroidectomy and anemia and showed that thyroid extract abolishes the anemia. In some early investigations, the anemia developing after thyroidectomy in animals was described as macrocytic and hyperchromic [127, 354, 537]. The later experiments of Crafts [128] on adult rats revealed a decrease in the mean cell volume without any change in the mean hemoglobin concentration in the cell. The total volume of the red blood cells in the rats 20–30 days after thyroidectomy was reduced by 20% of its normal level; later it became stabilized and showed no further change. The hemoglobin concentration and hematocrit index fell by the same percentage [191, 624].

Similar results were obtained in dogs, in which hypothyroidism was produced by destruction of the thyroid gland with radioiodine. Anemia developed in all the experimental animals and the hematocrit index fell by 13–35% below the control; some decrease in the mean cell volume occurred in most animals. The total volume of red cells was reduced by 22–52%, on the average by 38%. The plasma volume was reduced, but by a lesser degree. Similar results were obtained by Hollander et al. [279], who showed that after daily administration of thyroxine to hypothyroid dogs for 3 months the total red cell volume returned to normal.

Whereas in adult dogs a relatively mild anemia develops after thyroidectomy, depression of thyroid function in newborn rats (by the intraperitoneal injection of radioiodine) leads to a severe and progressive microcytic anemia acompanied by marked hypoplasia of the bone marrow [11]. Kunde et al. [354] found severe anemia after thyroidectomy in experiments on rabbits aged 2–3 weeks. Thus, the degree of anemia developing after thyroidectomy evidently depends on the age at which the operation was performed. Chemical thyroidectomy, by administration of antithyroid preparations, also leads to the development of anemia in animals. Hughes [287] found that retardation of growth and anemia appear immediately in rats receiving thiouracil daily after birth, but as a rule the anemia is mild in form. Consequently, suppression of thyroid activity in the animals (surgically or by means of drugs) leads to anemia, usually mild or only moderately severe, but if the thyroid function is suppressed immediately after birth, the anemia is more severe.

Thyroidectomy or administration of thiouracil to rats disturbs the rate of restoration of the blood picture after acute blood loss [234, 403], whereas the treatment of thyroidectomized rats with thyroxine stimulates the increase in the number of red cells and the rate of hemoglobin concentration after blood loss. The action of thyroxine on the hematopoietic effect of blood loss is more clearly manifested in thyroidectomized animals than in intact controls.

Thyroidectomy aggravates alimentary anemia in males but has no effect on the same condition in females. In males, meanwhile, an excess of protein in the diet abolishes or reduces the anemia caused by removal of the thyroid gland. Castration or injection of sex hormones does not abolish this difference between the sexes [31].

According to many clinical observations, the changes in the peripheral blood in thyrotoxicosis do not follow a regular pattern. Marked changes in the hemoglobin concentration or red cell count in patients with hyperthyroidism are rare [74, 296, 657]. Hartfall [261] described a microcytic anemia, whereas Biström [74] described mild macrocytic anemia in a few cases. True pernicious anemia is found less frequently in patients with hyperthyroidism than can be accounted for by simple coincidence, although it is not so common as in patients with hypothyroidism [604].

Whereas there is no disagreement in the literature that experimental hypothyroidism leads to the development of anemia, the results of investigation of hyperthyroidism caused by feeding animals with an excess of thyroid hormones are not always consistent. In rabbits with experimental hyperthyroidism, polycythemia develops first; as the administration of an excess of thyroid preparations continues, as a rule this gives way to anemia [354].

On the other hand, in analogous experiments no changes were found in the blood of rabbits [538] or cats [238]. Van Dyke et al. [624] measured the total red cell volume before and after administration of thyroid preparations to rats and found no change, although Evans et al. [167] described an increase in this parameter. Some workers [167, 416] found a direct correlation between red cell production and the initial oxygen consumption. In dogs receiving various doses of thyroid extract, an increase in the hematocrit index was found whenever the dose of extract was increased. The circulating red cell volume was increased both in absolute terms and when expressed per kilogram body weight. When the administration of thyroid preparations ceased, the parameters studied fell to their initial level [639]. Differences in the published results of the study of the effects of thyroid hormones on the total red cell volume in normal animals can be partly explained by species differences in reactivity and also by differences in the doses of thyroid hormones.

With these observations in mind, Ivleva [294] studied the volume and morphological composition of the peripheral blood after administration of thyroid extract with the food to rabbits in progressively increasing doses for various periods (7, 14, and 28 days). This led to loss of weight by 15–18% on the 14th day and by 25–30% of its initial level on the 28th day. By the 7th day of thyroid administration, some increase was observed in the hemoglobin concentration, the red cell count, and the hematocrit index. The mean red cell volume still remained unchanged after administration of thyroid from this period, but the red cell diameter was increased by 9%. The spherical index of the red cells was reduced by 20.5%, and this [340] could be evidence of the appearance of many young red cells in the peripheral blood. The relative and absolute numbers of reticulocytes were increased, mainly through an increase in the number of immature forms, while the number of mature (Group IV) reticulocytes, on the contrary, was reduced. Considering that the red cell count was slightly increased, this result can be explained by the more rapid maturation of the reticulocytes in the blood. A further increase in the hematocrit index was observed in the peripheral blood 14 days after the beginning of thyroid feeding (moderately severe thyrotoxicosis). Both the concentration and the absolute content of hemoglobin and red cells were increased.

On the 28th day of thyroid feeding, when severe toxicosis had developed, the hematocrit index in the peripheral blood was increased still further, i.e., hemoconcentration had occurred. The total circulating blood volume was reduced. The hemoglobin concentration and red cell count continued to rise. The absolute number of red cells also increased, but the absolute hemoglobin concentration remained at the same level as on the 14th day of thyroid administration. Despite the high count of erythrocytes in the peripheral blood, the reticulocyte counts suggest that erythropoiesis begins to be depressed in the late stages of thyrotoxicosis.

Clinical investigations revealed the same relations between the degree of activity of the thyroid gland and the red cell volume. In myxedema the plasma volume and total blood volume are usually reduced. In most cases these volumes increased considerably after treatment of hypothyroidism [78, 205]. The total red cell volume, calculated from the plasma volume and hematocrit index [433] or measured directly by labeling the erythrocytes with radioactive chromium [604], also increased after treatment of hypothyroidism. Conversely, in thyrotoxicosis the total red cell volume is constantly increased, falling as a result of suitable treatment [205, 433].

Morphological studies of rabbit bone marrow after various periods of thyrotoxicosis [295] showed that 7 days after the beginning of thyroid feeding increases were found in the number of undifferentiated cells (on account of an increase in the number of reticulum cells) and in the number of plasma cells. The total number of nonhemoglobin-containing erythroblasts also was increased. These changes are evidence of stimulation of the bone marrow and of intensified erythropoiesis. The differential erythroblast count revealed a decrease in the number of polychromatophilic and oxyphilic normoblasts, evidence of their utilization as a ready-prepared reserve of erythropoiesis.

Nevertheless, there are many facts to indicate that thyroid hormones are not the principal factor controlling erythropoiesis, and that they have no direct selective action on precursors of red cells in the bone marrow. Experiments in which animals were exposed to a reduced partial pressure of oxygen showed that thyroidectomy does not prevent the manifestation of the stimulant effect of hypoxia on red cell production. This phenomenon is seen in a more indirect form after removal of the pituitary, controlling thyroid gland activity, which likewise does not prevent the erythropoietic response to hypoxia. Thyroid hormones evidently do not play a decisive role in the regulation of erythropoiesis. This conclusion is supported by other facts. In particular, the anemia observed in myxedema differs in many respects from other dyshematopoietic anemias such as that observed in vitamin B_{12} deficiency [82]. The anemia in hypothyroid patients is rarely particularly severe; the bone marrow is hypoplastic; poikilocytosis and anisocytosis are rarely seen, and the initial cells of the erythroid series are not present in the circulating blood. Administration of an excess of thyroid hormones in the first phase can also increase red cell production above normal. This effect of thyroid hormones differs from the effect of administration of an excess of the more important hematopoietic factors such as cyanocobalamin and iron, which do not induce polycythemia and do not increase the red cell volume above its normal level.

Larsson [372] developed the view that the anemia in hypothyroidism arises through a disturbance of synthesis of proteins, including hemoglobin and transferrin. As support for his view he cited clinical evidence that in the treatment of hypothyroidism the hemoglobin concentration in the red cells recovers more slowly than its absolute content. He also reported that the blood serum iron concentration is low in most patients with myxedema regardless of whether they develop anemia or not. Other workers [604], however, found no decrease in the serum iron level in uncomplicated hypothyroidsm. The rapid initial hematological response to treatment of hypothyroid patients with iron, and also the normal utilization of iron by the red cells observed in hypothyroid patients with iron deficiency, do not support the view that thyroid hormones play a decisive and selective role in the regulation of iron metabolism.

Bomford [82] suggested that uncomplicated anemia in hypothyroidism is the result of a reduced rate of erythropoiesis which, in turn, can be explained by the reduced oxygen requirements of the tissues. Changes in the bone marrow *erythron* under the influence of the reduced oxygen requirement of the tissues and of their relative excess of oxygen in hypothyroidism were compared by Bomford with the depression of erythropoiesis caused by an excess of oxygen in the inspired air. From this standpoint the slow hematologic response of the bone marrow to replacement thyroid therapy observed in hypothyroid anemia ought to be explained by partial atrophy of the *erythron* in the bone marrow. By contrast, in the dyshematopoietic anemias developing as a result of cyanocobalamin deficiency, the ineffectively hyperplastic bone marrow produces a rapid response when the cyanocobalamin deficiency is made good. Bomford's hypothesis that erythropoiesis is linked with the tissue oxygen requirement was later clearly confirmed by data on the regulation of red cell production by erythropoietin liberated in the blood stream as the result of tissue anoxia. There is likewise important evidence that the total volume of circulating red cells and the rate of their production correlate directly with the level of the basal metabolism in man [433] and animals [167]. Muldowney et al. [433] further showed that regulation of the total red cell volume depends on changes in the basal oxygen consumption and not on the direct action of thyroid hormones on the bone marrow. DNP, for instance, increases the oxygen demand but does not simultaneously increase thyroid function [109]. After administration of DNP to patients with myxedema, the uptake of iodine by the thyroid gland is unchanged, but the total red cell volume rises considerably, parallel to the increase in basal metabolism [433]. In exactly the same way, administration of DNP to thyroidectomized rats restored both the total red cell volume and the basal metabolism to normal [167]. On the other hand, the opposite effect was described by Hollander et al. [279], who stated that administration of DNP to hypothyroid dogs for 3 months does not improve the course of the anemia.

There is also more direct evidence that thyroid hormones do not directly stimulate the bone marrow cells. When the isolated hind limb of a dog was perfused with blood containing triiodothyronine, erythropoiesis was not increased in the bone marrow of the limb, whereas perfusion with blood containing added erythropoietin led to a marked increase in the number of erythroid cells in the bone marrow [175]. There can be little doubt that the action of thyroid hormones on red cell production takes place indirectly through the influence of the hormones on the tissue oxygen consumption. Changes in erythropoiesis observed in isolated diseases of the thyroid gland are examples of the basic principle that the rate of erythropoiesis is controlled by the partial pressure of oxygen in the tissues. This, in turn, probably regulates the liberation of erythropoietin from the kidneys. There is no need to prove that thyroxine has any specific effect on the bone marrow cells. The increase in the total red cell volume in hyperthyroidism may reflect hypertrophy of the *erythron* as a manifestation of the ordinary physiological reaction to an increased oxygen demand by the tissues; the anemia in myxedema is the result of the reduced demands made by the body on the oxygen-transporting capacity of the blood.

At the beginning of the present century considerable attention was paid to the possible diagnostic importance of changes in the number of circulating leukocytes in thyroid diseases. In 1908 Kocher described changes which he regarded as pathognomonic of thyrotoxicosis: leukopenia with a relative or absolute lymphocytosis and a moderate increase in the number of eosinophils. He attached not merely diagnostic, but also prognostic significance to the changes in the white blood cell count. In his opinion, a return to the normal white cell count and formula indicated successful treatment. Although such changes can be observed in thyrotoxicosis, they do not arise constantly and they are not, of course, of prognostic significance.

Most workers agree that a relative or absolute lymphocytosis is often present in the blood of thyrotoxic patients but the deviations from normal as a rule are very small. In addition, there is no connection between the degree of lymphocytosis and the severity of the hyperthyroidism [74, 238, 392, 657]. The number of lymphocytes in the bone marrow of patients with thyrotoxicosis rises, sometimes to 30–40% of the total number of leukocytes in the film, even when the blood lymphocyte count is not increased [44]. Sometimes a slight decrease in the number of granulocytes is described, but, as a rule, leukopenia is not found in thyrotoxicosis.

Although the leukocyte count in thyrotoxicosis, as has already been emphasized, is of neither diagnostic nor prognostic importance, mention must be made of the interesting observations of Biström [74] who found a correlation between the degree of lymphocytosis in the blood and the degree of lymphocytic infiltration of the thyroid gland. In thyrotoxicosis the lymphoid tissue may be enlarged all over the body, including in the spleen and thymus. Careful investigation of the thymus [86] showed that, except for leukemia, the only disease in which the mean dimensions of the thymus were greater than normal was exophthalmic goiter. Administration of thyroxine to guinea pigs leads to hyperplasia of the lymph glands [159].

After thyroidectomy for thyrotoxicosis, the differential white cell count returns to normal, and the lymphocyte count falls [238, 392, 657]. After thyroidectomy on euthyroid subjects (for severe heart disease), no change was found either in the total white cell count or in the differential count [44]. One of the earliest communications describing a decrease in the lymphocyte count in animals after thyroidectomy was that of Kishi [331]. Later some workers described similar changes in rabbits [537] and rats [33, 127, 649]. Thyroidectomy in rats also led to a marked decrease in the eosinophil count, and this could be prevented by simultaneous removal of the adrenals [32]. Other workers, however, found no constant or considerable changes in the total white cell count or differential count in rats [234] or dogs [550] after thyroidectomy.

Treatment of schizophrenics with thyroxine gave rise to severe lymphocytosis with no change in the other blood cells [284]. The lymphocyte count was raised in cats [238] and rats [288] receiving thyroxine.

Action on the Liver and Gastrointestinal Tract

The liver is one of the important organs whose function is affected by thyroxine. Many of the metabolic disturbances characteristic of hyperthyroidism take place as a result of stimulation or of qualitative changes in individual functions of the liver. Many clinical and pathological investigations have demonstrated frequent functional and morphological disturbances of the liver in hyperthyroidism. Lesions of the liver caused by infections, poisons, and other factors follow a particularly severe course if hyperthyroidism is simultaneously present.

According to many investigations, administration of thyroid hormones leads to a marked increase in the rate of metabolic processes in the liver. Surviving liver tissue of mice, dogs, rabbits, and guinea pigs receiving thyroid preparations for a long time by mouth assimilated more oxygen than tissue from healthy control animals. In patients with hyperthyroidism the oxygen consumption of the liver is considerably increased. The stimulation of respiration by thyroxine is more marked in the liver tissue. For instance, in the liver tissue of rats receiving thyroxine daily for 4 days, the oxygen consumption was increased by 60%, in the kidney tissue by 40%, but in the muscles and heart, with equal doses of thyroxine, the increase in respiration was relatively slight, and in the brain, testes, and spleen no increase whatever in the oxygen consumption took place [298]. If thyroid function was blocked by thyrostatic agents, leading to a decrease in the quantity of circulating thyroid hormones, the opposite picture was observed.

According to Milcu [420], in dogs with a biliary fistula and closure of the bile duct, injection of thyroxine reduced the quantity of bile and lowered the cholesterol level. In his opinion, this was due to inhibition of bile formation in the liver and a change in the water balance. An increase in the quantity of bile secreted in dogs with experimental hypothyroidism was observed by Badrutdinov [50].

The ability of the liver to synthesize glycogen from glucose is reduced in hyperthyroidism. After oral administration of thyroid preparations, the liver glycogen level falls, and all the glycogen may disappear. The liver glycogen likewise is not maintained after a carbohydrate diet; other hexoses do not have the required effect. The disappearance of glycogen from the liver produced by thyroxine can be delayed by the combined administration of fructose and insulin. The disappearance of glycogen takes place only in the liver and heart muscle. The glycogen of the striated muscles is unaffected by thyroid hormones and undergoes only very slight changes. Thyroid deficiency, on the other hand, leads to a decrease in the glycogen content. In thyroidectomized sheep and guinea pigs the liver glycogen content was only 40–50% of that in normal animals, whereas the muscle glycogen was unchanged. It can be concluded that normal quantities of thyroid hormone are optimal for maintenance of the glycogen balance of the liver. Galactose loading in hyperthyroidism often gives abnormal results, probably because of the faster rate of resorption of galactose in the intestine characteristic of hyperthyroidism. If choline is given at the same time, thyroxine reduces the lipid and cholesterol content in the liver [181].

In comparative studies of metabolic effects and the mechanism of action of thyroid hormones, much attention has been paid to changes in activity of the liver enzymes corresponding to different functional states of the thyroid gland. Lee and Lardy [377] showed increased activity of glycerophosphate dehydrogenase in the liver mitochondria, an enzyme limiting the rate of the glycerophosphate cycle, under the influence of thyroid hormones. Recently Nolte et al. [452] carried out extensive investigations of the spectrum of enzymes of the citric acid cycle and connected metabolic pathways in biopsy material from the liver of thyrotoxic and hypothyroid patients and control subjects. In thyrotoxicosis, glucokinase activity and the glucose tolerance were reduced. Meanwhile, the activity of the liver and muscle hexokinase was increased in thyrotoxic patients, possibly in connection with the increased metabolic rate. Activity of triose phosphate and malate dehydrogenases, phosphoenolpyruvate carboxykinase, and carnitine acetyltransferase, enzymes concerned with increasing the turnover of fatty acids in thyrotoxicosis in man, also was increased. Meanwhile mitochondrial glycerophosphate dehydrogenase of the liver and muscles, the activity of which is considerably increased in rats by the action of thyroxine, showed no appreciable change in thyrotoxic patients. These results confirmed the existence of definite species differences in the response of the liver enzyme spectrum to toxic doses of thyroid hormones.

To determine the state of the liver function in thyrotoxicosis, a number of function tests reflecting the degree and sequence of disturbances of metabolic processes in the liver tissue are used. Mandl' [402] suggested 10 different liver function tests for use simultaneously in thyrotoxicosis. He concludes that protein metabolism is the first to be disturbed in thyrotoxicosis, followed by carbohydrate metabolism and, finally, by the antitoxic function of the liver. Lipid and pigment metabolism is disturbed in severe forms of thyrotoxicosis. Stepanenko [582], who investigated the antitoxic function of the liver in various forms of goiter, also noted that the greatest degree of disturbance of the barrier function occurs in the hyperthyroid forms of goiter.

Damage to the parenchyma of the liver can give rise to important changes in the metabolism of thyroid hormone and, in certain cases, can increase the amounts of the hormones in the blood stream. This effect can be attributed to the accumulation of thyroid hormones and of their glucuronic compounds in the blood and to changes in the structure of the serum protein fractions associated with liver damage. Experiments carried out by Milcu et al. [423] on dogs with toxic hepatitis caused by carbon tetrachoride showed reduced ability of the liver to inactivate thyroxine. In these animals the accumulation of radioactive iodine in the liver also was reduced. The results suggest that the liver is concerned with the regulation of the content of thyroid hormones and iodine in the plasma and bile.

The role of the liver in the peripheral regulation of thyroid hormones has been studied in some detail by Vannotti and Béraud [625] and by Milcu et al. [423]. They investigated thyroid function and thyroxine metabolism with the aid of radioactive iodine in patients with liver diseases. They conclude from their investigations and from data in the literature that the liver may serve to regulate the elimination of thyroxine from the blood into the intestine either by its destruction by deiodination or its inactivation through the conjugation of thyroid hormones with glucuronic acid. On the other hand, in diseases of the liver, diffuse damage to the organ may cause changes in the structure of the plasma protein, and these may affect the transport of thyroxine in the blood and thus lead to changes in penetration of the hormone into the cell and, consequently, changes in its action in the tissues.

Disturbance of the deiodination of iodotyrosines in the liver was found in animals with thyrotoxicosis produced by administration of thyroid extract. Marked inhibition of the deiodination of labeled MIT and DIT and of the conjugation of thyroxine and triiodothyronine with sulfuric and glucuronic acids in liver slices from rats fed with thyroid extract was demonstrated by Mirakhmedov [425]. He also investigated thyroid function during the development of cirrhosis of the liver in rats poisoned with the hepatotoxic alkaloid, heliotrine. In the initial period of poisoning, a sharp increase was observed in ^{131}I uptake, in the rate of hormone formation, and in the content of iodothyronines in the thyroid gland; this increase was followed by a decrease in all the parameters of thyroid activity studied.

An excess in the content of thyroid hormones in the body often leads to gastrointestinal disorders. Various lesions of the digestive organs have been observed in more than 30% of patients with thyrotoxicosis. Some workers also distinguish a special gastrointestinal form of thyrotoxicosis [329, 521, 541, 597]. Meanwhile, the pathogenetic connection between the disturbance of the functions of the gastrointestinal tract and thyrotoxicosis has been inadequately studied, and the corresponding data are at times contradictory.

Many investigations of the gastric secretion of hydrochloric acid in hypothyroidism have confirmed the presence of achlorhydria in this disease. In 1932 Lerman and Means [384] first described the results of a test involving histamine stimulation of gastric secretion in patients with thyroid pathology. The mean hydrochloric acid production in 17 patients with hypothyroidism was much less than in a group of healthy persons of the same age, and achlorhydria was observed in nine of them. Anemia was found more often among hypothyroid patients with achlorhydria than among patients with the normal ability to secrete hydrochloric acid. However, judging from the basal metabolism, the presence of achlorhydria did not correlate with the severity of the hypothyroidism.

Other workers have described the unusually low acid secretion in cases of severe myxedema. During thyroxine treatment no appreciable change was found in the acidity of the gastric juice. In 1960, Tudhope and Wilson [604] published the results of their investigation of gastric secretion by means of a more powerful histamine test in 52 patients with spontaneous hypothyroidism. Achlorhydria was found in 24 patients (46%). Thus, in patients with spontaneous primary hypothyroidism, achlorhydria is often present, and the absence of acid secretion is evidently a stable disturbance, not abolished by adequate treatment of the hypothyroidism for several years.

Other investigators have studied the effect of an excess of thyroid gland activity on gastric secretion. The high incidence of achlorhydria in patients with hyperthyroidism has often been described; according to Berryhill and Williams [69] it was found in 68% of patients with thyrotoxicosis, and according to most other workers, in 30–40%. Lerman and Means [384], for example, found achlorhydria in 19 of 50 patients. Williams and Blair [647] showed that complete achlorhydria is relatively frequent in patients with thyrotoxicosis, especially in those over 40 years of age, and that treatment does not lead to any permanent changes in the secretion of hydrochloric acid. In agreement with the earlier findings of Berryhill and Williams [69] and also of McElroy et al., these workers found no correlation between the achlorhydria and the severity or duration of the disease. Furthermore, Bock and Witts [79] found achlorhydria in four of 46 euthyroid patients after being cured of thyrotoxicosis. The high frequency of complete achlorhydria cannot be explained by disturbance of equilibrium in the autonomic innervation. The connection between thyrotoxicosis and disappearance of the acidity of the gastric juice evidently does not reflect any direct dependence of the achlorhydria on the hyperthyroidism, and it is a result of simple coexistence of lesions of the stomach and diseases of the thyroid gland. This connection is usually seen in elderly patients. The conclusion is supported by the study of biopsy material from the gastric mucosa. Most workers thus describe a decrease in the secretion of acid in the stomach of patients with thyrotoxicosis and, at least in some patients, these changes are evidently reversible after treatment of the thyrotoxicosis.

Experiments on animals also confirmed the view that an excess of thyroid hormone directly or indirectly modifies gastric function and reduces hydrochloric acid secretion. More than 40 years ago it was shown that feeding dogs with thyroid gland tissue inhibits gastric secretion [111, 256, 601]. Later experiments on dogs [436] and rats [76, 229, 530] also showed that administration of thyroid hormone leads to a marked decrease in the volume of gastric juice and in the total quantity of hydrochloric acid secreted, but with no structural changes in the gastric mucosa. The results of experiments on rats with ligation of the pylorus, described by Blair et al. [76], were unexpected in the sense that the gastric secretion, inhibited initially by administration of thyroxine, returned to normal after a few weeks despite the continued administration of thyroxine.

Thyroidectomy in animals produces variable results. In the experiments of Chang and Sloan [111] on dogs, a marked increase was observed in both the volume and the acidity of the gastric juice. On the other hand, Abrams and Baker [8] found that thyroidectomy in rats leads to a marked decrease in gastric secretion and a decrease in the total pepsin activity of the gastric juice.

Gastritis progressing to severe atrophy of the gastric mucosa and total achlorhydria is found more often in patients with thyrotoxicosis than can be accounted for by pure coincidence. The similarity of the histological picture of the gastric mucosa in such patients with that found characteristically in pernicious anemia must be taken into account in any analysis of the causes of the frequent discovery of pernicious anemia or latent pernicious anemia in patients with disturbances of thyroid function.

Research into the study of the motor–evacuatory function of the stomach in the presence of an excess of thyroid hormones has been conducted on a relatively small scale, and results obtained by different workers are extremely contradictory. Some investigators [59, 324, 593], for instance, observed lowered gastric tone, increased peristalsis, and a low relief of the gastric mucosa and rapid emptying in a high proportion of patients with thyrotoxicosis, while others [92, 235] found normal gastric tone and peristalsis and delayed or uneven emptying. These contradictions are evidently attributable to the fact that different workers used different tests to assess the evacuatory function of the stomach. Changes in the evacuatory function of the stomach in thyrotoxicosis are independent of the acidity of the gastric juice. No precise correlation likewise is found between the rate of emptying of the stomach and the severity and duration of the thyrotoxicosis. The excretory function of the stomach in most patients with thyrotoxicosis is inhibited [291, 293, 454, 546]. It must also be pointed out that the changes in the secretory, motor–evacuatory, and excretory functions of the stomach found in thyrotoxicosis are reversible in character. After appropriate treatment of the underlying disease they are largely restored to normal.

Relationship between the Thyroid Gland and Other Glands of Internal Secretion

Interaction between the thyroid gland and other glands of internal secretion has several aspects: the effect of thyroid hormones on the function and morphology of other endocrine glands; changes arising in those glands in thyrotoxicosis or hypothyroidism; the regulatory effect of the products of other glands on the parameters of thyroid function; interaction between thyroid and other hormones in producing their physiological effects in the intact organism and during their action on metabolic processes at different levels. All these aspects of interaction between internal secretions have recently been the subject of much experimental research. However, relations between the endocrine glands in the regulation of physiological function and metabolism and possible interaction between various hormones have not yet been adequately studied.

After thyroidectomy the whole endocrine apparatus is disturbed: The development of the gonads is delayed, the thymus atrophies, and the anterior lobe of the pituitary and adrenal cortex hypertrophy. After injection of thyroid hormones into experimental animals, hyperplasia of the adrenals develops. In hyperthyroid rabbits, Larina [369] found a marked increase in hydrocortisone biosynthesis in the adrenals, accompanied by an increase in weight of the glands. In patients with thyrotoxicosis of differing severity, Shamakhmudov [535] found a marked decrease in the 17-ketosteroids in the urine. The adrenals of patients with Basedow's disease were relatively insensitive to the action of ACTH.

Mikulaj and Nemeth [419] determined the adrenocortical reserves in thyrotoxic patients by studying the 17-hydroxycorticoid level after administration of ACTH. They concluded that the secretory power of the adrenal cortex in thyrotoxic patients is usually adequate in the case of maximal stimulation by ACTH. However, during prolonged stimulation with submaximal doses of ACTH, this adequate response was replaced by a phase of diminished secretion. Komissarenko [338] also studied the functional state of the adrenal cortex by determining the 17-ketosteroid and 17-hydroxycorticosteroid levels in patients with thyroid diseases before and after treatment. He found that adrenocortical function in hyperthyroidism as regards glucocorticoid synthesis is not depressed, but in most cases is actually increased.

The investigation of Roche et al. [502] *in vitro* showed that after the addition of 3,5,3′-triiodothyroacetic acid and T_3 to slices of adrenal cortex incubated in Krebs's solution the corticosteroid secretion increases. The action of thyroid hormones is particularly increased in the presence of ACTH, which selectively increases the secretion of corticosterone but not of 11-dehydrocorticosterone. Similar results were obtained in investigations on rats [501]. According to Roche et al., thyroid hormones stimulate the secretion of adrenocortical hormones and, in particular, of mineralocorticoids.

Larina [368, 370] observed an increase in the internal secretory zones of the adrenal cortex and a decrease in their content of cholesterol and ascorbic acid in rabbits with experimental thyrotoxicosis, evidence of increased secretion of hormones. The concentration of hydrocortisone in blood flowing from the adrenals was sharply increased, and this was accompanied by an increase in weight of the gland. Yates et al. [661] reported that triiodothyronine increases while thyroidectomy decreases the general ability of the liver to reduce the A ring of cortisone. They consider that this takes place as a result of a decrease in the activity of the enzyme Δ^4-4-steroid dehydrogenase or a deficiency of the coenzyme reduced NADP and that this is the enzymic basis of the change in the biological half-life period of corticosteroids in hyper- and hypothyroidism. A study of the metabolism of endogenous hydrocortisone and exogenous labeled 4-^{14}C-hydrocortisone in euthyroid subjects and patients with spontaneous hyperthyroidism and myxedema showed considerable changes in the formation and course of metabolism of this hormone [269]. An absolute increase in the formation of the hormone in the adrenals and in its conversion into 11-ketone metabolites was found in hyperthyroidism, while in myxedema the endogenous formation of the hormone was reduced and its conversions into 11-hydroxy derivatives were increased.

There have been many investigations of adrenocortical function in diseases of the thyroid gland. The function of the adrenal cortex is considered to be depressed in the hyperthyroid state, while thyroid function is increased if the quantity of available adrenocorticoids is reduced. Many clinical observations and experimental investigations have been devoted to the study of this problem [508, 622].

Jacobson [297] found increased excretion of 17-hydroxycorticosteroids and 17-ketosteroids in patients with thyrotoxicosis. With the restoration of normal thyroid function after administration of iodine or thiouracil or after operative treatment, the excretion of corticosteroids was reduced. However, many investigations yielded no evidence of changes in the production or metabolism of corticosteroids in patients with hyperthyroidism or in animals receiving thyroid hormones [326, 353, 524]. This problem has recently been investigated further. The reaction of the adrenal cortex to corticotropic hormone is evidently modified in different functional states of the thyroid gland, which suggests a disturbance of the pituitary–adrenocortical system in thyroid disease. Data on the inhibition of biosynthesis of catecholamines in the adrenals in thyrotoxicosis were cited above [309, 313].

The effect of stimuli arising from other endocrine glands on the function of the thyroid gland itself and on the peripheral action of the thyroid hormones is another important aspect of endocrine interrelationships. Regulation of the functions of the glands of internal secretion by the hypothalamus and pituitary occupies a central position in the neurohumoral connections of the endocrine glands. In 1940 Barron [60] demonstrated the action of the diencephalohypophyseal system on thyroid activity. In his opinion, the anterior zones of the hypothalamus, lying close to the supraopticohypophyseal tract, participate in the control of the thyroid gland. The paraventricular nuclei of the hypothalamus are an essential component in the mechanism of hypothalamic regulation of the thyrotropic function of the pituitary and of the thyroid gland. Only if these nuclei are injured is the goitrogenic effect of methylthiouracil abolished and the compensatory hypertrophy after unilateral thyroidectomy prevented [162]. Hormone formation in the thyroid gland undergoing compensatory hypertrophy after unilateral thyroidectomy, like the weight of the gland, is evidently under the control of the anterior hypothalamus, and the paraventricular nuclei are an essential component in this regulation. To examine the direct role of the individual hypothalamic nuclei, especially the paraventricular nucleus, in the regulation of the function of the thyroid gland and growth of its parenchyma, Demidenko and Mamina [137] destroyed this hypothalamic nucleus and studied the state of the thyroid parenchyma under these conditions. The results confirm that destruction of the paraventricular nucleus is accompanied by depression of thyroid function and by weakening of its regeneration. This observation was confirmed in dogs treated with propylthiouracil after destruction of the supraoptic and paraventricular nuclei by Ford [181a] in 1960.

It has now become clear that regulatory influences of the hypothalamus reach the thyroid gland, gonads, and adrenal cortex only through the intermediary of the appropriate organotropic hormones of the anterior pituitary and that connections between the components of the hypothalamus–pituitary–peripheral endocrine gland system are effected entirely by humoral factors. In particular, transmission of the effective impulse from the hypothalamus to the anterior pituitary in the system hypothalamus–pituitary–thyroid gland is brought about by thyrotropin-releasing factor, stimulating the secretion of thyrotropic hormone, and this in turn activates the thyroid gland [17, 55]. All these matters are fully examined in the section on the regulation of thyroid function.

Despite the exceptional position of thyrotropin in the regulation of the functions of the thyroid gland, other hormones also influence its activity. Growth hormone and ACTH, which evidently participate in the peripheral action of thyroid hormones also, exert a significant effect on thyroid function. Evans et al. [166] showed that growth hormone increases calorigenesis in hypophysectomized rats. This action probably takes place through stimulation of thyroid function, as the morphological and functional tests show. The anterior pituitary also influences the thyroid gland through ACTH, which exerts its action indirectly by increasing the output of adrenal steroids. ACTH and the glucocorticoids of the adrenals possess a calorigenic effect in hypophysectomized and thyroidectomized animals. Many workers assert that more than one factor acting on the thyroid gland is produced in the anterior pituitary. Beck [64], in his exeriments, found an increase in the liberation of ^{131}I from the thyroid gland under the influence of corticotropin. This effect also was observed in hypophysectomized rats. Cortisone had no effect on the acceleration of ^{131}I liberation produced by corticotropin. In Beck's opinion this unexpected phenomenon may depend on a direct effect of ACTH on the thyroid gland. Skebel'skaya [554] reached the same conclusion by demonstrating the action of ACTH on thyroid function after adrenalectomy.

Voitkevich [635] studied the reaction of the thyroid epithelium of puppies to cortisone and ACTH and obtained morphological evidence of stimulation of the thyroid gland. He found intensive local transformation of thyroid cells and whole follicles into pale islands of parafollicular cells when secretory activity was increased by the action of cortisone. In some experimental animals differentiation and the formation of new follicles in the thyroid tissue were stimulated by ACTH. Anderson et al. [26] observed a decrease in the PBI level in adrenalectomized rats and its return to normal values after hydrocortisone replacement therapy.

By contrast with these observations, Nikolaichuk and Rodkina [448] showed that ACTH does not stimulate the thyroid gland, but during prolonged administration of TSH the formation of corticotropic hormone is stimulated (hypertrophy of the adrenals takes place), inhibiting excitation of the thyroid gland by thyrotropic hormone. Cortisone and ACTH depress the uptake of ^{131}I in response to the action of thyrotropic hormone but have no effect on growth of the gland cells. Besides a decrease in ^{131}I uptake, a decrease in its excretion with the urine and feces also was observed in adrenalectomized rats receiving maintenance doses of deoxycorticosterone in response to the action of cortisone [418]. The ^{131}I concentration in the blood was increased. No difference was found in the ratio between the fraction of iodinated components in the gland between this group of rats and normal or adrenalectomized rats. However, Ackerman et al. [9] found no change in the PBI concentration in blood flowing from the thyroid gland after administration of cortisone. It did not affect the excretion of PBI when increased by the action of TSH. In patients with bilateral adrenalectomy, after the discontinuation of cortisone therapy both the absorption of ^{131}I by the thyroid gland and the blood PBI level were increased. With the resumption of cortisone therapy the uptake of ^{131}I and the blood PBI level fell again.

According to Abe [3], after injection of ACTH and cortisone into rats, the iodide and monoiodotyrosine content in the thyroid gland was increased but the diiodotyrosine, thyroxine, and triiodothyronine content was reduced, indicating a reduced rate of thyroid hormone formation. These differences of opinion can evidently be explained by the different relations established between the thyroid gland and adrenal cortex under normal conditions and when the functions of these glands are disturbed. As Vereckei [630] states on the basis of a study of the PBI and excretion of 17-ketosteroids in various pathological states of the thyroid and adrenal glands, when there is hypertrophy of one of these glands the function of the other is reduced, while in hypofunction of one gland the function of the other changes correspondingly.

New investigations have confirmed these findings. Broder et al. [90], for instance, determined the PBI and the metabolic rate in adrenalectomized rabbits maintained with 1.2 mg cortisone daily. When this dose was reduced to 0.15–0.3 mg, the metabolic rate rose considerably, but without any corresponding change in the PBI level. Kruskemper and Doering [350] studied the effect of cortisone on normal rats and showed that by itself cortisone does not affect the accumulation of iodine by the thyroid gland or the blood PBI concentration, but if given to a rat maintained on TSH, the stimulant action of TSH on ^{131}I accumulation is reduced.

The method of action of steroids on the assimilation of radioactive iodine by the thyroid gland is not yet known. They may act either directly or indirectly—through the pituitary. On the other hand, during cortisone therapy, the iodine clearance of the kidney is known to be increased. However, this alone cannot evidently explain the marked decrease in the absorption of iodine by the thyroid gland under the influence of ACTH and cortisone. There is evidence to show that these agents inhibit the liberation of thyrotropic hormone from the gland. In hypophysectomized rats and rabbits, ACTH caused no decrease in the rate of liberation of iodine by the already depressed gland, but it inhibited the secretion of radioiodine from the gland in response to exogenous TSH.

Colle and Elewant [121] showed that if TSH and hydrocortisone were added simultaneously to the incubation medium containing fragments of thyroid gland, the secretion of thyroid hormones was increased. Data obtained in Brown-Grant's laboratory [93] also confirmed the hypothesis that ACTH and cortisone depress thyroid function by inhibiting the secretion of thyrotropic hormone. After injecting cortisone, Halmi and Barker [250] discovered morphological changes characteristic of its increased activity in the cells of the thyroid gland. Consequently, the reduced activity of the thyroid gland after administration of cortisone observed by many investigators is due, not to the inhibition of TSH production, but to other factors possibly including changes in the extrathyroid iodine metabolism, inhibition of ^{131}I assimilation by the thyroid gland, or true antithyroid (thiouracil-like) activity. This explanation coincides with the views of Skebel'skaya. Her experimental data [553], as well as those of Éskin and Skebel'skaya [163], show that the action of ACTH on the thyroid gland is biphasic in character: Initially the thyrotropic hormone content in the pituitary is reduced, after which the reactivity of the thyroid gland to thyrotropic hormone is weakened. Later Skebel'skaya [554] showed that ACTH also acts after adrenalectomy. Consequently, ACTH may exhibit a direct action on the tissues of the thyroid gland without the participation of the adrenal cortex. Skebel'skaya concludes that the adrenal cortex does not play an essential role in the reaction of the thyroid gland to exogenous or endogenous ACTH.

Regarding the effects of the adrenal cortex on the peripheral action of thyroid hormones, the view has been expressed that cortisone inhibits the conversion of thyroxine into triiodothyronine, which possesses greater hormonal activity in peripheral tissues. Thus, data in the literature with respect to the action of corticosteroids on thyroid gland function show that both the function of the gland (reflected in hormone production) and the biological effect of the available thyroid hormones on tissue metabolism are inhibited. This conclusion is confirmed by clinical observations in which patients with thyrotoxicosis were treated with ACTH and cortisone. For instance, the onset of thyroid insufficiency has been reported during the prolonged treatment of some patients with corticosteroids [498].

There is also evidence of interaction between adrenalin and the thyroid gland. Under the influence of adrenalin the iodine content was increased sharply in the thyroid gland and appreciably in the blood. Injection of adrenalin into rats, according to several investigators, leads to a decrease in the assimilation of ^{131}I by the thyroid gland. The same treatment gives opposite effects in adrenalectomized animals.

An increase in the concentration of catecholamines in the adrenals is found in experimental hyperthyroidism. Two facts must be remembered when this phenomenon is discussed. First, the decrease in the catecholamine concentration in the adrenal tissue may to some extent be due to an increase in weight of the adrenals through hypertrophy of their cortex, as has been conclusively demonstrated in hyperthyroidism [369]. Second, the decrease in the catecholamine concentration in the adrenals in the presence of an excess of thyroid hormones can be interpreted either as the result of increased liberation of catecholamines into the blood stream or as a result of inhibition of their biosynthesis. The discovery of degenerative changes in the adrenal medulla in histological investigations of rats receiving large doses of thyroid hormones with their diet [388] did not help to elucidate the problem. Hokfelt [278] studied the effect of feeding rabbits with thyroid gland on the reaccumulation of adrenalin in the adrenals after their adrenalin content had been reduced in response to insulin hypoglycemia. No difference in the rate of accumulation of adrenalin in the adrenals could be found in the animals of the experimental and control groups. According to other investigations, a thyrostatic preparation did not affect the rate of reaccumulation of adrenalin in the adrenals after hypoglycemia. These two series of experiments thus demonstrated the activation of catecholamine biosynthesis in hyperthyroidism.

Utevskii and But studied the effect of thyroid extract on adrenalin metabolism in skeletal muscles and showed that prolonged administration of the preparation leads to the disappearance of reversibly oxidized forms of adrenalin-like substances in the muscles. Recently Sellers et al. [527] investigated the interaction between the thyroid gland and adrenal medulla in rats at a low temperature. They found that in hypothyroidism, because of the development of hypothermia, the rats died in the cold despite a sharp increase in the output of noradrenalin. The content of catecholamines in the adrenals of rats with hypothyroidism fell sharply at 4°C. Under these conditions the rats receiving thyroxine excreted less adrenalin, noradrenalin, and their metabolites in the urine than did the hypothyroid and control rats. At 24°C hyperthermia was observed in the hyperthyroid rats, their condition worsened, their excretion of noradrenalin in the urine was doubled, but the noradrenalin concentration in the heart was reduced.

Conquilhem and Malan [124] reported that the excretion of catecholamines in the urine of thyroidectomized hamsters during hibernation was much higher than that of intact animals. Injection of thyroxine restored the normal values of catecholamine excretion in the thyroidectomized animals: At temperatures of between 4 and 28°C the excretion of catecholamines in the urine was considerably higher than in intact animals.

In a recently published paper, Lorscheider and Reineke [391] described a study of the possible relations between the thyroxine level in the blood and the prolactin level in lactating rats. They found a decrease both in the thyroxine concentration in the serum and in the rate of secretion of T_4 during the period of lactation, a time usually associated with considerable losses of iodine with the milk and a relative deficiency of the element. Admittedly, a tenfold increase in the iodine content of the diet did not cause any increase in the serum thyroxine level. Exogenous prolactin did not lower the T_4 level in the serum of lactating or nonlactating rats. These workers concluded that the increase in the secretion of prolactin is not the cause of the lowered serum thyroxine level during lactation.

The anterior pituitary hormone prolactin, if injected into newts, increased the assimilation of ^{131}I by the thyroid gland, and this was accompanied by an increase in thyroxine formation and in the ^{131}I-PBI level in the blood serum [232].

Singh and Chaikoff [551] found an increase in the ^{131}I incorporation into thyroid tissue and into iodine-containing amino acids under the influence of insulin. However, insulin did not change the content of iodide-^{131}I in the gland into which tapazole (1-methyl-2-mercaptoimidazole) was injected. Presumably insulin increases the incorporation of ^{131}I into protein-bound mono- and diiodotyrosine and T_4 by activating the supply of iodide.

The role of the pineal gland in intrathyroid iodine metabolism is discussed in a few communications. Miline and Seepovic [424] injected pineal extracts into rats and observed a marked decrease in the blood PBI, the basal metabolic rate, and the metabolic effect of T_4 as well as a decrease in the degree of thyroid hyperfunction caused by TSH. Structural changes were also found in the follicles of the thyroid gland. The effect of the pineal gland on the structure and function of the thyroid gland was studied by Aulov, Islambekov, and Turakulov [42] in pinealectomized rats. The thyroid function was determined from the uptake of radioactive iodine and also by counting the activity of the gland tissue *in vitro* and by autoradiography. In rats undergoing the operation before reaching sexual maturity, a marked decrease in the uptake of radioactive iodine, an increase in weight of the thyroid by 30–40%, and lower fixation of iodine in the follicles of the thyroid gland were observed. In the thyroid gland of rats pinealectomized after reaching sexual maturity, no significant changes were found compared with the control animals. These results point to a role of the pineal gland in the regulation of thyroid function. The mechanism of this effect is not yet clear and requires further study.

Continuing the study of the connection between these two glands, Aulov showed a decrease in the content of thyroxine and triiodothyronine and an increase in the iodotyrosines and inorganic iodine in the thyroid gland and blood of pinealectomized animals. These findings were confirmed by the investigations of Baschieri et al. [62], who demonstrated the inhibitory effect of the active principle of the pineal gland (Melatonin) on the thyroid gland. Dillman and Cady [141] showed rapid uptake of thyroxine by pineal slices and its rapid deiodination.

In healthy volunteers, Read et al. [495] demonstrated a constant but slight decrease in the uptake of radioiodine by the thyroid gland during infusion of vasopressin. Under these circumstances the blood TSH level was not significantly raised. These results show that vasopressin does not stimulate thyroid function or TSH secretion.

The relations between the thyroid gland and the gonads have attracted the attention of many investigators for a long time. There is experimental evidence that athyroid female rabbits develop ovarian follicles but cannot ovulate. According to data in the literature, thyroxine does not change the gonadotropic activity of the pituitary. Special experiments have shown that hypothyroidism reduces the sensitivity of mice to estrone and that hyperthyroidism has the opposite effect, but the response to estradiol was not changed.

As a result of many experiments and analyses of the PBI level in the blood of pregnant women, the opinion has been formed that thyroid activity is increased and the blood PBI level is raised during pregnancy [147, 251, 267]. In a recent paper, however, Galton [193] published some rather different data. An increase both in thyroid gland activity and in thyroxine metabolism was found in pregnant rats. This depended, at least partly, on the action of estrogens. On injection of estradiol benzoate, the rate of deiodination of thyroxine and the rate of excretion of ^{131}I in the urine were increased and the serum ^{131}I-thyroxine concentration was lowered. However, estradiol had no effect on the fixation of thyroxine by serum proteins, although it increased the uptake of ^{131}I by the thyroid gland of both normal and hypophysectomized rats. This suggests that estrogens exert their action on the thyroid gland without the intervention of the pituitary. However, despite many investigations into this problem, there is as yet no general agreement regarding the effect of estrogens on the thyroid gland function. The suggestion has been made that estrogens may affect the thyroid gland in several ways: by inhibiting the liberation of TSH, by potentiating the action of TSH at the thyroid gland level, by reducing the peripheral utilization of thyroxine, and by increasing the rate of secretion of thyroid hormones.

Both male and female gonads and hormonal products are known to be able to modify thyroid gland function. Gannong and Hildegard [194] observed a marked decrease in the uptake of ^{131}I by the thyroid gland of castrated dogs. Aron et al. [29] observed a decrease in thyroid gland activity in the spring and summer, and the mean activity in castrated rats was lower than in intact animals. Ogawa et al. [453] found various changes in ^{131}I uptake by the thyroid gland after castration: The iodine uptake was increased in castrated male rats but reduced in castrated females. According to some reports, a decrease in ^{131}I uptake by the thyroid gland is observed only in the first few weeks after castration, after which it returns to its initial level [26]. It is stated that estradiol, estrone, and diethylstilbestrol inhibit the uptake of radioiodine by the thyroid gland of rats kept on a diet with a low iodine content. Testosterone, estrone, progesterone, and other steroids also led to a decrease in the accumulation of ^{131}I by the thyroid gland. Ogawa et al. [453] injected various hormones into rats and reached similar conclusions. However, directly opposite results have also been obtained. Gzerniak et al. [248], for instance, observed an increase in the uptake of ^{131}I by the thyroid gland in women with disturbances of thyroid-ovarian character after administration of estrogens.

In experiments on rats the ovaries were removed and sex hormones administered. According to Moon and Turner [429], the rate of ^{131}I secretion fell by 33% in the first six days after the operation. In their opinion estrogens stimulate the liberation of TSH, which increases the secretion of thyroxine.

Recent investigations have shown that administration of large doses of estrogens to nonpregnant women causes a simultaneous increase in the serum PBI concentration and in the thyroxine-binding power of the serum. These changes were quantitatively similar to the increase in these characteristics during pregnancy. Meanwhile, under the influence of estrogens the production of thyroid hormones is also increased. Grosvenor and Turner [244], for instance, found an increase in the rate of T_4 secretion in rats after administration of estradiol, in a daily dose of 3.6 μg.

Similar results were obtained by Alexander and Marmarston [18], who found an increase of 1.7–2.1 μg% in the blood PBI with no sign of thyrotoxicosis in men and women receiving two synthetic estrogens. At the same time, on the basis of an increased goiter development in rats receiving propylthiouracil in addition to progesterone and estrogens, De Witt [140] concluded that estrogens have the opposite effect on the pituitary-thyroid system. Merkulov [417] found in experiments on rabbits that sex hormones of the same sex modify iodine metabolism in the thyroid gland but have no effect on thyroid function in the opposite sex. For example, diethylstilbestrol reduces the ability of females to assimilate iodine and slows the excretion of the isotope from the thyroid gland. Testosterone has a similar action on males. Neither preparation has any effect on the gland of the opposite sex. The results of investigations *in vitro* showed that estradiol and progesterone in high concentrations reduce the uptake of ^{131}I by thyroid gland slices and the formation of organically bound iodine. The oxygen consumption of the slices is reduced, but small concentrations of estradiol accelerate this process slightly, and progesterone has no action on it.

Consequently, estrogens affect thyroid gland activity and thyroxine metabolism, but this effect is not entirely due to changes in the binding of thyroxine in the serum.

Interaction between the thymus and thyroid glands is described in a paper by Cherdyntsev [113], who states that thyroid activity in rabbits is reduced after removal of the thymus. In his opinion, the functional link between the thymus and thyroid glands is effected through the cerebral hemispheres.

As these results show, the question of interaction between the thyroid gland and other endocrine glands is still far from being solved. Information is more complete for the relations between the thyroid and pituitary glands, but as regards the other endocrine glands, it is only fragmentary and not always consistent.

Evidence of functional interaction between the thyroid hormones and calcitonin, secreted by the thyroid gland, has recently been published. Cure et al. [130] showed that the secretion of calcitonin from the thyroid gland is stimulated by calcium and glucagon. A definite connection has been established between thyroxine and calcitonin in the regulation of calcium metabolism in the body. Cherny et al. [115], for example, observed a marked anabolic action of large doses of thyroxine on skeletal calcium metabolism in growing rats, together with an increase in the uptake of Ca^{++} by the kidneys, muscles, and other tissues under these conditions. Single doses of thyroxine increased, but repeated doses reduced the hypocalcemic effect of thyrocalcitonin. According to the observations of Collignon et al. [122] on rats kept on an iodine-free diet for a long time, the degree of osteolysis fell sharply. This was acompanied by a decrease in the action of exogenous calcitonin. Injection of thyroxine restored the normal level of osteolysis, indicating that thyroid function is essential for the effects of calcitonin on calcium metabolism.

Thyroid Hormones and Resistance of the Organism

The importance of the thyroid gland for the resistance of the organism depends, first, on the effect of thyroid hormones themselves on metabolism and on the state of the organs and tissues and, second, on interaction between the thyroid and the other endocrine glands and, in particular, the adrenal cortex with its important role in adaptation of the body to unfavorable conditions of existence [529].

Many workers [94, 553, 555, 556, 567] have found a decrease in thyroid gland activity during stress, with a decrease in the concentration of protein-bound iodine in the blood and the uptake of ^{131}I by the gland tissue. Schambaugh and Beisel [536] found a decrease in ^{131}I uptake by the thyroid gland and a low rate of excretion of hormonal iodine in rats with pneumococcal infection, although the blood thyrotropin level remained normal. Conflicting views are expressed in the literature on the thyroid function in infectious disease. For instance, after administration of typhoid vaccine, some workers found inhibition [95], others [37] an initial inhibition followed by potentiation of thyroid gland function. Thyroid function was reduced by pulmonary infection and increased by experimental rheumatic fever [38, 289]. Babare et al. [609] injected an adsorbed tetravaccine into rats and showed that it affected the hormonal activity of the thyroid gland both directly and also via the hypothalamohypophyseal system. The sharp decrease in thyroid gland function was regarded as the result of the action of the vaccine as a stressor and of the development of the immunological process. On the basis of their findings, these workers suggested that stressors may have a direct inhibitory action on the thyroid gland.

Other workers [52, 246, 290], however, consider that the response of the hypothalamus–pituitary–thyroid gland system to stress may be of the greatest importance in adaptation to unfavorable conditions. The response of the thyroid gland depends on the character of the stimulus and of the direction of its action [359, 532, 600]. After exposure to a single dose of the harmful agent, inhibition of thyroid function decreases rapidly and is followed after only 24 h by a compensatory increase in ^{131}I uptake by the gland. A stimulus acting on an animal already exposed to stress may actually stimulate thyroid gland activity. A chronic stimulus (extensive surgical trauma, for example) induces prolonged hypofunction of the thyroid parenchyma, as reflected in its morphological changes. The activation of the thyroid gland observed in response to the action of a weak stimulus is followed by inhibition of its function if the pathological factor is intensified [532, 600].

Changes in the serum protein-bound iodine concentration have been found after pyrexial and electric shock therapy [442]. Badrick et al. [49] investigated the uptake of ^{131}I by the thyroid gland of rats after they had been made to swim in water at 15 or 40°C for 10–15 min after electric shock and also after intraperitoneal injection of adrenalin. All these procedures evoked a decrease in the uptake of ^{131}I by the thyroid gland both in intact rats and in hypophysectomized and adrenalectomized rats. Inhibition of thyroid gland function after electric shock and injection of adrenalin was temporary and passed off quickly. These workers showed that the ^{131}I uptake is reduced only *in vivo*, and they were unable to find any change in the uptake of iodine *in vitro* by thyroid gland slices.

Some investigators have observed species differences in the response of the thyroid gland to stress. Gerwing et al. [203], for instance, showed that injections of bacterial endotoxin reduce the rate of elimination of ^{131}I by the thyroid gland in rats, mice, and rabbits but increase the secretion of thyroid hormones in guinea pigs and monkeys. However, Brown-Grant and Pethers [95] found that a variety of procedures (noise, electric shock, diphtheria toxin, typhoid vaccine, etc.) depress thyroid gland function in guinea pigs in precisely the same way as in rats and rabbits.

Other workers state that there is no change in thyroid gland activity or that it is actually stimulated during stress. In particular, the effect of muscle contractions on the blood levels of thyroid hormones and on the rate of excretion of injected thyroxine has been investigated in healthy human subjects [373]. Determination of the butanol-extractable iodine in the serum and the PBI and radioactivity of the serum showed that muscular contraction caused no clear changes in the concentration of the hormone in the serum; i.e., walking for long distances or swimming for 13 min had no appreciable effect on the thyroxine utilization by the tissues, as was reflected in the peripheral concentration of the hormone. The same workers showed that muscular exertion in young persons causes no change in the concentration of thyroid hormones in the blood or in the rate of disappearance of injected labeled hormone from the blood. However, experiments on thyroidectomized rats showed that muscular exertion accelerates the disappearance of thyroxine from the blood and organs of the gastrointestinal tract [161]. This observation evidently reflects the actual changes more correctly. Surgical intervention, trauma, or emotional stress may actually increase the plasma hormonal iodine concentration.

Falconer [169, 170] and also Falconer and Hetzel [171] observed an increase in the PBI concentration in blood flowing from the thyroid gland of sheep starting 12–20 min after emotional stress (barking of a dog, gunfire) and continuing for 2 h. Similar investigations by Mason et al. [411]

showed that the level of butanol-extractable iodine rose to twice its initial value and remained high for two to three weeks. Harrison et al. [258] showed in experiments on monkeys exposed every 20 sec to electric shock that most of the experimental animals developed neurotic responses with an increase in the PBI and butanol-extractable iodine levels. The effect of emotional stress, activating the thyroid gland, has also been demonstrated by the high relative importance of psychic trauma among the causes of toxic goiter in man.

Investigations have shown phasic changes in thyroid gland activity under the influence of external stimuli [139, 185, 209]. According to Goldenberg et al. [227, 228], thyroid gland function is initially increased in response to stress (surgical trauma). However, the activation of adrenocortical activity subsequently inhibits the secretion of thyroid hormones. At the same time, as was pointed out above, by no means all investigators have found regular changes in thyroid gland function in stress. Many workers who have investigated the state of the thyroid gland during exposure to a diversity of unfavorable factors (starvation, hypoxia, shock, poisoning, etc.) have obtained contradictory results.

To sum up, therefore, it has not yet been proved that the thyroid gland responds by uniform changes of activity to exposure to all types of stimuli (as, for example, does the adrenal cortex). It therefore seems doubtful that the thyroid gland is concerned in the formation of the adaptation syndrome—the standard set of responses of the body to the action of a stressor as such, i.e., a stimulus with no qualitative specificity. More likely the type of response of the thyroid gland is determined by the type or quality of the factor inducing the response. However, the sphere of participation of thyroid hormones in the adaptive responses of the body is considerable. Administration of thyroid hormones to animals stimulates phagocytosis [323], and phagocytic activity is reduced when thyroid function is deficient. Thyroid extract stimulates antibody formation [10].

Administration of an excess of thyroid hormones, leading to an increase in the intensity or a change in direction of tissue metabolism and disturbing the vitamin balance, increases the sensitivity of the body to poisons and infections. In rats with hyperthyroidism, for instance, sensitivity to ergotamine is sharply increased; thyroxine reduces the resistance of mice and rabbits to Shiga dysentery toxin and in guinea pigs to diphtheria toxin. Injection of thyroid hormones into guinea pigs increases their susceptibility to typhoid infection.

Thyroidectomy has the opposite direction, i.e., it increases resistance to pharmacological agents, toxins, and infections. For example, thyroidectomy reduces the sensitivity of guinea pigs to pharmacological poisons and also to adrenalin and histamine. It increases the resistance of dogs to diphtheria toxin and increases the resistance of rabbits to infection with *Shigella shigae*. Many workers have found that preliminary thyroidectomy reduces the sensitivity of rabbits and guinea pigs to sensitization and anaphylaxis; injection of thyroid hormones in the period of sensitization restores the susceptibility of thyroidectomized animals. As regards the effect of thyroidectomy on the formation of various antibodies (hemolysins, agglutinins, precipitins, antitoxins), workers using different species of animals (horses, dogs, rabbits) have obtained contradictory results, and reliable conclusions cannot be drawn.

As long ago as 1910, Asher et al. [34] found that thyroidectomized animals, because of their lowered basal metabolism and oxygen consumption, are less susceptible to to anoxia than normal animals. This was later confirmed by many other workers [154, 173]. Hyperfunction of the thyroid gland or administration of an excess of thyroid hormones, on the other hand, reduces the resistance of the body to anoxia [134, 564].

Animals receiving thyroid extract are more susceptible to shock [344, 474], probably because of the circulatory disturbances and tissue anoxia developing in shock. Krushinskii and Dobrokhotova [349] studied the effect of the functional state of the thyroid gland in rats on mortality from shock and hemorrhagic states produced by intensive acoustic stimulation and showed that hyperthyroidization increased the mortality level eightfold. In the overwhelming majority of thyroidized rats, symptoms of a severe state of shock developed from the first minute of action of the acoustic stimulus, ending with the early death of the animal. Removal of the thyroid gland reduced the mortality. Similar results were obtained by Kovach et al. [342]. In these workers' experiments, the survival after shock was considerably shortened if the animals were fed for the previous 1–3 weeks with minced thyroid gland or if they received preliminary thyroxine (100 μg/100 g body weight). The addition of methylthiouracil to the diet for three weeks, on the other hand, prolonged survival after shock. Other investigations [612] showed a decrease in the resistance of animals to shock-inducing factors whether thyroid gland function was increased or decreased.

Thyroid hormones play an important role in the outcome of terminal states and, together with other hormones, they evidently determine the course of compensatory processes and the restoration of vital functions in the early postresuscitation period as well as the eventual results of resuscitation. Ladygin [362] studied the effect of pharmacological inhibition of thyroid gland function and saturation of the body with thyroid hormones on dying (clinical death was produced by exsanguination) and revival. Administration of thyroid extract shortened the dying period in rabbits and cats, and after clinical death it impaired the restoration of the bodily functions. In animals treated with methylthiouracil, the duration of dying was unchanged but restoration of cardiac activity and spontaneous respiration was greatly facilitated; during resuscitation the arterial pressure was higher and more stable. Prolongation of the times of clinical death under experimental conditions by thyrostatic agents was also observed by Voss and Schoen [636].

Efremova [154], working in Negovskii's laboratory, showed in experiments on dogs that a deficiency of thyroid hormones is accompanied by delay in dying processes and by improved changes of survival after prolonged clinical death, preceded by a short period of dying. An excess of thyroid hormones in the body adversely affected the restoration of vital functions after only a short period of dying. Full and effective resuscitation was possible under these conditions only after clinical death from blood loss and only in some animals.

Thyroid hormones have a particularly important role in thermoregulation and adaptation of the body to various environmental temperature conditions. If the external environmental temperature is lowered, thyroid gland function is increased in several animals and man, and the production of thyroid hormones rises [126, 259, 260, 261, 563]. Exposure of laboratory animals to cold stimulates thyroid gland function [578]. The secretion of the thyroid gland is stimulated by cooling, when the demand for increased metabolism arises. Watanabe et al. [640] demonstrated a decrease in the PBI level in both men and women in the winter and autumn seasons, possibly on account of the more rapid metabolism of the thyroid gland hormones.

The effect on temperature of the thyroid gland has been demonstrated both by histological methods, based on the increase in height of the follicular cells, and by the increased absorption and circulation of radioiodine. Experiments on animals after dividing the brain stem demonstrated that the stimulus acts on the temperature control center in the mesencephalon [617]. Animals under cold conditions require more thyroxine to prevent the goitrogenic action of thiouracil than under hot conditions; this may reflect the increased requirements of the hormone by the peripheral tissues [138]. The need thus observed is manifested as stimulation of the thyroid gland via the mesencephalon and pituitary. Regular activation of the thyroid gland during exposure to cold is one basis for excluding its reactions from the general adaptation syndrome for, as we have seen, the thyroid gland responds to most other factors in the opposite way.

In rats kept for several days at a low temperature, hyperplasia of the thyroid gland is found [528], and, judging from the incorporation of radioactive iodine into circulating thyroid hormones [93], and also from the increase in the oxygen demand [590], the synthesis and secretion of thyroxine are increased. Activation of a feedback mechanism between the blood hormone level and the hypothalamohypophyseal centers of regulation, secreting thyrotropin-releasing factor and thyrotropic hormone, probably plays the decisive role in the stimulation of thyroid gland function in response to cold. Adaptation to cold is in fact accompanied by increased metabolism of thyroid hormones in the tissues [658], and this could lead to an initial decrease in their blood concentration. The relations between the times of the change in the blood thyroxine concentration and activation of the higher centers of regulation of the thyroid gland during exposure of the organism to cold have evidently not yet been sufficiently investigated. By analogy with other stress situations, a mechanism of plus–minus interaction must evidently be considered to have a subordinate role under these conditions. Increased activity of the hypothalamic centers regulating the thyroid gland and secretion of thyrotropin from the anterior pituitary is determined chiefly by ascending nervous impulses. Otherwise it would be difficult to understand the prolonged elevation of the blood thyroid hormone level during adaptation to cold.

The increased secretion of these hormones is the main reason why animals can survive in a low external environmental temperature, for thyroidectomized animals die if exposed to less severe cooling or sooner after the beginning of cooling [528] than control animals, and the administration of thyroid preparations restores their normal ability to survive in cold [80]. Laties and Weiss [374] taught rats to create the required temperature in a chamber by pressing on a pedal and showed that when the air temperature was lowered to 2°C, thyroidectomized animals created a higher environmental temperature than intact animals. Injection of triiodothyronine restored the normal heat requirements of the rats. The role of thyroid hormones in acclimatization to cold is also confirmed by the fact that an increased oxygen demand in response to cold arises only in tissues whose oxidative processes are accelerated by thyroxine. The brain, spleen, testes, and ovaries do not increase their oxygen demand during cooling of the animals; this likewise does not happen after administration of thyroid hormones [642]. An excess of these hormones gives rise to better adaptability to cold, but at the same time it reduces the animal's ability to withstand high temperatures. The characteristic subfebrile temperature of clinical thyrotoxicosis and the raised temperature of animals receiving large doses of thyroid preparations also point to a disturbance of thermoregulation in thyroid gland dysfunction.

The effects of deep hypothermia on thyroid function have recently been investigated under experimental conditions. Andjus studied the uptake of radioiodine by the thyroid gland of rats while the body temperature was maintained at between 16 and 39°C and showed that the lower the body temperature, the lower the rate of iodine uptake by the thyroid gland [41]. Most of the fixed iodine was found in the organically bound form, mainly in monoiodotyrosine and diiodotyrosine.

Similar results were obtained by Verzar et al. [629] and Mach et al. [396] using rats in hypoxic hypothermia. When the body temperature was 15–20°, the thyroid gland could not assimilate radioactive iodine. At a temperature of 25–28°C the activity of the gland was slightly reduced. The environmental temperature also affected the serum PBI concentration. According to Kassenaar et al. [320], the serum PBI level in thyroidectomized rats maintained with a daily dose of 6 μg thyroxine was much lower at 4°C than at 21 and 36°C, whereas in normal rats the serum PBI level was higher at the low temperature than at the high temperature.

A study of oxygen absorption in thyroidectomized rats receiving thyroxine and adrenalin at temperatures of 10, 18, and 30°C showed that thyroxine at low temperatures stimulates the calorigenic action of adrenalin, and that this is the main role of the thyroid hormone in adaptation to cold [396]. Sultanov [586] found that after rats had been heated in a hot chamber to 45°C, the rate and degree of uptake of ^{131}I by the thyroid gland were reduced. The decrease in the radioiodine level in the gland took place on account of both inorganic and organic iodine [478].

Woods and Carlson [658] studied the effect of prolonged cooling on thyroxine secretion and on the rate of circulation of thyroid hormones in rats kept for between 1 and 180 days at 5°C. After a stay of only two weeks at the low temperature, the thyroxine secretion was increased considerably, and so also was the rate of circulation of thyroid hormones. The thyroid gland has a definite regulatory effect on the oxygen consumption at a lowered temperature. For example, removal of the thyroid gland from rats kept at 5°C reduced the oxygen consumption to a minimum on the 8th day, and in rats kept at 28°C on the 12th day [286].

Like the effect of thyroid hormones on other processes, their role in adaptation to changes in temperature conditions of existence is closely interwoven with the effects of other hormones, and at present it is very difficult to distinguish the independent role of thyroid hormones *in vivo*. The facts described above do, however, indicate the undoubted importance of thyroid hormones in determining the resistance of the organism to many unfavorable factors. This role is evidently affected by a change in the general metabolic rate, accompanied by a change in the oxygen demand of the body cells and in the temperature conditions under which they function. Any attempt to explain the "molecular" mechanism of action of the thyroid hormones must therefore take into account their effect not only on oxidative metabolism, but also on the heat balance of the cell.

Data on the action of whole-body irradiation on thyroid gland function are also to be found in the literature. An increase in the uptake of ^{131}I was observed 2 h after irradiation in a dose of 800–1000 R; this increase lasted for 24 h and was then followed by a decrease. Larger doses of irradiation also increased the radioiodine uptake; however, there was a small initial decrease which can be explained by increased secretion of adrenocortical hormones.

Local X-ray irradiation of the rat thyroid gland, according to Tuzhilkova [611], led to prolonged depression of thyroid function, after a transient increase in activity. Ablyaeva [7] investigated the formation of thyroid hormones and their transport by the blood after local X-irradiation of the gland and also after whole-body irradiation. She found stimulation of thyroid function during the first days after both whole-body and local irradiation, followed by inhibition on subsequent days. Changes in the uptake of iodine and the synthesis of thyroid hormones are fluctuating in character and determine the blood protein-bound iodine level.

Finally, it is interesting to note that exposure of mice to darkness stimulates thyroid function, as is shown by an increase in size of the gland and in the absorption of ^{131}I, whereas exposure to light had the opposite effect. Guzek and Mach [247] found an increase in the blood iodine concentration in rabbits kept for a long time in darkness, while the iodine content in the thyroid gland was reduced.

REFERENCES FOR PART II

1. Abbot, A. J., and Van Buskirk, F. W. *Am. J. Med. Sci. 182*:610, 1931.
2. Abdurakhimov, F. A. *Probl. Éndokrinol., 1965* (11):6.
3. Abe, T. *Ref. Zh. Biol. Khim. 210*:226, 1961.
4. Abelin, J. In: *Fermente, Hormone, Vitamine und die Beziehungen dieser Wirkstoffe zumeinander*, vol. 2 (Hormone), Stuttgart, 1960, p. 77.
5. Abelin, J., and Kürsteiner, P. *Biochem. Z. 198*:19, 1928.
6. Abelin, J., and Ryser, H. *Helv. Med. Acta 24*:321, 1957.
7. Ablyaeva, N. Kh. *Effect of Co^{60} γ-rays on the formation and transport of thyroid hormones.* Author's abstract of candidate's dissertation, Tashkent, 1970.
8. Abrams, G. D., and Baker, B. L. *Gastroenterology 27*:462, 1954.
9. Ackerman, W. G., Smith, R. W., Jr., and Miller, J. M. *Metabolism 10*:27, 1961.
10. Adamov, A. K., and Nikolaev, N. I. *The Molecular and Cellular Basis of Immunology* (in Russian), Saratov University Press, Saratov, 1966.
11. Adams, A., and Doljanski, F. *Endocrinology 62*:129, 1958.
12. Aebi, H., and Abelin, J. *Biochem. J. 324*:364, 1953.
13. Aiyar, A. S., Sulebele, G. A., Rege, D. V., and Sreenivasan, A. *Nature 184*:1867, 1959.
14. Aizenshtein, F. A. *Proceedings of the First Conference of Morphologists and Endocrinologists* (in Russian), Moscow, 1960.
15. Aizenshtein, F. A. *Probl. Éndokrinol. Gormonoter. 13*:84, 1967.
16. Akishina, N. I., Lutsenko, G. S., and Markova, E. V. In: *Proceedings of a Conference on Cortico-Visceral Relations and Hormonal Regulation* (in Russian), Khar'kov, 1963, p. 8.
17. Aleshin, B. V. *Probl. Éndokrinol. 16*:108, 1970.
18. Alexander, R. W., and Marmarston, J. *J. Clin. Endocrinol. Metabol. 21*:243, 1961.
19. Aliev, M. N., and Gaidina, G. A. *Byull. Éksp. Biol. Med. 3*:42, 1973.
20. Allousi, A., and Mallow, S. *Am. J. Physiol. 206*:603, 1964.
21. Althousen, T. L. *J. Am. Med. Assoc. 115*:101, 1940.
22. Althousen, T. L., and Stockholm, M. *Am. J. Physiol. 123*:577, 1938.
23. Altschule, M. D. *N. Engl. J. Med. 233*:265, 1945.
24. Ambrus, G., and Ambrus, L. *Orgosok Lapja 3*:865, 1947.
25. Anan'eva, K. A. In: *Problems in Goiter and Thyrotoxicosis* (in Russian), Moscow, 1955, p. 62.
26. Andersen, R. R., Grossie, J. A., and Turner, C. W. *Proc. Soc. Exp. Biol. Med. 107*:571, 1961.
27. Antopol, W., Tuchman, L., and Schifrin, A. *Proc. Soc. Exp. Biol. Med. 36*:46, 1937.
28. Antopol, W., Schifrin, A., and Tuchman, L. *Proc. Soc. Exp. Biol. Med. 38*:363, 1938.
29. Aron, C., Gender, R., and Asch, L. *C. R. Soc. Biol. 151*:2193, 1957.

30. Arslanov, A. S., and Gasanov, S. G. *Byull. Eksp. Biol. Med., 1967*(12):38.
31. Aschkenasy, A. *Sang 27*:97, 1956.
32. Aschkenasy, A. *Sang 23*:89, 1952.
33. Aschkenasy, A. *Sang 28*:485, 1957.
34. Asher, L., and Flack, M. *J. Physiol. (London) 24*:211, 1910.
35. Asling, W., Simpson, M., and Evans, H. In: *Transactions of the 3rd Conference on Metabolic Interrelations*, New York, 1951, p. 125.
36. Asper, S. P., Selenkow, H. A., and Plamorklon, C. *Bull. Johns Hopkins Hosp. 93*:164, 1953.
37. Ass-Babich, B. T. *Formation of Antibacterial Immunity and the Thyroid Gland.* Author's abstract of candidate's dissertation, Khar'kov, 1967.
38. Astrauskas, V. I. *The Hypothalamo-Hypophyseo-Adrenal System and Reactivity of the Organism.* Author's abstract of doctoral dissertation, Vilnius, 1968.
39. Asu, J. M. In: *Vitamins and Hormones*, Vol. 21, New York, 1963, p. 113.
40. Aub, J. C., Bauer, W., Heath, C., and Ropes, M. *J. Clin. Invest. 7*:97, 1929.
41. Andjus, R., Lachives, F., and Olivereau, M. *C. R. Acad. Sci. 238*:838, 1954.
42. Aulov, D. M., Islambekov, R. K., and Turakulov, Ya. Kh. *Abstracts of Proceedings of an Annual Scientific Session of the All-Union Institute of Experimental Endocrinology* (in Russian), Moscow, 1961.
43. Awwad, H., and Coolden, A. W. *Clin. Sci. 20*:113, 1961.
44. Axelrod, A. R., and Berman, L. *Blood 6*:436, 1951.
45. Azimov, G. M. *Zh. Éksp. Biol. Med. 8*:85, 1927.
46. Babichev, V. N. *Electrophysiological Characteristics of the Transmission of Excitation in Sympathetic Ganglia Depending on the Hormone Content of the Thyroid Gland.* Dissertation for the degree of candidate of biological sciences, Leningrad, 1964.
47. Babichev, V. N. *Probl. Éndokrinol. 13*:108, 1967.
48. Bachmann, K., and Griese, M. *Med. Welt 28*:1464; *29–30*:1500, 1961.
49. Badrick, F. E., Brimblecombe, R. W., Reiss, S. M., and Reiss, M. J. *Endocrinology 11*:305, 1954.
50. Badrutdinov, M. G. *Probl. Éndokrinol. Gormonoter. 8*:3, 1962.
51. Baikle, A. G., and Lawson, N. *Lancet 1*:86, 1965.
52. Balze, F. A., Socolsky, R. C., Yanches, M., De Paoli, Y. C., Funes, Y., and Goldberg, V. *Folia Endocrinol. 21*:611, 1968.
53. Baranov, V. G. *Diseases of the Endocrine System and Metabolism* (in Russian), Medgiz, Leningrad, 1965.
54. Baranov, V. G. In: *Textbook of Internal Medicine in Several Volumes* (in Russian), Meditsina, 1966, pp. 9–178.
55. Baranov, V. G., Loskutova, E. A., and Propp, M. V. *Probl. Éndokrinol. 16*:43, 1970.
56. Baranov, V. G., Speranskaya, E. N., and Tendler, D. S. *Probl. Éndokrinol. Gormonoter. 1*:28, 1955.
57. Bargoni, N., Luzzati, A., Rinando, M. T., Rossini, L., and Strumia, E. *J. Physiol. Chem. 326*:65, 1961.
58. Barker, S. B., and Lewis, W. J. *Proc. Soc. Exp. Biol. Med. 91*:650, 1956.
59. Barkov, V. D. In: *Problems in Clinical Medicine.* Transactions of Perm' Medical Institute, No. 28, Perm', 1958, p. 81.
60. Barron, D. H. *J. Neurophysiol. 3*:403, 1940.
61. Baru, I. M. In: *Proceedings of the First Congress of Endocrinologists of the Ukrainian SSR* (in Russian), Khar'kov, 1965, p. 53.
62. Baschieri, L., and Campanacci, L. *Folia Endocrinol. 10*:489, 1957.
63. Beaven, M. A., Costa, E., and Brodie, B. B. *Life Sci. 4*:241, 1963.
64. Beck, R. N. *Endocrinology 62*:347, 1958.

65. Benetato, G., Oprishu, K., Rozenfel'd, E., and Vasilesku, V. *Probl. Éndokrinol. Gormonoter.* *5*:43, 1959.
66. Benua, R. S., Leeper, R. D., Kumaoka, S., Rawson, R. W. *Ann. N. Y. Acad. Sci.* *86*: 563, 1960.
67. Berezovskaya, B. M. *The Velocity of the Blood Flow (the Circulation Time) in Cardiovascular Patients.* Dissertation, Odessa, 1940.
68. Berg, H. *Arch. Exp. Pathol. Pharmakol.* *185*:359, 1937.
69. Berryhill, W. R., and Williams, H. A. *J. Clin. Invest.* *11*:753, 1932.
70. Betheil, J. J., and Lardy, H. A. *J. Nutr.* *37*:495, 1949.
71. Beznak, M. *Can. J. Biochem. Physiol.* *40*:1647, 1962.
72. Bhagat, B., and Lockett, M. F. *J. Endocrinol.* *23*:227, 1961.
73. Biggs, J. C., and Witts, L. J. *Isr. Med. J.* *22*:294, 1963.
74. Biström, O. *Acta Chir. Scand.* *94* (Suppl. 114):1, 1946.
75. Bixler, D., Muhler, I. C., Webster, R. C., and Shater, W. G. *Proc. Soc. Exp. Biol. Med.* *94*:521, 1957.
76. Blair, D. W., Williams, M. F., Carr, A. J., and Kilpatrick, S. J. *Gut.* *6*:343, 1965.
77. Blum, K. U., and Schols, A. *Klin. Wschr.* *45*:516, 1967.
78. Blumgart, H. L., Cargill, S. L., and Gilligan, D. R. *J. Clin. Invest.* *9*:91, 1931.
79. Bock, O. A. A., and Witts, L. J. *Br. Med. Bull.* *11*:20, 1963.
80. Bodansky, M., Pilcher, L. F., and Duff, V. B. *J. Exp. Med.* *63*:523, 1936.
81. Boekelman, A. J. *Presse Méd.* *56*:23, 1948.
82. Bomford, R. *Q. J. Med.* *7*:495, 1938.
83. Bondarenko, M. F. *Probl. Éndokrinol., 1967*(1):67.
84. Borimskaya, A. R. *A Study of Metabolism in the Heart during Disturbances of Its Function.* Candidate's dissertation, Kiev, 1953.
85. Botkin, S. P. *Clinical Lectures, 1885* (in Russian), Moscow, 1952.
86. Boyd, E. *Am. J. Dis. Child.* *43*:1162, 1932.
87. Boyd, G. S. In: *Hormones and Atherosclerosis.* Academic Press, New York, 1959, p. 49.
88. Bradley, P. B., Eayrs, J. T., and Schmalbach, R. E. E. *J. Clin. Neurophysiol.* *12*:467, 1960.
89. Bressler, R., and Wittels, B. *J. Clin. Invest.* *45*:34, 1966.
90. Broder, I., Langer, B., Ezrin, C., and Horsey, W. I. *Endocrinology* *68*:559, 1961.
91. Bronshtein, M. E., and Negovskaya, A. V. *Byull. Éksp. Biol. Med., 1971*(2):25.
92. Brown, R. B., Pendergrass, E. P., and Burdick, E. D. *Surg. Gynecol. Obstet.* *73*:766, 1941.
93. Brown-Grant, K. *J. Physiol. (London)* *131*:52, 1956.
94. Brown-Grant, K., Harris, G. W., and Reichlin, S. *J. Physiol. (London)* *126*:29, 1954.
95. Brown-Grant, K., and Pethers, G. *J. Physiol. (London)* *151*:40, 1960.
96. Buccino, R. A., Spann, J. E., Pool, P. E., Sonnenblick, E. H., and Braunwald, E. *J. Clin. Invest.* *46*:1669, 1967.
97. Bülbring, E. *Br. J. Pharmacol.* *4*:234, 1949.
98. Burn, J. H., *Br. Med. J.* *1*:784, 1952.
99. Burton, S. D., Robbins, E. D., and Byers, S. O. *Proc. Soc. Exp. Biol. Med.* *92*:272, 1958.
100. Bussel', G. A. *The Hemodynamics in Basedow's Disease* (in Russian), Tashkent, 1949.
101. Buso, R., Olavarrieta, S. T., and Suarez, R. M. *J. Clin. Endocrinol.* *18*:501, 1958.
102. Byere, S. O., Rosenman, R. H., Friedman, M., and Biggs, M. W. *J. Exp. Med.* *96*:513, 1952.
103. Byrot, F. B., *Clin. Sci.* *1*:273, 1933–1934.
104. Byshevskii, A. Sh. *Probl. Éndokrinol., 1960*(3):62.
105. Canal, N., and Maffei-Faccioli, A. *Chem. Abstr.* *54*:16631, 1960.
106. Canzanelli, A., Guild, R., and Rapport, D. *Endocrinology* *41*:108, 1947.

107. Cereijo-Santalo, R., Dinella, R., Park, C. R., and Park, I. H. *Endocrinology 69*:422, 1961.
108. Carr, C. W., and Woods, K. R. *Arch. Biochem. Biophys. 55*:1, 1955.
109. Castor, C. W., and Beierwaltes, W. . *J. Clin. Endocrinol. 16*:102, 1956.
110. Challoner, D. R. *Am. J. Physiol. 216*:905, 1969.
111. Chang, H. C., and Sloan, J. H. *Am. J. Physiol. 80*:732, 1927.
112. Chatagner, F., and Gautheron, D. *Biochim. Biophys. Acta 41*:544, 1960.
113. Cherdyntsev, S. G. *Probl. Éndokrinol. Gormonoter. 8*:30, 1962.
114. Chernogorov, I. A. *Disturbance of the Cardiac Rhythm* (in Russian), Medgiz, Moscow, 1962.
115. Cherny, S. N., Chausmer, A. B., Bellavia, J. V., and Wallach, S. *Endocrinology 86*:1337, 1970.
116. Chilson, O. P., and Sacks, J. *Proc. Soc. Exp. Biol. Med. 101*:331, 1959.
117. Christophe, J., and Mayer, J. *Endocrinology 65*:475, 1959.
118. Cline, M. J., and Berlin, N. I. *Am. J. Physiol. 204*:415, 1964.
119. Cloche, R., Azerad, E., and Stuhe, L. *Ann. Endocrinol. (Paris) 19*:103, 1958.
120. Coggeshall, H. C., and Greene, I. A. *Am. J. Physiol. 105*:103, 1933.
121. Colle-Vandecelde, A., and Elewant, A. *C. R. Acad. Sci. 273*:894, 1971.
122. Collignon, G., Badhidantz, A., Baret, A., Maura, Anne-Marie, and Blanquet, P. *C. R. Acad. Sci. 271*:1552, 1970.
123. Condon, I. V., Becka, R., and Gibbs, T. A. *J. Clin. Endocrinol. 14*:1511, 1954.
124. Conquilhem, B., and Malan, A. *Arch. Sci. Physiol. 25*:517, 1971.
125. Cope, C. L., and Wolff, B. *Biochem. J. 35*:413, 1942.
126. Cottle, W. H. *Fed. Proc. 19*(Suppl. 5):59, 1960.
127. Crafts, R. C. *Endocrinology 29*:596, 1941.
128. Crafts, R. C. *Endocrinology 53*:235, 1953.
129. Crispell, K. R., Parson, W., and Hollifield, G. *J. Clin. Invest. 35*:164, 1956.
130. Cure, A. D., Bates, R. F. L., Philippo, M., Lequin, R. W., Hackeng, W. H. Z., Barlet, J. P., and Larvor, P. *J. Endocrinol. 48*:667, 1970.
131. Cutting, W. C., and Tainter, M. L. *Proc. Soc. Exp. Biol. Med. 31*:97, 1933–34.
132. Dagaeva, L. N. In: *Proceedings of the 4th All-Union Conference of Pathophysiologists* (in Russian), Tbilisi, 1964, p. 39.
133. Dayton, S., Dayton, I., Drimmer, F., and Kendall, F. A. *Am. J. Physiol. 199*:71, 1960.
134. Debias, A. *Fed. Proc. 25*:1227, 1966.
135. Deineka, I. Ya., and Serkov, F. N. In: *Problems in Physiology* (in Russian), vol. 7, Kiev, 1954, p. 81.
136. Deitrich, R. A., and Smith, D. L. *Biochem. Pharmacol. 3*:85, 1960.
137. Demidenko, N. S., and Mamina, V. V. In: *Physiology, Biochemistry, and Pathochemistry of the Endocrine System* (in Russian), Kiev, 1969, p. 42.
138. Dempsey, E. W., and Astwood, E. B. *Endocrinology 32*:509, 1943.
139. Dewhurst, K. E., Elkabir, D. I., Harris, J. W., and Mandelbrote, B. M. *Confin. Neurol. 30*:161, 1968.
140. De Witt, M. *Endocrinology 69*:2, 1961.
141. Dillman, R. O., and Cady, P. *Endocrinology 8*:198, 1971.
142. D'Lorio, A., and Plaut, A. W. E. *Arch. Biochem. Biophys. 41*:153, 1952.
143. D'Lorio, A., Marvides, C. *Adv. Enzyme Regul. 1*:97, 1963.
144. Domino, E. F., and Mcas, B. *Arch. Int. Pharmacodyn. 94*:225, 1953.
145. Dozorets, Yu. A. *Probl. Éndokrinol. 6*:62, 1960.
146. Dow, D. S., and Allen, C. E. *Can. J. Biochem. Physiol. 39*:981, 1961.
147. Drill, V. A. *Physiol. Rev. 23*:355, 1943.
148. Du Bois, E. F. *Basal Metabolism in Health and Disease,* London, 1936.

149. Duncan, C. H., and Best, M. M. *Endocrinology 63*:169, 1958.
150. Durie, D. S., Micic, S. V., and Simic, N. *Acta Med. Iugosl. 17*:37, 1963.
151. Dutoit, C. H. In: *Phosphorus Metabolism,* vol. 1. Baltimore, 1951, p. 597.
152. Eaton, P., Steinberg, D., and Thompson, R. *J. Clin. Invest. 44*:247, 1965.
153. Efimov, A. S. In: *Problems in Neuroendocrine Pathology* (in Russian), Gor'kii, 1961, p. 30.
154. Efremova, N. M. *Effect of the Functional State of the Thyroid Gland on the Development of the Terminal State and Outcome of Resuscitation.* Candidate's dissertation, Moscow, 1970.
155. Eiler, J. J., Althausen, T. L., and Stokholm, M. *Am. J. Physiol. 140*:699, 1944.
156. Emerson, G. A. *Proc. Soc. Exp. Biol. Med. 70*:392, 1949.
157. Épel'baum, S. E., and Dergousova, E. A. In: *Abstracts of Proceedings of the 1st Urals Conference of Physiologists, Biochemists, and Pharmacologists* (in Russian), Sverdlovsk, 1956, p. 79.
158. Eriksson, S. *Proc. Soc. Exp. Biol. Med. 94*:582, 1957.
159. Ernström, U., and Gullensten, L. *Acta Pathol. Microbiol. Scand. 47*:243, 1959.
160. Ershoff, B. N. *Arch. Biochem. Biophys. 15*:365, 1947.
161. Escobar, R. F., and de Escobar, M. G. M. *Acta Endocrinol. 24*:393, 1956.
162. Éskin, I. A., and Samsonova, V. M. *Probl. Éndokrinol. 13*:56, 1967.
163. Éskin, I. A., and Skebel'skaya, Yu. B. *Proceedings of a Joint Session of the All-Union and Ukrainian Institutes of Experimental Endocrinology* (in Russian), Medgiz, Moscow, 1952.
164. Estabrook, R. W., Neufeld, H. A., and Mason, W. B. *Fed. Proc. 13*:205, 1954.
165. Éster, K. M., and Kandror, V. I. *Byull. Éksp. Biol. Med. 60*:118, 1965.
166. Evans, E. S., Miram, E., and Hervert, M. E. *Endocrinology 63*:836, 1958.
167. Evans, E. S., Rosenberg, L. L., and Simpson, M. E. *Endocrinology 68*:517, 1961.
168. Faber, M. *Acta Med. Scand. 114*:59, 1943.
169. Falconer, Y. R. *J. Endocrinol. 26*:241, 1963.
170. Falconer, Y. R. *J. Physiol. (London) 177*:215, 1965.
171. Falconer, Y. R., and Hetzel, B. S. *Endocrinology 75*:42, 1964.
172. Fatterpaker, P., Marfatia, V., and Sreenivasan, A. *Nature 176*:165, 1955.
173. Filatova, L. G. In: *Scientific Reports of the Faculty of Biology and Soil Science, Kirghiz University* (in Russian), Frunze, 1955, p. 68.
174. Filinovskaya, I. G. *Probl. Éndokrinol. Gormonoter. 11*:13, 1965.
175. Fisher, Y. W., Roh, B. L., Couch, C., and Nightingale, W. O. *Blood 23*:87, 1964.
176. Fletcher, K., and Myant, N. B. *J. Physiol. (London) 144*:361, 1958.
177. Fletcher, K., and Myant, N. B. *J. Physiol. (London) 154*:145, 1960.
178. Fogel'son, L. I. *Diseases of the Heart and Vessels* (in Russian), Moscow, 1958.
179. Fol'b, I. L. *Muscular Disturbances in Thyrotoxicosis in the Light of Some Biochemical Indices and Data of Electromyography.* Author's abstract of candidate's dissertation, Minsk, 1964.
180. Follis, R. H. *Bull. Johns Hopkins Hosp. 92*:405, 1953.
181. Forbes, I. C. *Endocrinology 35*:126, 1944.
181a. Ford, D. H. *Acta Anat. 43*:97.
182. Ford, D. H., and Rhines, R. *Brain Res. 6*:481, 1967.
183. Fraenkel-Conrat, J., and Greenberg, D. M. *Proc. Soc. Exp. Biol. Med. 63*:537, 1946.
184. Fränko, O. *Acta Anat. 16* (Suppl.):17, 1952.
185. Franksson, C., Hastad, K., and Larson, L. G. *Acta Chir. Scand. 118*:264, 1960.
186. Fridberg, D. I. *Klin. Med. 7*:51, 1954.
187. Fridberg, D. I. *Motor Disturbances in the Clinical Picture of Thyrotoxicosis and Their Pathogenesis.* Author's abstract of doctoral dissertation, Moscow, 1963.

188. Friedberg, C. K. In: *Diseases of the Heart.* Philadlephia, 1956.
189. Friedberg, F., and Greenberg, D. M. *J. Biol. Chem. 168*:405, 1947.
190. Frieden, E. *Am. Zool. 1*:115, 1961.
191. Friedlander, M., Laskey, N., and Silbert, S. *Endocrinology 19*:342, 1935.
192. Gaidina, G. A., Gol'ber, L. M., and Kryzhanovskii, G. N. *Byull. Éksp. Biol. Med. 74*(9): 24, 1972.
193. Galton, V. A. *Endocrinology 88*:976, 1971.
194. Gannong, W. F., and Hildegard, I. J. *Endocrinology 56*:105, 1955.
195. Ganzha, O. N. *Changes in Metabolism of some Energy-Yielding Substances in Experimental Thyrotoxicosis and Hyperthyroidism.* Candidate's dissertation, Kiev, 1954.
196. Gemmil, C. L. In: *Metal-Binding in Medicine* (Seven, M. I., ed.). Philadelphia, 1960, p. 321.
197. Genes, S. G. *The Nervous System and Internal Secretion* (in Russian), Medgiz, Moscow, 1955.
198. Genes, S. G. *Usp. Sovrem. Biol. 44*:186, 1957.
199. Genes, S. G., and Lesnoi, N. G. *Probl. Éndokrinol. 2*:38, 1956.
200. Georgieva, S. A., and Kuz'mina, K. A. In: *Problems in Physiology and Pathology of the Thyroid Gland* (in Russian), Saratov, 1962, p. 15.
201. Gershberg, H., and Kuhl, W. J. *J. Clin. Invest. 29*:1625, 1950.
202. Gershoff, S. N., Vital, J. J., Antonowicz, I., Nakamura, M., and Hellerstein, E. E. *J. Biol. Chem. 231*:849, 1958.
203. Gerwing, J., Long, D. A., and Pitt-Rivers, R. *J. Physiol. (London) 144*:229, 1958.
204. Gibbs, F. A., and Gibbs, E. L. *Atlas of Electroencephalography,* Cambridge, 1941.
205. Gibson, J. G., and Harris, A. W. *J. Clin. Invest. 18*:59, 1939.
206. Gimlette, T. M. D. *Br. Med. J. 2*:1143, 1959.
207. Gitman, L., Greenblatt, I. G., and Mitchell, N. *Proc. Soc. Exp. Biol. Med. 71*:179, 1949.
208. Glants, R. M. *Effect of the Thyroid Gland on Intensity of the Cholinergic Reactions of the Organism.* Candidate's dissertation, Khar'kov, 1949.
209. Glants, R. M. In: *Experience of the Use of Isotopes in Medicine* (in Russian), Kiev, 1955, p. 92.
210. Glock, G. E., and McLean, P. *Biochem. J. 61*:390, 1955.
211. Gol'ber, L. M. *The Role of the Spleen in the Regulation of Some Metabolic Functions of the Liver.* Doctoral dissertation, Riga, 1947.
212. Gol'ber, L. M. *Some New Data on Relations between the spleen and Liver in Metabolism* (in Russian), Riga, 1948.
213. Gol'ber, L. M., Anan'eva, K. A., Kandror, V. I., Kryukova, I. V., and Negovskaya, A. V. *Byull. Éksp. Biol. Med. 67*:23, 1969.
214. Gol'ber, L. M., Gaidina, G. A., and Ignatkov, V. Ya. *Probl. Éndokrinol. Gormonoter. 15*:77, 1969.
215. Gol'ber, L. M., Gaidina, G. A., and Ignatkov, V. Ya. *Dokl. Akad. Nauk SSSR 196*:987, 1971.
216. Gol'ber, L. M., Gaidina, G. A., Zhukova, N. I., and Ignatkov, V. Ya. In: *Mechanisms of Regulation of the Vital Activity of the Organism under Pathological Conditions* (in Russian), Baku, 1970.
217. Gol'ber, L. M., and Kandror, V. I. In: *Abstracts of Proceedings of the First All-Union Biochemical Congress* (in Russian), no. 2, Izd. AN SSSR, 1964, p. 295.
218. Gol'ber, L. M., and Kandror, V. I. In: *Textbook of Pathological Physiology in Several Volumes* (in Russian), vol. 4, Meditsina, Moscow, 1966, p. 219.
219. Gol'ber, L. M., and Kandror, V. I. *Kardiologiya 7*:53, 1967.
220. Gol'ber, L. M., and Kandror, V. I. In: *Abstracts of Proceedings of Symposia at the 2nd All-Union Biochemical Congress* (in Russian), Tashkent, 1969, p. 142.

221. Gol'ber, L. M., Kandror, V. I., and Dagaeva, L. N. *Patol. Fiziol. Éksp. Ter. 10*:16, 1966.
222. Gol'ber, L. M., Kandror, V. I., and Éster, K. M. In: *Physiology and Pathology of the Endocrine System* (in Russian), Khar'kov, 1965, p. 129.
223. Gol'ber, L. M., Kandror, V. I., and Éster, K. M. *Cor Vasa 9*:3, 1967.
224. Gol'ber, L. M., Kandror, V. I., Kryukova, I. V., and Zhukova, N. I. In: *Proceedings of the 2nd Endocrinological Conference of the Belorussian, Latvian, and Lithuanian SSRs* (in Russian), Vilnius, 1966, p. 23.
225. Gol'ber, L. M., Kandror, V. I., Salakhova, N. S., and Shakhnarovich, V. M. *Kardiologiya 10*:98, 1970.
226. Gold, M., Scott, I., and Spitzer, I. *Am. J. Physiol. 213*:239, 1967.
227. Goldenberg, I. S., Lutwak, L., and Rosenbaum, P., and Hayes, M. A. *J. Clin. Endocrinol. 15*:227, 1955.
228. Goldenberg, I. S., Rosenbaum, P. J., White, C., and Hayes, M. A. *Surg. Gynec. Obstet. 104*:295, 1957.
229. Goldsmith, D. P. J., and Nasset, E. S. *Am. J. Physiol. 197*:1, 1959.
230. Goldstein, M. S. *J. Biol. Chem. 199*:923, 1952.
231. Golovach, A. P. *Some Aspects of Serotonin and Catecholamine Metabolism in Diseases of the Thyroid Gland.* Candidate's dissertation, Khar'kov, 1969.
232. Gona, A. G., Perlman, T., and Etkin, W. *J. Endocrinol. 48*:585, 1970.
233. Goodall, M. *Acta Physiol. Scand. 24* (Suppl.):85, 1951.
234. Gordon, A. S., Kadow, P. C., and Finkelstein, G. *Am. J. Med. Sci. 212*:385, 1946.
235. Gordon, O. L., Khvorov, V. V., and Chernya, Yu. I. *Probl. Éndokrinol. 6*:117, 1941.
236. Gorkin, V. Z. *The Nature of Mitochondrial Monoamine Oxidases.* Doctoral dissertation, Moscow, 1964.
237. Gorkin, V. Z., Kandror, V. I., Krivchenkova, R. S., and Shakhnarovich, V. M. *Probl. Éndokrinol. 13*:64, 1967.
238. Gottlieb, R. *J. Lab. Clin. Med. 19*:371, 1934.
239. Gould, R. C., Leroy, G. V., Okita, G. T., Kabara, J. J., Keegan, P., and Bergenstal, D. M. *J. Lab. Clin. Med. 46*:372, 1953.
240. Graettinger, J. S., Muester, J. J., Selverstone, L. A., and Campbell, J. A. *J. Clin. Invest. 38*:1316, 1959.
241. Grashchenkov, N. I., *The Hypothalamus and Its Role in Physiology and Pathology* (in Russian), Moscow, 1964.
242. Grawer, R. C., Starkey, W. F., and Saler, E. *Endocrinology 30*:474, 1942.
243. Grigor'ev, P. Ya. *Ter. Arkh. 1965*(6):91.
244. Grosvenor, C. E., and Turner, C. W. *Proc. Soc. Exp. Biol. Med. 101*:194, 1959.
245. Günter, H. Cited by Rajmon, J. *Zbl. Chir. 83*:2329, 1958.
246. Gurevich, G. M., and Mastbaum, I. S. *Thyrotoxicosis and Its Surgical Treatment* (in Russian), Meditsina, Moscow, 1968.
247. Guzek, J. W., and Mach, L. *Patol. Pol., 1957*:265.
248. Gzerniak, P., and Itelson, I. *Sem. Hôp. Pathol. Biol. 8*:1889, 1960.
249. Halevy, S., and Avivi, L. *Biochim. Biophys. Acta 30*:198, 1958.
250. Halmi, N. S., and Barker, S. B. *Endocrinology 51*:127, 1952.
251. Halnan, K. E. *Clin. Sci. 17*:281, 1958.
252. Hamburgh, M., and Flexner, L. B. *J. Neurochem. 1*:279, 1957.
253. Hamburger, V., Smith, R., and Miller, V. *Metabolism 12*:821, 1963.
254. Hamolsky, M. W., Michel, R., Carnicero, H., and Roche, J. *Biochim. Biophys. Acta 69*:420, 1963.
255. Handler, P. *J. Biol. Chem. 173*:295, 1948.
256. Hardt, L. L. J. *Am. J. Physiol. 40*:314, 1916.
257. Harrison, T. S. *Lancet 11*:1311, 1961.

258. Harrison, R. S., Silver, D. M., and Luidema, J. D. *Endocrinology 78*:685, 1966.
259. Hart, J. S. *Fed. Proc. 71*:1045, 1958.
260. Hart, J. S. *Fed. Proc. 19*(Suppl. 5):15, 1960.
261. Hartfall, S. Y. *Br. Med. J. 1*:136, 1934.
262. Hawkins, R. D., Nishikawara, M., and Mendel, B. *Endocrinology 43*:167, 1948.
263. Herrlich, H. C., Raab, W., and Gigce, W. *Arch. Int. Pharmacodyn. 129*:201, 1960.
264. Hegglin, R., Ruteschauser, W., Kaufmann, G., Luthy, E., and Scheu, H. *Kreislaufdiagnostik mit der Farbstoffverdünnungsmethode,* Stuttgart, 1962.
265. Heimberg, M., Park, J. H., Isaacs, A., and Pitt-Rivers, R. *Endocrinology 57*:756, 1955.
266. Heinbecker, P., Rolf, D., and White, H. I. *Am. J. Physiol. 139*:545, 1943.
267. Heineman, M., Johnson, C. E., and Man, E. *J. Clin. Invest. 27*:91, 1948.
268. Hellegers, A., Okuda, K., Nesbitt, R. E. L., Smith, D. W., and Chow, B. F. *Am. J. Clin. Nutr. 5*:327, 1957.
269. Hellman, L., Bradlow, H. L., Zumoff, B., and Gallagher, T. F. *J. Clin. Endocrinol. Metabol. 21*:1231, 1961.
270. Heroux, O. *Fed. Proc. 19*(Suppl. 5):82, 1960.
271. Hill, S. R., Barker, S. B., McNeill, J. H., Tingley, Y. O., and Hibbet, L. L. *J. Clin. Invest. 39*:523, 1960.
272. Hoagland, H., Rubin, M. A., and Cameron, D. E. *J. Neurophysiol. 2*:170, 1939.
273. Hoch, F. L. *Physiol. Rev. 42*:605, 1962.
274. Hoch, F. L., and Lipmann, F. *Proc. Nat. Acad. Sci. (Washington) 40*:909, 1954.
275. Hoffman, B., and Cranefield, P., *Electrophysiology of the Heart* (Transl. from Russian), Moscow, 1962.
276. Hoffman, F., and Hoffman, E. G. *New Physiological Aspects of Hyperthyreosis,* Santiago, 1944.
277. Hoffman, F., Hoffman, E. G., and Talesnik, G. *Am. J. Physiol. 148*:689, 1947.
278. Hökfelt, B. *Acta Physiol. Scand. 25*(Suppl.):92, 1951.
279. Hollander, C. S., Thompson, R. H., Barrett, P. V. O., and Berlin, N. I. *J. Clin. Invest. 45*:1024, 1966.
280. Holtz, P., Stock, K., and Westerman, E. *Arch. Exp. Pathol. Pharmakol. 228*:322, 1956.
281. Hopsu, V. K. *Acta Endocrinol. 1960* Suppl. 48.
282. Horstmann, W., and Martinius, J. *Arch. Kinderheilk. 170*:56, 1964.
283. Horvath, A. *Nature 179*:968, 1957.
284. Hoskins, R. G., and Yellinek, E. M. *Endocrinology 16*:455, 1932.
285. Howitt, G., Rowlands, D. J., Leung, D. Y. T., and Logan, W. F. *Clin. Sci. 34*:485, 1968.
286. Hsieh, A. C. L., and Carlson, L. D. *Am. J. Physiol. 188*:40, 1957.
287. Hughes, A. M. *Endocrinology 34*:69, 1944.
288. Hung, L. V. *C. R. Soc. Biol. 153*:1007, 1959.
289. Ignotene, G. K. *Functional and Morphological State of the Endocrine Glands in Experimental Rheumatism.* Author's abstract of candidate's dissertation, Vilnius, 1967.
290. Il'ina, N. A., and Shtul'man, D. R. *Probl. Éndokrinol. Gormonoter. 5*:44, 1960.
291. Il'yasov, Sh. Sh. *Med. Zh. Uzb. 1958* (10):20.
292. Issekutz, B. V., Leinzinger, M., and Issekutz, B. *Arch. Exp. Path. Pharmak. 185*:673, 1937.
293. Ivanova-Tikhvinskaya, E. L. In: *Collected Scientific Papers of Ivanovo Medical Institute* (in Russian), no. 17, 1958, p. 188.
294. Ivleva, V. V. *Patol. Fiziol. Éksp. Ter. 1959*(5):63.
295. Ivleva, V. V. *Byull. Éksp. Biol. Med. 68*(9):35, 1969.
296. Jackson, A. S. *J. Am. Med. Assoc. 197*;1954, 1931.
297. Jakobson, T. *Acta Endocrinol. 27*:432, 1958.
298. Jeanrenaud, B. *Metabol. Clin. Exp. 10*:535, 1961.

299. Johnson, D. C. *Acta Physiol. Scand. 65*:337, 1956.
300. Johnson, R. M., and Baumann, C. A. *J. Biol. Chem. 171*:513, 1947.
301. Jonas, V., and Horejsi, I. *Cas. Lek. Cesk. 72*:378, 1005, 1061, 1068, 1933.
302. Jones, G. B., Thèse pour le doctorat en médicine, Université de Toulouse, 1958.
303. Kakhana, M. S. *Proceedings of a Scientific Conference on Functional Relations between Different Systems of the Body under Normal and Pathological Conditions* (in Russian), Ivanovo, 1962, p. 420.
304. Kakushkina, E. A., and Tatarko, T. T. *Dokl. Akad. Nau. SSSR 55*:363, 1947.
305. Kamel, T., Michel, R., and Roche, J. *C. R. Soc. Biol. 156*:7, 1962.
306. Kandror, V. I. *Probl. Éndokrinol. 2*:88, 1965.
307. Kandror, V. I. In: *Problems in Neuroendocrine Pathology* (in Russian), Gor'kii, 1965, p. 133.
308. Kandror, V. I. In: *The Molecular Basis of Disease* (in Russian), Meditsina, Moscow, 1965, p. 21.
309. Kandror, V. I. In: *The Biogenic Amines. Transactions of the I. M. Sechenov First Moscow Medical Institute* (in Russian), Moscow, 1967, p. 295.
310. Kandror, V. I. *On Mechanisms of Cardiovascular Disorders in Thyrotoxicosis (Experimental Investigation)*. Doctoral dissertation, Moscow, 1968.
311. Kandror, V. I., and Éster, K. N. In: *The Thyroid Gland* (in Russian), Tartu, 1966, p. 58.
312. Kandror, V. I., and Kryukova, I. V. *Probl. Éndokrinol. 1966* (5):102.
313. Kandror, V. I., Men'shikova, V. V., Bol'shakova, T. D., and Lukicheva, T. I. *Probl. Éndokrinol. 1967* (2):70.
314. Kandror, V. I., and Salakhova, N. S. *Abstracts of Sectional Proceedings of the Second All-Union Biochemical Congress. Biochemistry of Hormones* (in Russian), Tashkent, 1969, p. 43.
315. Kandror, V. I., and Salakhova, N. S. *Byull. Éksp. Biol. Med. 69*(4):47, 1970.
316. Kandror, V. I., and Shapiro, G. A. *Probl. Éndokrinol. 1966*(6):101.
317. Kardashev, V. L., Kubli, S. Kh., and Nevstrueva, V. S. *Probl. Éndokrinol. 1964*(10):95.
318. Karp, A., and Stetten, D. *J. Biol. Chem. 179*:819, 1949.
319. Kasbekar, D. K., Lavate, W. V., Rege, D. V., and Sreenivasan, A. *Biochem. J. 72*:374, 1959.
320. Kassenaar, A. A., Laweyer, L. D. F., and Querido, A. *Acta Endocrinol. 21*:37, 1956.
321. Kassil', G. N., and Plotitsina, T. T. *Fiziol. Zh. SSSR 32*:681, 1946.
322. Kazaryan, G. A., and Arutyunyan, G. K. In: *Cortico-Visceral Relations and Hormonal Regulation* (in Russian), Khar'kov, 1963, p. 116.
323. Kebadze, I. I. *Transactions of the Institute of Experimental and Clinical Surgery* (in Russian), no. 7, Tbilisi, 1967.
324. Keder-Stepanova, I. A. *The Role of Iono-Hormonal Relations in the Onset and Development of Vagal Inhibition of the Heart.* Candidate's dissertation, Moscow, 1949.
325. Kekki, M. *Acta Endocrinol. 45* (Suppl.):91, 1964.
326. Kellen, J. *Z. Gesamte Inn. Med. 12*:139, 1957.
327. Kennedy, R. L. I. In: *Practice of Pediatrics. Vol. I.* Hagerstone, 1944, Ch. 38.
328. Kessler and Gelhorn. *Ann. Endocrinol. 22*:203, 1961.
329. Khavin, I. B., and Shtegeman, I. A. *Probl. Éndokrinol. Gormonoter. 7*:1, 1961.
330. Kibyakov, A. V., and Pen'kina, Z. I. *Byull. Éksp. Biol. Med. 34*(1):7, 1954.
331. Kishi, K. *Virchows Arch. Pathol. Anat. Physiol. 176*:260, 1904.
332. Kleine, D. *Endocrinology 45*:596, 1949.
333. Klyachko, V. R. *Probl. Éndokrinol. 2*(11):31, 1956.
334. Klyachko, V. R., Frenkel', G. M., and Dobrzhanskaya, A. K. *Probl. Éndokrinol. Gormonoter. 11*(6):25, 1965.
335. Kochakian, C. D., and Bartlett, M. N. *J. Biol. Chem. 176*:243, 1948.

336. Kogan-Yasnyi, V. M. *Ter. Arkh. 15*(2):195, 1937.
337. Koludin, J. S. *Acta Biol. Med. Ger. 8*:238, 1962.
338. Komissarenko, I. V. *Vrach. Delo 1962*(4):67.
339. Konge, L. A. *Abstracts of Proceedings of a Conference on the Evolutionary Physiology of the Nervous System* (in Russian), Leningrad, 1956, p. 87.
340. Kost, E. A. In: *Textbook of Internal Medicine in Several Volumes* (in Russian), vol. 6, Meditsina, Moscow, 1962, p. 56.
341. Koudelkova, Z., and Vik, J. *J. Plzen. Lekar. Sb. 19*:75, 1962.
342. Kovach, A. B., Tahacs, L., Mohacsi, A., Kaldoi, V., and Kolmar, L. *Acta Physiol. Acad. Sci. Hung. 11*:181, 1957.
343. Kovalev, G. G. *Khirurgiya 1960*(6):63.
344. Kovishkov, F. I. In: *Problems in Reactivity and Shock* (in Russian), Moscow, 1952, p. 176.
345. Krasnogorskii, N. I. *Zh. Vyssh. Nerv. Deyat. 1*(6):793, 1951.
346. Kreezer, G. *Am. J. Dis. Child. 81*:233, 1951.
347. Kritchevsky, D. *Metabolism 9*:784, 1960.
348. Krump, J. E. *Verhandl. Dtsch. J. Inn. Med. 66 Kongr., Wiesbaden, 25–28 April, 1960.* Munich, 1965, p. 389.
349. Krushinskii, L. V., and Dobrokhotova, L. P. *Byull. Éksp. Biol. Med. 44*(8):46, 1957.
350. Kruskemper, H. L., and Doering, P. *Acta Endocrinol. 30*:205, 1959.
351. Kryukova, I. V. *Role of Parasympathetic Influences in the Genesis of Disturbances of the Cardiac Rhythm in Rabbits with Experimental Thyrotoxicosis.* Candidate's dissertation, Moscow, 1967.
352. Kryukova, I. V., Frolov, V. A., Abinder, A. A., and Kandror, V. I. In: *The Thyroid Gland. Proceedings of the 6th Republican Conference of Endocrinologists* (in Russian), Tartu, 1966, p. 82.
353. Kubacki, J. *Pol. Tyg. Lek. 16*:703, 1961.
354. Kunde, M. M., Green, M. F., and Burus, G. *Am. J. Physiol. 99*:469, 1932.
355. Kunkel, H. O., and Crawford, W. P. *Fed. Proc. 16*:207, 1957.
356. Kuschke, H. J. *Br. Med. J. 1*:1656, 1960.
357. Kuschke, H. J., Weruze, H., and Igata, A. *Lancet 11*:360, 1962.
358. Kuz'menko, G. I. *Uch. Zap. Leningr. Med. Inst. 9*(4):215, 1938.
359. Kuz'mina, V. E. *Response of the Thyroid Gland to Simple and Combined Stresses and the Role of the Central Nervous System in Its Mechanism.* Candidate's dissertation, Saratov, 1967.
360. Labouesse, J., Chatagner, F., and Jollec-Bergeret, B. *Biochim. Biophys. Acta 39*:372, 1960.
361. Lachance, J. P., and Page, E. *Endocrinology 52*:57, 1953.
362. Ladygin, V. I. *Effects of the Functional State of the Thyroid Gland on Death and Resuscitation after Lethal Blood Loss.* Candidate's dissertation, Moscow, 1966.
363. Lang, G. F. *Diseases of the Circulatory System. Textbok of Internal Diseases* (in Russian), Medgiz, Moscow, 1958.
364. Laraia, P. J., and Reddy, W. J. *Biochim. Biophys. Acta 117*:189, 1969.
365. Lardy, H. A. In: *The Thyroid.* Brookhaven Lab., Upton, 1954, p. 90.
366. Lardy, H. A., and Feldott, G. *Ann. N. Y. Acad. Sci. 54*:636, 1951.
367. Lardy, H., and Kent, A. B. In: *The Biochemical Aspects of Hormone Action,* Boston, 1964, p. 127.
368. Larina, M. A. *Probl. Éndokrinol. Gormonoter. 8*(2):26, 1962.
369. Larina, M. A. *Biosynthesis of Corticosteroids in the Adrenals of Rabbits with Experimental Thyrotoxicosis.* Candidate's dissertation, Moscow, 1962.
370. Larina, M. A. *Probl. Éndokrinol. 1964*(3):118.
371. Larionova, T. I. *Vopr. Med. Khim. 2*(5):378, 1956.

372. Larsson, S. O. *Acta Med. Scand. 157*:349, 1957.
373. Lashof, J. C., Bondy, P. K., Sterling, K., and Man, E. B. *Proc. Soc. Exp. Biol. Med. 86*: 233, 1954.
374. Laties, V. G., and Weiss, B. *Am. J. Physiol. 197*:1028, 1959.
375. Lawson, J. D. *N. Engl. J. Med. 259*:761, 1958.
376. Leak, D. *Acta Endocrinol. 43*:131, 1963.
377. Lee, X. P., and Lardy, H. A. *J. Biol. Chem. 240*:1427, 1965.
378. Leeper, R. D., Mead, A. W., Money, W. L., and Rowson, R. W. *Clin. Pharmacol. Therap. 2*:3, 1961.
379. Lehninger, A. L. *Physiol. Rev. 42*:467, 1962.
380. Leites, S. M. *The Pathophysiology of the Thyroid and Parathyroid Glands* (in Russian), Moscow, 1965.
381. Leithold, S. L., David, D., and Best, W. R. *Am. J. Med. 24*:534, 1958.
382. Leonard, S. L. *Am. J. Phys. Med. 34*:297, 1955.
383. Leonard, S. L., and Ringler, I. *Endocrinology 55*:212, 1954.
384. Lerman, J., and Means, J. H. *J. Clin. Invest. 11*:167, 1932.
385. Leven, R. J., and Smith, D. H. *J. Physiol. (London) 169*:755, 1963.
386. Levey, G. S., Skelton, C. L., and Epstein, S. E. *Endocrinology 85*:1004, 1969.
387. Levine, R. J., Oates, J. A., Vendsalu, A., and Goerdema, A. *J. Clin. Endocrinol. 22*:1242, 1962.
388. Lhotka, J. K., McArthur, L. G., and Hellbaum, A. A. *Anat. Rec. 133*:406, 1959.
389. Lindsley, D. B., and Rubinstein, B. B. *Proc. Soc. Exp. Biol. Med. 35*:558, 1937.
390. Lipsky, S. R., Bondy, P. K., Man, E. B., and McGuire, J. S. *J. Clin. Invest. 34*:950, 1955.
391. Lorscheider, L., and Reineke, E. P. *Proc. Soc. Exp. Biol. Med. 138*:1116, 1971.
392. McCullagh, E. P., and Dunlap, Y. H. *J. Lab. Clin. Med. 17*:1060, 1932.
393. McDowall, R. G. S. *J. Physiol. (London) 104*:392, 1946.
394. McElroy, J. S., Schuman, E. B., and Ritchey, J. O. *Ann. Int. Med. 12*:106, 1938.
395. McGuire, J. S., and Tomkins, G. M. *J. Biol. Chem. 234*:791, 1959.
396. Mach, Z., Toczycki, T., and Zygulska-Machowa, H. *Pol. Tyg. Lek. 12*:1571, 1957.
397. Maclagan, N. F., and Rundle, F. F. *Q. J. Med. 1940*:215.
398. McMillan, W. H., and Rand, M. *J. Pharm. Pharmacol. 14*:257, 1962.
399. Maley, G. F. *Am. J. Physiol. 188*:35, 1957.
400. Malyugin, N. S. In: *Abstracts of Proceedings of the Annual Scientific Session of the First Moscow Medical Institute* (in Russian), Moscow, 1956, p. 94.
401. Mandel'shtam, M. E. *Paroxysmal Tachycardia* (in Russian), Leningrad, 1940.
402. Mandl', S. F. *Probl. Éndokrinol. Gormonoter. 2*(1):37, 1956.
403. Mansfeld, G., and Sos, J. *Klin. Wschr. 17*:386, 1938.
404. Marchi, P., and Mayer, J. *Experientia 15*:359, 1959.
405. Marits, A. M. *Fiziol. Zh. SSSR 47*:1235, 1961.
406. Marits, A. M. *Fiziol. Zh. SSSR 49*:434, 1963.
407. Marits, A. M. In: *The Evolution of Functions* (in Russian), Moscow, 1964, p. 140.
408. Martius, C. *Arch. Biochem. Biophys. 33*:486, 1951.
409. Marx, W., Gustin, S. T., and Levi, C. *Proc. Soc. Exp. Biol. Med. 83*:143, 1953.
410. Mascitelli-Coriandoll, E., and Boldrini, R. *Experientia 15*:229, 1959.
411. Mason, J. W., Mougey, E. H., Brady, V., and Tolliver, G. A. *Psychosom. Med. 30*:682, 1968.
412. Mattonet, C. *Z. Gesamte Exp. Med. 90*:237, 1933.
413. Matyushin, I. F., Vogralik, M. V., and Kolokol'tsev, E. F. In: *Problems in Clinical Biochemistry. Proceedings of the First Scientific Conference* (in Russian), Gor'kii, 1965, p. 42.
414. Mazel', Ya. I. *Klin. Med. 16*:1035, 1938.

415. Meerson, F. Z. *The Myocardium in Hyperfunction, Hypertrophy, and Failure of the Heart* (in Russian), Meditsina, Moscow, 1965.
416. Meinike, H. A., and Crafis, R. C. *Proc. Soc. Exp. Biol. Med. 102*:121, 1959.
417. Merkulov, M. F. *Transactions of the All-Union Society of Physiologists, Biochemists, and Pharmacologists* (in Russian), 1958, No. 4.
418. Migeon, C. J., Gardner, J. I., Cligler, J. F., and Wilkins, L. *Endocrinology 51*:117, 1952.
419. Mikulaj, L., and Nemeth, S. *J. Clin. Endocrinol. Metabol. 18*:539, 1958.
420. Milcu, S. M. *Stud. Cercet. Endocrinol. 8*:243, 1957.
421. Milcu, S. M., Brosteano, E., Nicolescu-Cataragi, A., and Jonesko, B. *Rev. Neurol. 94*: 853, 1956.
422. Milcu, S. M., and Demetrescu, M. *Fiziol. Norm. Patol. 1956*(3):211.
423. Milcu, S. M., Vajsler, L., and Kostiner, E. *Probl. Éndokrinol. Gormonoter. 4*(5):24, 1958.
424. Miline, L., and Seepovic, M. *Ann. Endocrinol. 2*:511, 1959.
425. Mirakhmedov, M. M. *Metabolism of Thyroid Hormones in the Liver in Thyrotoxicosis.* Author's abstract of candidate's dissertation, Tashkent, 1966.
426. Mirsky, I. A., and Broh-Kahn, R. H. *Am. J. Physiol. 117*:6, 1936.
427. Moltke, E. *Proc. Soc. Exp. Biol. Med. 88*:596, 1955.
428. Mongdal, N. Sreenivasan, V., and Sarma, P. *J. Nutr. 61*:97, 1957.
429. Moon, R. C., and Turner, C. W. *Proc. Soc. Exp. Biol. Med. 103*:66, 1960.
430. Mori, G. *Arch. Klin. Chir. 199*:29, 1940.
431. Morrison, G. W., and Cunningham, B. *Comp. Psychol. 31*:413, 1941.
432. Mudge, G. H. *Lancet 73*:166, 1953.
433. Muldowney, F. P., Crooks, J., and Wayne, E. *J. Clin. Sci. 16*:309, 1957.
434. Munro, D. S., Renschler, H., and Wilson, G. M. *Metabolism 7*:124, 1958.
435. Nahum, L. H., and Hoff, H. E. *J. Am. Med. Assoc. 105*:254, 1935.
436. Nasset, E. S., Logan, V. W., Kelley, M. L., and Thomas, M. *Am. J. Physiol. 196*:1262, 1959.
437. Naumova, V. I. *Pediatriya 38*(3):72, 1960.
438. Necheles, T. F. *Fed. Proc. 20*:67, 1961.
439. Necheles, T., and Beutler, E. *J. Clin. Invest. 38*:788, 1959.
440. Negoescu, J., Stancu, H., Chivu, V., Balan, M., Petrescu, C., and Dragomirescu, M. In: *Omagiu bui C. J. Parhon.* Bucharest, 1966, p. 333.
441. Negovskaya, A. V. *Data on the Pathogenesis and Experimental Treatment of Disturbances of Fat and Lipid Metabolism in Thyrotoxicosis.* Candidate's dissertation, Moscow, 1969.
442. Nemeth, S. *Schweiz. Med. Wschr. 88*:242, 1958.
443. Nersimal, O., Roth, B., Smykal, V., and Soumar, J. *Cr. Neural. 25*:243, 1962.
444. Nevstrueva, V. S., Dolina, L. A., and Sokolova, E. A. *Probl. Éndokrinol. Gormonoter. 11*(4):83, 1965.
445. Nielson, R., Loizzi, R., and Klitgaard, H. *Am. J. Physiol. 200*:55, 1961.
446. Nieman, E. A., *Br. Med. J. 5131*:1204, 1959.
447. Nikkila, E. A., and Pittkanen, E. *Acta Endocrinol. 31*:573, 1959.
448. Nikolaichuk, S. P., and Rodkina, B. S. Effect of corticotropic hormone on the thyroid gland and adrenal cortex, *Vrach. Delo 1947*(1):15.
449. Nikolova, F. A., In: *Problems in the Physiology and Pathology of the Endocrine Glands* (in Russian), Khar'kov, 1962, p. 136.
450. Noback, C., Barnett, J., and Kupperman, H. *Anat. Rec. 103*:49, 1949.
451. Noda, Tacuo. *Bull. Kobe Med. Coll. 19*:841, 1960.
452. Nolte, J., Pette, D., Bachmaier, B., Kiefhaber, P., Schneider, H., and Scriba, P. C. *Eur. J. Clin. Invest. 2*:141, 1972.

453. Ogawa, E., Tobe, M., Machido, J., Sunaga, J., and Shibata, K. *Endocrinol. Jpn. 5*:27, 1958.
454. Ogorodova, N. N. *State of the Skeletal Musculature in Toxic Goiter* (*Clinical and Electrophysiological Investigation*), Candidate's dissertation, Moscow, 1967.
455. Okuda, K., and Chow, B. F. *Endocrinology 68*:607, 1961.
456. Olivier, M. P., and Boyd, G. S. *Lancet 1*:124, 1957.
457. Oliverau, M., and Serfaty, A. *Ann. Endocrinol. 16*:749, 1955.
458. Olson, R., and Piatnek, D. *Ann. N. Y. Acad. Sci. 72*:467, 1959.
459. Olson, R. E., and Vester, J. W. *Physiol. Rev. 40*:677, 1960.
460. Osinskaya, V. O., In: *Problems in the Physiology and Pathology of the Endocrine Glands* (in Russian), Khar'kov, 1962, p. 144.
461. Ostrovskii, Yu. M., and Larin, F. S. *Abstracts of Proceedings of the Second All-Union Conference of Endocrinologists* (in Russian), Moscow, 1962, p. 247.
462. Page, I., and McCubbin, J. W. *Circulation 5*:390, 1952.
463. Paik, W. K., and Cohen, P P. *J. Gen. Physiol. 43*:683, 1960.
464. Panachin, E. F., and Kandror, V. I. *Byull. Éksp. Biol. Med. 72*(7):33, 1971.
465. Pashkov, A. V. *Functional State of the Kidneys in Thyrotoxicosis.* Candidate's dissertation, Moscow, 1966.
466. Passauant-Fontaine, T., Flandive, C., and Mauche, D. *C. R. Soc. Biol. 147*:1158, 1953.
467. Pasternak, L., and Page, S. *Biochem. Z. 274*:122, 1934.
468. Patek, A. J., and Haig, C. *Proc. Soc. Exp. Biol. Med. 57*:343, 1961.
469. Pekarskii, D. E. *Functional State of the Kidneys in Patients with Thyrotoxic Goiter in Connection with Operative Treatment under Different Types of Anesthesia.* Condidate's dissertation, Moscow, 1963.
470. Pekkarinen, A., Kovusalo, M., and Pyorala, K. *Acta Endocrinol. 6*:233, 1951.
471. Pencea, V., and Zbrance, E. T. *Med. Int.* (*Bucharest*) *20*:1211, 1968.
472. Pende, N. *Endocrinology. Pathology and Clinical Features Relating to the Organs of Internal Secretion* (Transl. from Russian), Moscow, 1937, p. 504.
473. Peters, R. A., and Rossiter, R. J. *Biochem. J. 33*:1140, 1939.
474. Petrov, I. R. In: *Shock and Therminal States* (in Russian), Leningrad, 1960, p. 75.
475. Petrova, M. K. *Tr. Fiziol. Lab. im. I. P. Pavlova 12*(1):49, 1945.
476. Piatnek, D. A. *Fed. Proc. 15*:145, 1956.
477. Pickens, J., and Lockett, M. F. *J. Endocrinol. 23*:231, 1961.
478. Pittman, J. *N. Engl. J. Med. 267*:861, 1962.
479. Pittman, C. S., and Barker, S. B. *J. Clin. Invest. 41*:696, 1969.
480. Plesch, I. *Z. Exp. Pathol. Ther. 6*:380, 1909.
481. Ponirovskii, N. G. *Vrach. Delo 7*:315, 1924.
482. Portugal'skaya, E. A. *Nauch. Izv. Kazakh. Med. Inst. 1958*(15):126.
483. Portugal'skaya, E. A. In: *Vitamins* (in Russian), Izd. Akad. Nauk Ukr. SSR., vol. 4, 1958, p. 78.
484. Prasad, A. S., Flink, E. B., and McCollister, R. *J. Lab. Clin. Med. 58*:531, 1961.
485. Preobrazhenskii, A. P., and Turkel'taub, M. S. *Probl. Éndokrinol. 2*:512, 1937.
486. Pribytkova, G. N., *Byull. Éksp. Biol. Med. 22*:117, 1936.
487. Pugachev, A. G. *Byull. Éksp. Biol. Med. 487*(7):1, 1953.
488. Quadramagna, C., Massari, N., and Bertollini, A. M. *Acta Vitamin.* (*Milan*) *1958*(12):77.
489. Raab, W. J. *Pharmacol. Exp. Ther. 82*:330, 1944.
490. Rachev, R. R. *Mitochondria and the Thyroid Hormones* (in Russian), Meditsina, Leningrad, 1969.
491. Raiskina, M. E. *Biochemistry of Nervous Regulation of the Heart* (in Russian), Medgiz, Moscow, 1962.
492. Rajmon, J. *Zbl. Chir. 83*:2329, 1958.

493. Rawson, R. W., Rall, J. E., Pearson, O. H., Robbins, J., Popell, H. F., and West, C. D. *Am. J. Med. Sci. 226*:405, 1953.
494. Rawson, R. W., Rall, J. E., and Sonenberg, M. *The Hormones* (G. Pincus, K. K. Thimann, eds.), vol. 3, Academic Press, New York, 1955, p. 433.
495. Read, D. G., Hershman, J. P., and Pittman, J. A. Jr. *J. Clin. Endocrinol. Metabol. 29*: 1496, 1969.
496. Redding, T. W., and Johnson, P. C. *Proc. Soc. Exp. Biol. Med. 109*:153, 1962.
497. Reid, E. *Mem. Soc. Endocrinol. 9*:130, 1960.
498. Reinberg, A., and Sidi, E. *Ann. Endocrinol. 20*:541, 1959.
499. Reuter, H. *Klin. Wochenschr. 41*:737, 1963.
500. Roch, S., Bierman, E. L., and Schwalts, I. L. *J. Clin. Invest. 38*:275, 1959.
501. Roche, J., Michel, R., Jouan, P., and Wilf, W. *C. R. Acad. Sci. 241*:1880, 1955.
502. Roche, J., Michel, R., and Jouan, P. *Bull. Soc. Chim. Biol. 41*:1163, 1959.
503. Rohmer, F., Wackenheim, A., and Kurtz, D. *Rev. Neurol. 100*:297, 1959.
504. Root, A. W., Oski, F. A., Bongiovonni, A. M., and Eberlein, W. R. *Pediatrics 70*:369, 1967.
505. Rosenman, R. H., Byers, B. O., and Friedman, M. *J. Clin. Endocrinol. 12*:1287, 1952.
506. Rosner, Yu. *Fiziol. Zh. SSSR 44*(5):473, 1958.
507. Ross, D. A., and Shwab, R. S. *Endocrinology 25*:75, 1939.
508. Rossano, P. *Boll. Soc. Ital. Biol. Sperim. 35*:1609, 1959.
509. Rozanov, L. P. *Tr. Belorussk. Univ. (Minsk) 1925*(8):10.
510. Rubin, M. A., Cohen, L. H., and Hoagland, H. *Endocrinology 21*:536, 1937.
511. Rupp, J., Paschkis, K. E., and Cantarow, A. *Endocrinology 44*:449, 1949.
512. Sager, O. *The Diencephalon* (in Russian), Bucharest, 1962.
513. Saidkhanov, A. *Some Hemodynamic Indices and the Functional State of the Kidney in Patients with Thyroid Gland Pathology before and after Operation.* Candidate's dissertation, Moscow, 1963.
514. Salakhova, N. S. *The Contractile Function of the Myocardium and Its Supply of Structural Materials in Thyrotoxicosis when an Additional Load Is Placed on the Heart.* Candidate's dissertation, Moscow, 1970, p. 310.
515. Salakhova, N. S., and Kandror, V. I. *Probl. Éndokrinol. 1969*(6):100.
516. Salei, A P., and Stepanova, V. S. *Byull. Éksp. Biol. Med. 60*(12):35, 1965.
517. Salganik, R. I. *Biokhimiya 17*(5):649, 1952.
518. Samoilova, Z. T. *Zh. Vyssh. Nervn. Deyat. 2*:2, 1952.
519. Saralidze, G. N. *Soobshch. Akad. Nauk Gruz. SSR 25*(2):225, 1960.
520. Scaif, J. F., and Migikowsky, B. B. *Can. J. Biochem. Physiol. 35*:15, 1957.
521. Scarf, M. *J. Lab. Clin. Med. 21*:1253, 1936.
522. Schneiberg, P., Sted, E. A., Brannon, E. S., and Warren, J. S. *J. Clin. Invest. 29*:1139, 1950.
523. Schumann, H. *Z. Gesamte Exp. Med. 105*:577, 1939.
524. Schwartz, I. L., and Debons, A. F. *Physiologist 2*:104, 1959.
525. Scott, J., Finkelstein, L., and Spitzer, J. *Am. J. Physiol. 203*:482, 1962.
526. Scow, G., Baer, P., and Boeri, E. *Arch. Sci. Biol. 22*:142, 1936.
527. Sellers, E. A., Flattery, K. V., Shun, A., and Johason, G. E. *Can. J. Physiol. Pharmacol., 1971.*
528. Sellers, E. A., and Yeu, S. A. *Am. J. Physiol. 163*:81, 1950.
529. Selye, H. *The Story of the Adaptation Syndrome* (Russian translation), Medgiz, Moscow, 1960.
530. Sessions, J. T., Rand, T. S., Hiestand, F. C., Hardy, I. M., and Fand, S. B. *Clin. Res. 9*: 155, 1961.
531. Severin, S. E. *Usp. Sovrem. Biol. 48*:123, 1959.
532. Shaitanov, M. *Eksp. Med. Morfol. 4*(3):175, 1965.

533. Shakhnarovich, V. M. *Role of the Autonomic Nervous System in the Genesis of some Symptoms of Thyrotoxicosis (Experimental Investigation)*. Candidate's dissertation, Moscow, 1970.
534. Shakhnarovich, V. M., and Kandror, V. I. *Dokl. Akad. Nauk SSSR 185*:1386, 1969.
535. Shamakhmudov, Sh. Sh. *Tr. Inst. Kraevoi Ėksp. Med. Akad. Nauk Uzb. SSR* (Tashkent) *1961*(1):149.
536. Shambaugh, G. E., and Beisel, W. R. *Endocrinology 79*:511, 1906.
537. Sharpe, J. C., and Bisgard, J. D. *J. Lab. Clin. Med. 21*:347, 1936.
538. Sharpe, J. C., and Bisgard, J. D. *J. Lab. Clin. Med. 23*:219, 1937.
539. Sheets, R. F., and Struck, H. C. *Science 96*:408, 1942.
540. Shepotin, B. M., and Mil'ko, V. I. In: *Physiology and Pathology of the Endocrine Glands* (in Russian), Khar'kov, 1965, p. 541.
541. Shereshevskii, N. A., In: *Clinical Endocrinology* (in Russian), Moscow, 1957, p. 20.
542. Sheveleva, V. S. *Interneuronal Transmission of Excitation in Sympathetic Ganglia* (in Russian), Medgiz, Moscow, 1961.
543. Sheves, G. S. *Biokhimiya 23*:80, 1958.
544. Shitkova, T. A. *Probl. Ėndokrinol. 6*(2):18, 1960.
545. Shnitser, I. S. *Klin. Med. 34*(11):3, 1956.
546. Shtel'makh, N. I. *Ter. Arkh. 30*:16, 1958.
547. Shurygin, D. Ya. *Changes in Hematopoiesis in Patients with Basedow's Disease in Connection with Methylthiouracil Therapy*. Candidate's dissertation, Leningrad, 1951.
548. Silberberg, M., and Silberberg, R. *Arch. Pathol. 36*:512, 1943.
549. Silverman, S. H., and Gardner, L. I. *N. Engl. J. Med. 250*:938, 1954.
550. Simms, E., Preiffenbergen, M., and Heinbecker, P. *Endocrinology 49*:45, 1951.
551. Singh, V. N., and Chaikoff, L. *Endocrinology 78*:339, 1966.
552. Skanse, B., and Nyman, G. E. *Acta Endocr. 22*:246, 1956.
553. Skebel'skaya, Yu. B., *Probl. Ėndokrinol. Gormonoter.* 1956(6).
554. Skebel'skaya, Yu. B. *Probl. Ėndokrinol. Gormonoter. 3*(6):32, 1957.
555. Skebel'skaya, Yu. B. *Probl. Ėndokrinol. 9*(1):111, 1963.
556. Skebel'skaya, Yu. B., and Bagramyan, E. T. *Probl. Ėndokrinol. 8*(6):27, 1962.
557. Skhodnitskii, B. S. In: *Collected Scientific Papers of Chernovtsy Medical Institute* (in Russian), Number 11, Chernovtsy, 1960, pp. 71–73.
558. Skow, R. *Endocrinology 49*:522, 1951.
559. Skuratovskaya, L. N. *Some Aspects of Myocardial Metabolism in Experimental Thyrotoxicosis*. Candidate's dissertation, Moscow, 1969.
560. Slukhai, Yu. M. *Med. Radiol. 12*(5):67, 1967.
561. Smart, G. A., and Robson, A. M. *Lancet 1*, 1963.
562. Smelser, G. K., and Ozanics, V. *J. Cell. Comp. Physiol. 43*:107, 1954.
563. Smith, R. E., and Hoijer, D. J. *Physiol. Rev. 42*:60, 1962.
564. Smith, W. W., and Smith, F. *Am. J. Physiol. 165*:651, 1951.
565. Smith, R. H., and Williams-Ashman, H. G. *Biochim. Biophys. Acta 7*:295, 1951.
566. Smyk, M. M., and Fishchenko, L. Ya. Disturbance of urea formation in experimental thyrotoxicosis. In: *Goitrous Disease* (in Russian), Kiev, 1956.
567. Soffer, L. J., Cohn, C., Grossman, E. B., Jacobs, M. D., and Sobatka, H. *J. Clin. Invest. 20*:429, 1941.
568. Sokoloff, L., Campbell, P. L., Francis, C. M., and Kleem, C. B. *Biochim. Biophys. Acta 76*:329, 1963.
569. Sokoloff, L., and Kaufman, S. *Science 129*:569, 1959.
570. Sokoloff, L., and Kaufman, S. *J. Biol. Chem. 236*:795, 1961.
571. Sorokin, V. M., and Turakulov, Ya. Kh. In: *Proceedings of a Tashkent Conference on the Peaceful Uses of Atomic Energy* (in Russian), vol. 3, Tashkent, 1961, p. 156.
572. Spang, K., and Korth, C. *Arch. Kreislaufforsch. 4*:189, 1939.

573. Spinks, A., and Burn, J. H. *Br. J. Pharmacol. 271*:93, 1952.
574. Spiro, M. J., and Ball, E. G. *J. Biol. Chem. 231*:31, 1958.
575. Spirtes, M. A., Medes, G., and Weinhouse, S. *J. Biol. Chem. 204*:705, 1953.
576. Sribner, I. M. In: *Abstracts of Proceedings of the Second All-Union Conference of Endocrinologists* (in Russian), Moscow, 1962, p. 371.
577. Staehelin, M. *Helv. Physiol. Acta 13*:50, 1955.
578. Starr, P., and Roskelley, R. *Am. J. Physiol. 130*:549, 1949.
579. Stasilli, N., Krog, R., and Nemith, P. *Endocrinology 68*:1068, 1961.
580. Stein, O., and Gross, J. *Proc. Soc. Exp. Biol. Med. 109*:817, 1962.
581. Stenram, U. *Exp. Cell. Res. 3*:147, 1952.
582. Stepanenko, A. P. *Probl. Éndokrinol. Gormonoter. 2*(1):35, 1956.
583. Stern, B., and Altschule, M. *J. Clin. Invest. 15*:633, 1936.
584. Sternheimer, R. *Endocrinology 25*:899, 1939.
585. Stoilov, L. D., Klyachkov, V. R., and Shapiro, G. A. In: *Proceedings of an All-Union Scientific Conference on the Biogenic Amines* (in Russian), Moscow, 1967, p. 265.
586. Sultanov, F. F. *Probl. Éndokrinol. Gormonoter. 8*(4):51, 1962.
587. Sure, B., and Easterling, L. *J. Nutr. 42*:221, 1950.
588. Svyatkina, O. B. *Dynamics of Protein and RNA Renewal in the Myocardium in Experimental Thyrotoxicosis.* Dissertation, Moscow, 1968.
589. Svyatkina, O. B., and Kandror, V. I. *Probl. Éndokrinol. 14*(1):83, 1968.
590. Swanson, H. E. *Endocrinology 60*:205, 1957.
591. Tabachnick, I. I. A., Bonnycastle, D. D., and Salter, W. T. *J. Endocrinol. 10*:302, 1954.
592. Tabatadze, P. D. In: *Abstracts of Proceedings of a Scientific Session of the Institute of Clinical and Experimental Cardiology* (in Russian), Tbilisi, 1956, p. 18.
593. T'ang Weng-Chang. *Functional State of the Stomach in Thyrotoxicosis.* Candidate's dissertation, Moscow, 1964.
594. Tapley, D. F. *Bull. Johns Hopkins Hosp. 96*:274, 1955.
595. Taylor, S. *J. Clin. Endocrinol. 14*:1412, 1954.
596. Timiras, P. S., and Woodbury, D. M. *Endocrinology 58*:181, 1956.
597. Tinker, M. B. *J. Am. Med. Assoc. 97*:515, 1931.
598. Travina, O. B. *Probl. Éndokrinol. 3*(1):58, 1938.
599. Trendelenburg, M. *Br. J. Pharmacol. 8*:454, 1953.
600. Trofimov, V. K. *Uch. Zap. Stavrop. Gos. Med. Inst. 12*:38, 1963.
601. Truesdell, C. *Am. J. Physiol. 76*(1):20–27, 1926.
602. Tucek, S., Diepold, F. *Physiol. Bohemoslov. 12*:258, 1963.
603. Tudhope, G. B. *The Thyroid and the Blood.* London, 1969.
604. Tudhope, G. R., and Wilson, G. M. *Q. J. Med. 29*:513, 1960.
605. Turakulov, Ya. Kh. *The Biochemistry and Pathochemistry of the Thyroid Gland* (in Russian), Tashkent, 1963.
606. Turakulov, Ya. Kh., Abidov, A. A., and Rakhimdzhanova, T. *Dokl. Akad. Nauk Uzbek. SSR 1972*(3):48.
607. Turakulov, Ya. Kh., Khamidov, D. Kh., Mirakhmedov, A. K., and L'vovich, N. A. *Uzbek. Biol. Zh. 1972*(3):6.
608. Turakulov, Ya. Kh., Mirakhmedov, M. M., and Rakhmatullaev, M. M. *Byull. Éksp. Biol. Med. 72*(11):19, 1971.
609. Turakulov, Ya. Kh., Nigmatov, N. N., Furdui, F. I., Babare, G. M., and Kuvatbekova, D. A. In: *Proceedings of the Institute of Zoology, Academy of Sciences of the Moldavian SSR* (in Russian), Kishinev, 1972, p. 3.
610. Turchetto, E., Sanguinetti, F., and Rossi, C. A. *Boll. Soc. Ital. Biol. Sper. 31*:1324, 1955.
611. Tuzhilkova, T. N. *Probl. Éndokrinol. Gormonoter. 9*(4):35, 1963.

612. Tyan Hiu. *Role of the Functional State of the Thyroid Gland in the Development of Traumatic Shock.* Candidate's dissertation, Leningrad, 1959.
613. Udel'nov, M. G. *The Nervous Regulation of the Heart* (in Russian), Moscow University Press, Moscow, 1961.
614. Ugoleva, S. V. *Probl. Éndokrinol. Gormonoter. 11*(4):3, 1965.
615. Ugol'nikov, V. A. *Probl. Éndokrinol. Gormonoter. 11*(5):97, 1965.
616. Uono, J. *Med. Progr. Jpn. 42*:120, 1955.
617. Uotiba, U. *Endocrinology 26*:129, 1940.
618. Utevskii, A. M. In: *Mechanisms of Action of Hormones* (in Russian), Kiev, 1959.
619. Utley, H. G. *Endocrinology 75*:975, 1964.
620. Uzhanskii, Ya. G. In: *Textbook of Pathological Physiology in Several Volumes* (in Russian), vol. 3, Meditsina, Moscow, 1966, p. 11.
621. Val'kov, A. V. *Russk. Fiziol. Zh. 1924*(7):324.
622. Val'kov, A. V. *Collection in Celebration of the 75th Birthday of Academician I. P. Pavlov* (in Russian), 1925, p. 363.
623. Vallejos, F., Benitez, D., Meddleton, S., and Talesnik, J. *Bol. Soc. Biol. (Santiago, Chile) 8*:66, 1950.
624. Van Dyke, D. C., Contopoules, A. N., Williams, B. S., Simpson, M. E., Lawrence, J. H., and Evans, H. M. *Acta Haematol. 11*:203, 1954.
625. Vannotti, A., and Béraud, T. *Bull. Schweiz. Acad. Med. Wiss. 14*:214, 1958.
626. Vartapetov, B. A., Gladkova, A. I., Kalmykova, K. M., Kuz'menko, E. S., Novikova, M. V., and Trandofilova, G. M. In: *Cortico-Visceral Relations and Hormonal Regulation* (in Russian), 1963, p. 79.
627. Vasil'ev, G. A. *Proceedings of the 7th Conference on Problems in Higher Nervous Activity, in Memory of I. P. Pavlov* (in Russian), Leningrad, 1940, p. 13.
628. Vaughan, M. *J. Clin. Invest. 46*:1482, 1967.
629. Verzar, F. Vidovic, V., and Hajdukovic, S. *Endocrinology 10*:46, 1952.
630. Vereckei, J. *Z. Gesamte Inn. Med. 14*:488, 1959.
631. Vignais, P. V. *Exp. Cell Res. 13*:414, 1957.
632. Vitale, J. J., Hegeted, D. M., Nahamura, M., and Cannors, P. *J. Biol. Chem. 226*:597, 1957.
633. Vogralik, V. G. *The Heart in Neuro-endocrine Disturbances* (in Russian), Gor'kii, 1963.
634. Vogralik, M. V., and Mironova, G. V. *Probl. Éndokrinol. Gormonoter. 10*:32, 1964.
635. Voitkevich, A. A. *Probl. Éndokrinol. Gormonoter. 5*(1):31, 1959.
636. Voss, R., and Schoen, H. R. *Thoraxchir. Vask. Chir. 13*:3, 1965.
637. Voznesenskii, B. B., and Khitrov, N. K. *Byull. Éksp. Biol. Med. 55*(4):61, 1963.
638. Vuopio, P. *Scand. J. Clin. Lab. Invest. 15*(Suppl.):72, 1963.
639. Waldmann, T. A., Weissman, S. M., and Levin, E. H. *J. Lab. Clin. Med. 59*:926, 1962.
640. Watanabe, L., Uematsu, I., and Horii, K. *J. Endocrinol. Metabol. 23*:383, 1963.
641. Wayne, E. J. *Br. Med. J. 1*:78, 1960.
642. Weiss, A. K. *Fed. Proc. 19*(Suppl. 5):137, 1960.
643. Wertheimer, E., and Benter, V. *Metabolism 2*:536, 1953.
644. Wertheimer, E., Benter, V., and Wurzel, M. *Biochem. J. 56*:297, 1954.
645. Westerman, E. *Arch. Exp. Pathol. Pharmakol. 228*:159, 1956.
646. White, J. E., and Engel, F. L. *J. Clin. Invest. 37*:1556, 1958.
647. Williams, M. J., and Blair, D. W. *Br. Med. J. 1*:940, 1964.
648. Williams, R. H., Egana, E., Robinson, P., Asper, P., and Dutol, C. *Arch. Intern. Med. 72*:353, 1943.
649. Wilson, T. E. *Med. J. Aust. 1*:26, 1944.
650. Wilson, W. P., and Johnson, J. E. *Electroencephalogr. Clin. Neurophysiol. 16*:321, 1964.
651. Wilt, F. H. *Biochem. J. 73*:13, 1959.

652. Wise, B., and Hoff, H. *J. Pharmacol. Exp. Ther. 64*:217, 1938.
653. Wiswell, J. C., Hurwitz, G. E., Coronho, V., Bing, O. H., and Child, D. L. *J. Clin. Endocrinol. 23*:1102, 1963.
654. Wohl, M. G., Levy, H. A., Szutka, A., and Maldia, G. *Proc. Soc. Exp. Biol. Med. 105*: 523, 1960.
655. Wolff, J., and Wolff, E. C. *Biochim. Biophys. Acta 36*:387, 1957.
656. Wolternik, L. F., Cornwall, R. L., Vinson, C., and Cole, L. L. *Fed. Proc. 12*:158, 1953.
657. Woodruff, P. *Med. J. Aust. 11*:190, 1940.
658. Woods, R., and Carlson, L. D. *Endocrinology 59*:330, 1956.
659. Wurtman, R. G., Ropin, L., and Axelrod, G. *Endocrinology 73*:63, 1963.
660. Yasenchak, S. A. *Nauch. Zap. Uzhgorod. Gos. Univ. 32*:173, 1957.
661. Yates, F. E., Urquhart, J., and Herbst, A. L. *Am. J. Physiol. 195*:373, 1958.
662. Zavadovskii, B. M. *Proceedings of the Second All-Union Congress of Physiologists* (in Russian), Leningrad, 1926, p. 186.
663. Zavadovskii, B. M., and Zak, A. A. *Med.-Biol. Zh. 2*:15, 1928.
664. Zhangelova, M. B. *The Effect of Experimental Thyrotoxicosis on Activity of the Enzyme Monoamine Oxidase and Some Aspects of Pyrocatecholamine Metabolism.* Candidate's dissertation, Khar'kov, 1968.
665. Zhukova, N. I. *Investigation of the Metabolism of Heart Muscle in Experimental Hypo- and Athyroidism.* Candidate's dissertation, Moscow, 1966.
666. Ziffer, H., Gutman, A., Pasher, I., Sobotka, H., and Baker, H. *Proc. Soc. Exp. Biol. Med. 96*:229, 1957.

PART III

Molecular Mechanisms of Action of Thyroid Hormones

The Mechanism of action of any biologically active compound cannot be satisfactorily explained until at least two fundamental questions have been answered: First, what is the process that is changed *primarily* by the action of this compound and, second, how does the compound modify the process? A subsidiary problem is the discovery of the link between the *primary* changes in the cell and the whole series of visible, yet outwardly apparently disconnected, effects of the substance at the level of the organ, system, or organism as a whole. The inability to establish such a connection provides a basis for the postulated polyvalent character of the compound, the multiplicity of its points of action, and so on, still so widely held in physiology, pharmacology, and endocrinology.

It is only recently, as a result of the advances in biochemistry and molecular biology which provide a deep insight into the organization of cellular functions, that it has become possible to regard the effects of hormones on the systems of a minimal cell, i.e., on those constituting the essential condition for its existence, as their primary effects. These systems include the membranes, responsible for the autonomy of the cell and its organelles, the reproductive system of the cell and its component structures, and the system providing the cell with energy [77].

The fact that the state of virtually all organs and tissues of the body is altered by thyroid hormones and that these changes are manifested at different structural levels indicates that thyroxine and triiodothyronine act on certain fundamental cell functions, which are reflected in the oxygen consumption of the cell. It is still too early to identify with confidence the system on which thyroid hormones exert their primary effect.

As a result of extensive research in the last twenty years, much direct and indirect evidence has been obtained indicating that the action of many physiological agents, such as the thyroid hormones, is at the cellular and subcellular levels and is directly linked with their effect on metabolism and on energy in the mitochondria.

Since 1950 the generally accepted explanation of the mechanism of action of thyroid hormones has been their ability to uncouple the process of ATP synthesis from the transport of electrons along the mitochondrial respiratory chain, i.e., to uncouple oxidative phosphorylation. This effect of thyroid hormones has by no means been relegated to the background even today when the mechanisms whereby the thyroid hormones exert their effects are evaluated, despite the revision of the pharmacological and physiological aspects of the action of thyroid hormones recently undertaken by Tata and co-workers. According to the facts presented by this group of workers, the physiological manifestations of hormonal activity are brought about by activation of the genetic apparatus of the cell with the stimulation of biosynthesis of specific proteins in the cells of target tissues [256, 248–258]. However, it must be recognized that not all hormonal effects can be explained in terms of this concept [80, 90–96, 260].

On the other hand, it is possible that the diverse effects of thyroid hormones—changes in the permeability of mitochondrial membranes, stimulation of the biosynthesis of enzymes and other proteins, a direct effect on the catalytic activity of isolated enzymes and enzymes organized into complex groups, and so on—are not mutually exclusive but are successive or parallel stages in a multistage mechanism developing as the result of the triggering of some unique starting process in the mitochondria or other subcellular target [254]. However, there are also no serious theoretical or practical objections to double or multiple points of application of hormones. Before preference can be given to any one existing view of the mechanism of action of thyroid hormones, we must evidently examine the well-known effects of the biological activity of these hormones separately and then collectively.

Action of Thyroid Hormones on the Catalytic Activity of Isolated Enzymes and of Enzymes Organized into Groups

Action of Thyroid Hormones on Catalytic Activity of Enzymes

One way in which metabolism is controlled by thyroid hormones is through a change in the catalytic activity of enzymes. In some cases it is difficult to decide whether the effect of the hormone on enzymic activity is due to a change in the activity of the enzyme or in its amount. The final answer can be given only by directly measuring the quantity of the enzyme and its specific activity as, for example, in the case of the cytochromes [104] or the RNA-polymerase activity of nuclei [235].

Catalytic activity of enzymes can be regulated by thyroid hormones either directly by the removal of essential coenzymes or activators (for example, as a result of complex formation between the thyroid hormones and magnesium, calcium, zinc, copper, and other ions [90] or a change in the reactivity of the SH-groups of thiol enzymes [90, 259, 270]) or indirectly

Table XIII. Action of Thyroid Hormones on Catalytic Activity of Certain Enzymes

Enzyme	Characteristics of effect of hormones on enzyme activity	Investigation cited
Glutamate dehydrogenase	Mixed type of inhibition relative to substrate and $NADH_2$; noncompetitive inhibition relative to $NADPH_2$	90
Lactate dehydrogenase	Inhibition of soluble, purified, and crystalline enzyme of the mixed type	90, 151
Glucose-6-phosphate and 6-phosphogluconate dehydrogenases	2- to-3-fold activation *in vivo,* no effect *in vitro*	90
Isocitrate dehydrogenase (NADP-specific)	Inhibition	90
Transhydrogenase	Inhibition in partly purified preparations	90
Succinate dehydrogenase	Stimulation (7×10^{-7} M T_4) and inhibition (1.4×10^{-6} M T_4). Partly purified enzyme from sarcosomes in completely inhibited noncompetitively and irreversibly in the presence of 4×10^{-5} M T_4	90, 248
Malate dehydrogenase	Inhibition by thyroxine, ICN, and I_2 as a result of direct action on the sulfhydryl groups of the enzyme	270
Cytochrome c oxidase	Increase in the number of *cycles* in hypothyroidism and a decrease in hyperthyroidism	104
Ascorbate oxidase	Activation (1×10^{-5} M T_4) as a result of binding copper ions	90
Xanthine oxidase	50% inhibition obtained with 4.6×10^{-4} M T_3 or 5.6×10^{-5} M ICN. Possible action of I^+	169
Purified mitochondrial ATPase	Considerable inhibition of activity in the presence of uncoupling analogs of thyroxine	196
ATP-creatine transphosphorylase	Inhibition through the removal of soluble Mg^{++}	151

by their control over a reaction in which an inhibitor is formed or used up (for example, the thyroid hormones control the activity of the malate dehydrogenase reaction in the course of which oxaloacetic acid—a competitive inhibitor of succinate dehydrogenase—is formed).

Many facts pointing to the regulation of catalytic activity of enzymes by thyroid hormones have been published [90, 104, 151, 259, 270]. Some of these facts, given in Table XIII, demonstrate in particular the great diversity of ways in which thyroid hormones act on enzymic processes. In some cases the effect of thyroid hormones on the catalytic activity of enzymes is nonspecific in character. For example, in the case of ascorbate oxidase, thyroxine can be replaced by other chelating agents [90], and inhibition of xanthine oxidase and malate dehydrogenase is observed in the presence not only of thyroid hormones, but also of other iodine-substituted compounds, iodine cyanide and molecular iodine. There is also clear disparity between the action of the hormone on activity of an enzyme *in vivo* and *in vitro* [90, 104, 151, 248]. Nevertheless, there is a real possibility that such a pathway of regulation of metabolism exists, although it tells us little about the mechanism of hormonal action.

The action of thyroid hormones on the activity of enzymes organized structurally and functionally into systems is of very great interest. Examples of such systems are intact mitochondria, various types of submitochondrial particles (SMPs), oligoenzyme complexes of mitochondria, and so on.

Oxidative Phosphorylation and the Principal Pathways for the Transfer of Energy in Mitochondria

The initial stages of oxidation are catalyzed in the mitochondria of animal tissues by more than 20 specific dehydrogenases, using NAD, NADP, and flavins as coenzymes. Determination of the sequence of components of the respiratory chain and of their kinetic and physicochemical parameters is linked with the early investigations of Keilin and the more recent work carried out in the laboratories of Chance and Green [36, 37, 42, 76]. It is postulated that individual electron carriers in mitochondria are oriented in a definite manner relative to each other. This increases many times over the rate of interaction between the components of one respiratory chain by comparison with interaction between the components of different chains. This high degree of orderliness in the arrangement of respiratory carriers, coded according to some suggestions [76, 77] in a special structural protein template, leads to high efficiency of energy production in the mitochondria. A general scheme of the order of the components of the respiratory chain and the localization of the coupling points is given in

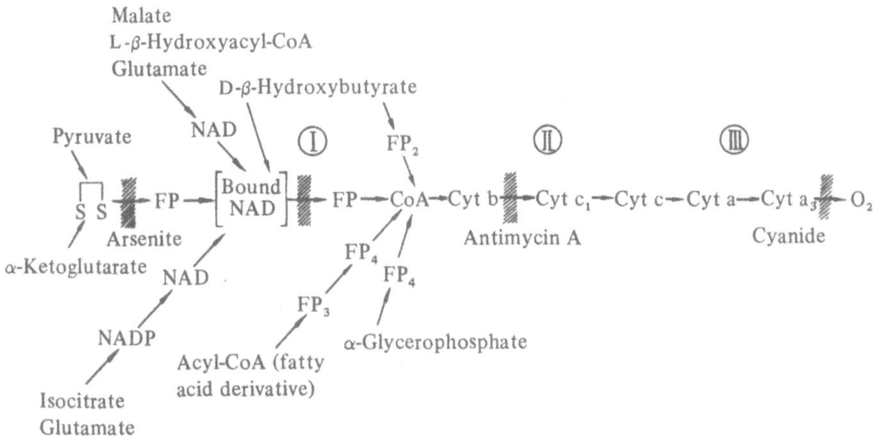

Fig. 7. Scheme of the respiratory chain according to Lehninger [142]. Hatched areas represent points of action of inhibitiors; I, II, III, points of phosphorylation.

Figure 7; the points at which the most frequently used inhibitors of electron transport act are also indicated.

There is as yet no general agreement regarding the molar relations between enzymes of the redox chain [61, 63, 76, 142]. The values of these ratios vary depending on the organ from which the mitochondria were isolated, and in most cases they are not 1:1.

An essential thermodynamic condition for the coupling of respiration with ATP synthesis is a change in the free energy ΔG at the corresponding site of the respiratory chain by an amount of not less than 9 kcal, corresponding to the free energy of hydrolysis of ATP (under physiological conditions). It follows from the redox potentials of the carriers of the respiratory chain that the necessary potential difference is provided at three sites of the respiratory chain (during oxidation through NAD): between NAD and FP_1, between cytochromes b and c, and between cytochrome c and oxygen. During oxidation of succinate only two coupling sites function. The presence of phosphorylation in precisely those sites which were predicted by thermodynamic calculations was brilliantly confirmed by the experiments of Chance using the *crossing points* method and incorporating the phenomenon of respiratory control [42].

The P/O and ADP/O ratios (since the equilibrium: HEC* + ADP + $P_{in} \rightarrow$ ATP is shifted to the right the ratios for ADP/O and P/O are approximately equal for firmly coupled mitochondria) reflecting the number of phosphorylations during the reduction of one atom of oxygen have the

*HEC, high-energy compound.

value of 3 for substrates oxidized through NAD but 2 for oxidation of succinate.

The mechanism of transformation of energy at the coupling points has been discussed now for two decades. In accordance with the original schemes of *chemical* coupling and some of their subsequent modifications [228], the primary high-energy bond is formed during interaction of the coupling components either with the oxidized form of the electron carrier or with its reduced form. The possibility that such a bond may also arise between the electron carrier and phosphate has also been admitted. Numerous attempts to convert these schemes to concrete reality have failed for various reasons [225–228].

As an alternative and more hopeful approach to the solution of the mechanism of energy transformation in mitochondria and chloroplasts, the chemo-osmotic theory of coupling formulated by Mitchell in 1961 must be examined [170]. Mitchell's theory was later modified, its details filled in, and its basic postulates proved experimentally [171–175, 229, 230, 291]. The basic principle of this theory is that respiration and phosphorylation are linked together through the electrochemical potential of hydrogen ions ($\Delta\mu_H$) on the mitochondrial membrane so that the phosphorylating mechanism utilizes the $\Delta\mu_H$ generated by the work of the redox chain. At one stage in the work of the phosphorylating mechanism the formation of a high-energy precursor of ATP (X~Y) from X^- and YO^- anions is assumed [229–230]:

$$X^- + YO^- + 2H^+ \rightleftarrows X{\sim}Y + H_2O$$

However, it is not this component but $\Delta\mu_H$ that must be identified with the universal intermediate substance X~Y postulated in the theory of chemical coupling and which is the source of the various ways for energy transfer in mitochondria (Figure 8). According to the illustrated scheme, hydrolysis of the primary high-energy compound X~Y can be reversed although equilibrium in the reaction given is strongly shifted to the left. The

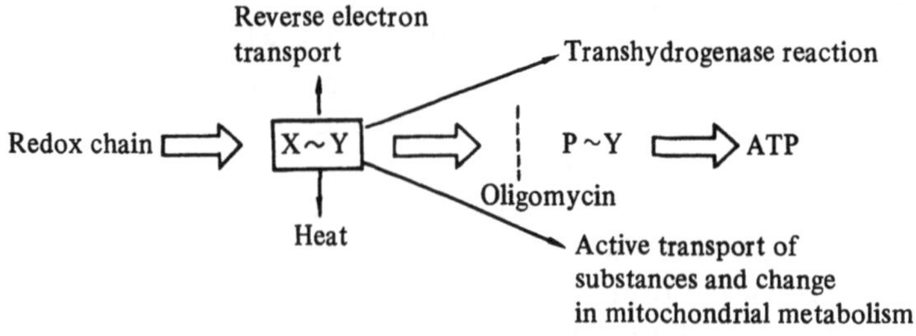

Fig. 8. Alternative pathways for the transfer of energy in mitochondria (after Skulachev [228]). The large arrows denote the main direction—the process of ATP synthesis.

hydrolysis of X∾Y can be reversed by an increase in the concentrations of X^-, YO^-, and H^+ and a decrease in X∾Y and H_2O, as a result of induced respiration, in the active center of the ATP synthetase. The necessary changes in concentrations, as Skulachev [229, 230] points out, are the result of interaction among several factors.

1. The increase in concentration of X^- and YO^- can take place through the electrophoresis of these anions in the internal membrane of the mitochondria. Mitchell postulated that the respiratory chain, localized in the membrane, carries negative charges (e^- or OH^-) inside the mitochondrion. The electric field thus formed, oriented across the membrane (with the negative charge inside the mitochondrion), can be used as the motive force for the transfer of X^- and YO^- inside the membrane. To explain the existence of three coupling points between $NADH_2$ and O_2 Mitchell postulated that the respiratory chain forms three *loops* in the membrane (the electrons move inward and the H^+ ions outward).
2. The high H^+ concentration outside can be maintained entirely by the same respiratory chain sharing the charges (the low permeability of the membrane for ions under the conditions favoring oxidative phosphorylation also contribute to this result).
3. The removal of X∾Y from the sphere of its formation, located nearer to the outer surface of the mitochondrial membrane, is catalyzed by a special enzyme known as X∾Y translocase, which transports X∾Y toward the inner surface of the membrane. It is here that ATP formation, coupled with X∾Y breakdown, takes place.
4. The water formed during the synthesis of X∾Y is removed from the membrane because of the hydrophobic properties of this part of the mitochondria.

The possibility of chemo-osmotic synthesis of ATP on account of the H^+ gradient was verified experimentally in principle in Mitchell's laboratory [202] on mitochondria and by Jagendorf and Uribe [102] on chloroplasts. Other workers [48, 49, 229, 230] have described ATP synthesis coupled with movement of cations along the concentration gradient in the mitochondria during the outflow of K^+ or Ca^{++}.

Experiments to reconstruct the system of energy transformation in the mitochondria [105, 198, 229, 230, 291] have confirmed the basic postulate of Mitchell's chemo-osmotic theory of the ability of two systems (oxidation-reduction and ATPase) to transform the chemical energy of redox conversions or ATP hydrolysis independently into the membrane electrochemical potential difference. If a portion of the respiratory chain (cytochrome c + cytochrome oxidase) and ATPase were introduced into lysosomal membranes simultaneously, these membranes were able to synthesize ATP on account of the energy of ascorbate oxidation [198]. An objective evaluation of the situation as it now stands in bioenergetics thus enables us, in the words of Skulachev [230], "... to use Mitchell's scheme as the only working hypothesis and to give it preference before the chemical and conformational concepts of oxidative phosphorylation."

Progress in the elucidation of the mechanisms participating in the main pathway of utilization of the energy produced by the respiratory chain (the pathway of ATP synthesis) has been largely due to the discovery of alternative pathways of energy utilization in the mitochondria in the 1960s (Figure 8). Among these alternative pathways are the energy-dependent transhydrogenase reaction, the reverse transport of electrons, active transport of materials and the changes in volume of the mitochondria associated with it, and the dissipation of energy as heat [142, 227, 272]. The common feature of all these alternative pathways of energy utilization is their dependence on intermediate HEC. The use of the $X{\sim}Y$ component in pathways alternative to the ATP-synthetase reaction is sharply inhibited under conditions where the transfer of energy along the phosphorylating pathway is impossible [228]. However, if ATP synthesis is blocked, for example, by the antibiotic oligomycin (which blocks the transfer of energy between $X{\sim}Y$ and $X{\sim}P$) or by a deficiency of ADP, all the energy can be directed into the channel of the alternative pathway (in particular, toward supplying energy for active transport of ions in isolated mitochondria). It must also be pointed out that the endergonic reactions mentioned above can be powered by energy produced in the mitochondria both by hydrolysis of ATP and by the work of the respiratory chain. In the first case, oligomycin completely blocks these processes, unlike in systems in which energy is provided by the work of the redox chain.

Action of Thyroid Hormones on Oxidative Phosphorylation in the Mitochondria

In 1951 three groups of workers independently described the effect of thyroxine on oxidative phosphorylation. Martius and Hess [159] found that thyroxine inhibits the esterification of inorganic phosphate. Niemeyer et al. [178] showed that respiratory control is lost in mitochondria isolated from the tissues of rats receiving large doses of thyroxine. Finally, Lardy and Feldott [129] found a decrease in the P/O ratio in tissue preparations from hyperthyroid rats and also after the addition of 1×10^{-5} M thyroxine to the tissues of control animals *in vitro*. Thyroxine and triiodothyronine increased the ATPase activity of the mitochondria. These results were later confirmed in many laboratories.

The decrease in the energy equivalent of tissue respiration in the mitochondria under the influence of large doses of thyroid hormones provided a sound basis for the understanding of the origin of symptoms of thyrotoxicosis such as loss of weight, muscular weakness, lowered working capacity, rapid onset of fatigue, and so on, which are difficult to explain from the standpoint of simple activation of biological oxidation. When phosphorylation is undisturbed, such activation could only lead to an increase in the energy resources of the body. Attention was therefore directed toward the chemical similarity between the molecules of thyroid hormone (an iodinated phenol) and the classical uncoupler of oxidative phosphorylation—2,4-dinitrophenol [178].

The only property common to all members of this class of uncouplers of oxidative phsophorylation is their ability to uncouple electron transport along the respiratory chain from energy production, accompanied by the inhibition of endergonic reactions in the mitochondria [8, 122, 147, 148, 228, 231].

Within the framework of the chemical hypothesis of coupling it is usually accepted that the uncoupling of oxidative phosphorylation is caused by interaction between the uncoupling agent and the primary high-energy compound:

$$AH_2 + B + I = A{\sim}I + BH_2$$

$$A{\sim}I + \Phi = A + \Phi{-}I$$

$$\Phi{-}I + H_2O \rightarrow \Phi + I$$

where $A{\sim}I$ is the primary high-energy compound, Φ the uncoupling agent, A and B are components of the respiratory chain, and I is the coupling component.

Depending on the stability of the $\Phi{-}I$ complex, either the inhibition of respiration (if the complex is stable) or the activation of respiration (if the complex is unstable) is observed. Even in the latter case, however, the reaction may be shifted toward complex formation through an increase in the concentration of the uncoupler. This could explain the inhibition of mitochondrial ATPase and respiration caused by an excess of uncoupler. In some cases, however, other causes of inhibition of respiration by uncouplers have undoubtedly been demonstrated, and these are analyzed in detail by Skulachev [228]. One possible way by which uncoupling agents can influence the rate of transport of electrons along the respiratory chain is by protonation of those groups of the dehydrogenases that are responsible for binding the substrate and are protected from H^+ ions of water by hydrophobic sites [220, 228]. In this case the ability of uncoupling agents to dissociate like weak acids and their ability to act as conductors of H^+ (protonophores) into the hydrophobic sites of the membranes, important for all the classical uncoupling agents, is clearly manifested. The action of uncoupling agents as weak lipid-soluble acids is not limited to protonation of dehydrogenases—in the undissociated form uncoupling agents, having penetrated into the hydrophobic sites of mitochondrial membranes, possibly protonate the nucleophilic coupling intermediate in the first place or bring about acid hydrolysis of the primary HEC and protonate dehydrogenases only in higher concentrations [200, 228]. Replacement of the only *dissociable* hydrogen atom in the highly active uncoupler tetrachloro-2-trifluoromethylbenzimidazole (TTFB) by a methyl group thus leads to the total loss of its uncoupling properties [10].

Another point of view on the mechanism of uncoupling has been developed by Van Damm and Slater (see [228]), who consider that a disturbance of the mechanisms of energy transfer in the presence of uncoupling agents is the result of the useless dissipation of energy in the cyclic active transport of the anion of the uncoupler within the mitochondrion. Racker, in turn, considers that classical uncouplers of the 2,4-dinitrophenol (DNP) type cause the spatial separation of the phosphorylation system from the respiratory chain and not hydrolysis of the primary HEC [196]. The different views about the mechanism of uncoupling, within the chemical concept of oxidative phosphorylation, are compared in recent publications [122, 228, 231], and there is therefore no need to dwell specially on this matter.

On the other hand, in accordance with the chemo-osmotic mechanism of oxidative phosphorylation, the action of uncouplers, which may include various substances, can be attributed to an increase in the conductance of the membrane. This leads to a decrease in the membrane potential difference necessary for ATP synthesis [171]. Ideal uncouplers are lipid-soluble substances with the ability to increase the conductance of the membrane for protons, i.e., substances which dissociate like acids. Nonideal uncouplers are carriers of any other ions (in this case alkali will accumulate on one side of the membrane and acid on the other). In fact, as Mitchell [174], showed, the chemical coefficient of conduction of hydrogen ions (C_M) for mitochondria under normal conditions is 0.110 ± 0.006 μg-ion H^+/sec · 1 pH · g protein, but after addition of DNP or *p*-trifluoromethoxycarbonylcyanidephenylhydrazone (FCP) the values of the coefficient C_M are 1.21 and 1.76, respectively. Consequently, because of their properties of a shunt with H^+-conductance, uncoupling agents cause a special kind of *short-circuiting* of the membrane potential difference, with the resulting uncoupling of oxidative phosphorylation, so that energy is dissipated.

It is interesting to note that the action of uncouplers of oxidative phosphorylation on artificial bimolecular phospholipid membranes (BPMs)

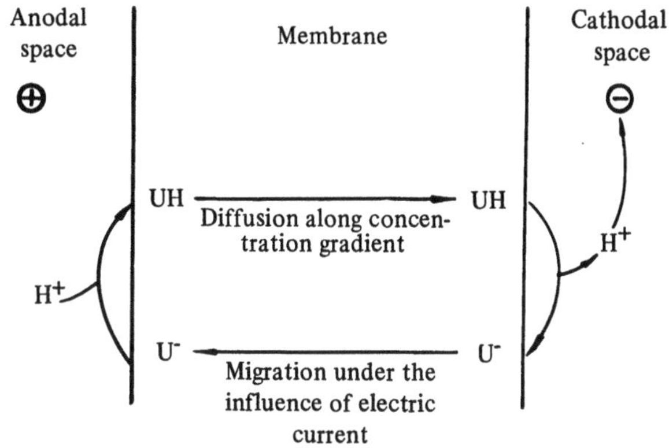

Fig. 9. Scheme illustrating the mechanism of increased proton conductance of membranes in the presence of classical uncouplers of oxidative phosphorylation (after Skulachev [228]).

is characterized by the same shunting property (Figure 9), a phenomenon first studied in detail in the laboratories of Lehninger, Liberman, and Skulachev [8, 12, 147, 220, 228]. The uncoupling activity of a wide range of compounds, both already known and predicted theoretically beforehand, also correlated strictly with their ability to increase the proton conductance of BPMs [147, 148, 228].

In order to answer the question whether thyroid hormones act on oxidative phosphorylation by the same mechanism as DNP and the other classical uncouplers, their effects must be compared on intact mitochondria and on more simplified systems, including artificial phospholipid membranes. Thyroid hormones disturbed the mechanism of energy coupling both *in vivo*, when administered to animals and oxidative phosphorylation was then studied in isolated mitochondria, and *in vitro*, when the thyroid hormones were added directly to mitochondria isolated from the tissues of normal animals [90, 97, 143, 194, 195, 212, 217, 218, 224, 248, 263].

Thyroid hormones bring about both complete and partial uncoupling [90, 248, 259]. This last fact is generally regarded as proof of the selective action of thyroid hormones on coupling sites. According to numerous observations, the first coupling site is most sensitive to thyroxine [194, 195, 259]. In particular, uncoupling of oxidative phosphorylation was demonstrated with $NADH_2$ as the donor and ferricyanide as the electron acceptor in the liver mitochondria in thyrotoxicosis. The effect of thyrotoxicosis on the transformation of energy linked with oxidation of reduced cytochrome c was only moderate [157]. To emphasize this feature, Rachev describes the first point of energy transformation as "labile," the second as "latent," and the third as "indifferent" [194, 195]. This selectivity is evidently due to the fact that the physical characteristics of the three phosphorylation points are different [196]. The molecular mechanism of the preferential action of thyroid hormones on the first phosphorylation point, in Lehninger's opinion [143, 144], is interaction with the bound form of NAD. Unequal activity at different coupling points has been demonstrated, incidentally, for many classical uncouplers, although the reasons for this phenomenon are not yet sufficiently clear [127, 199, 283].

As Racker [196] has shown, coupling of phosphorylation with oxidation is dependent on several soluble factors. The accessibility of these coupling factors, the relative rate of oxidation, and the other kinetic features which determine which factor plays the limiting role at each phosphorylation point can all influence the properties of the individual coupling sites and stages of phosphorylation.

The action of classical uncouplers, Ca^{++} ions, and ADP on a mitochondrial suspension is accompanied by oxidation of all respiratory carriers [34, 36, 38–40, 142]. However, the effect of thyroid hormones is a combination of two opposite effects: (1) activation of respiration linked with uncoupling of oxidative phosphorylation, (2) inhibition of electron transport manifested by reduction of flavin coenzymes [167]. There is evidence that both phenomena take place simultaneously but are independent and antagonistic. This combined action of the thyroid hormones on the system of oxidation and phosphorylation in the mitochondria is not an exception. For example, amytal, an inhibitor of electron transport in the NAD-oxidase branch of the respiratory chain (Figure 7), in high concentration inhibits oxidation of succinate and uncouples oxidative phosphorylation [196, 228]. The presence of uncoupling properties has also been demonstrated for inhibitors of respiration such as antimycin A [98], azide [196], and so on. Characteristically, mitochondria isolated from animals treated with thyroxine respond to the addition of amytal as if they contained an agent acting like amytal at the first coupling point [96]. Amytal is evidently an uncoupler of the type whose inhibitory action on respiration precedes its uncoupling effect proper. As Skulachev states, it is not so easy to demonstrate uncoupling in this case because phosphorylation is inhibited to the same degree as respiration, and the P/O ratio is virtually unchanged [228]. Inhibitory effects of this type no longer correlate with the efficiency of uncouplers as conductors of an electric current through artificial membranes, and they are manifested most sharply when the whole respiratory chain from NAD to oxygen is activated. In the case of thyroid hormones, the analysis of their effect on the respiratory chain is complicated by the possible simultaneous action of several factors:

a. the direct effect of the hormones on dehydrogenase activity and on components of the electron transport chain (Table XIII);

b. changes in the rate of electron transport through their influence on the coupled mechanism;
c. synthesis of new respiratory enzymes *in vivo*.

Just as with most other classical uncouplers, the effects of thyroid hormones can be conveniently analyzed by measuring parameters such as the respiration rate of mitochondria in state 3 (in the presence of ADP, P_{inorg}, oxidation substrate, and oxygen), and also in state 4 (the resting state after the completion of phosphorylation of ADP). The ratio between the respiration rates in these two metabolic states gives the value of what Chance [38, 42] describes as the respiratory control (RC), the parameter of the functional state of the mitochondria which changes most precisely in response to various factors. Another quantitative index of the efficiency of the coupling mechanism—the ADP/O ratio—is approximately equal to the P/O ratio, but in polarographic experiments ADP/O can be calculated only in the case of mitochondrial preparations with respiratory control (as defined by Chance) greater than 1. In the presence of thyroid hormones the value of the respiratory control of the mitochondria may be considerably reduced, down to a minimal value of 1, whereas the P/O ratio is virtually unchanged [90, 97, 99]. By contrast with *firmly* coupled preparations, such systems are usually described as *loosely* coupled [144]. The response of mitochondria to the action of thyroid hormones can be expressed not only as conversion into a state of loose coupling (Table XIV, experiment I), but also by complete loss of coupling (Table XIV, experiment II). It is noteworthy that in both cases respiration in state 4 (without acceptor) is sharply increased in thyrotoxicosis. Administration of DNP, pentachlorophenol, or other uncouplers to animals gives a similar effect [31, 90, 187]. Morphological and biochemical investigations of mitochondria isolated from the tissues of animals with different levels of thyroid hormones showed a parallel between the structural state of the mitochondria and functional changes in their metabolism.

Table XIV. Demonstration of "Loose" Coupling and Complete Uncoupling in Thyrotoxicosis (after Hoch [90])

	Experimental conditions	Rate of respiration – Acceptor	Rate of respiration + Acceptor	RC	P/O
I	Control	19	27	1.42	2
	Thyrotoxicosis	28	29	1.04	2
II	Control	19	32	1.7	1.4
	Thyrotoxicosis	25	27	1.08	0.2

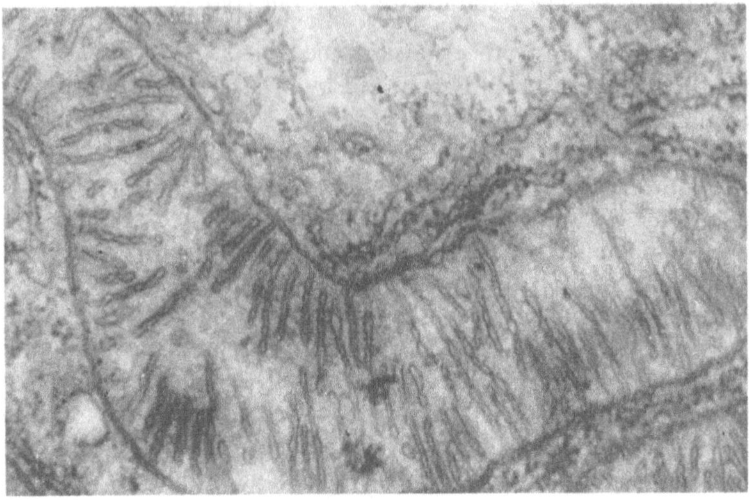

Fig. 10a

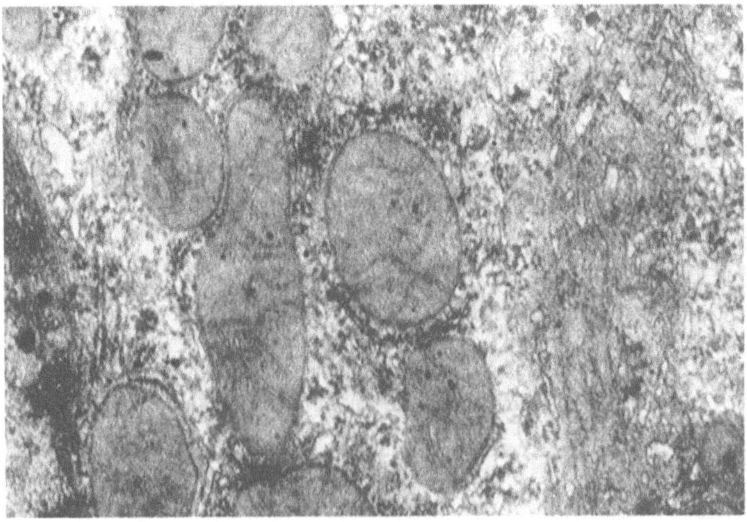

Fig. 10b

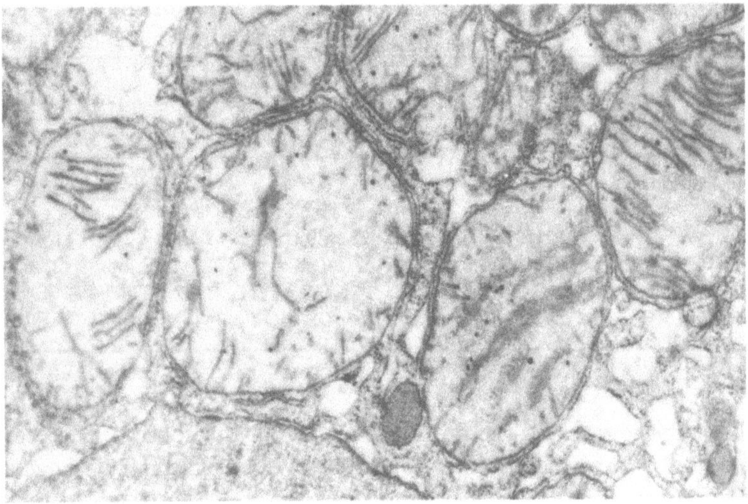

Fig. 10c

Fig. 10. Ultrastructure of the mitochondria in liver cells of rats: (a) hyperthyroidism, (b) hypothyroidism, (c) thyrotoxicosis.

A marked increase in the number of mitochondrial cristae and an increase in size of the mitochondria are observed in the liver cells in hyperthyroidism. The endoplasmic reticulum is firmly applied to the outer mitochondrial membrane and contains many ribosomes, frequently forming polyribosomal agglomerations (Figure 10a). A marked increase in size of the mitochondria and close contact with the granular endoplasmic reticulum are found in the liver cells of thyrotoxic rats. There is a marked increase in the number of ribosomes, especially on membranes adjacent to the mitochondria. The mitochondria of the liver cells in thyrotoxicosis are mainly of two types: (a) with the structure completely intact, (b) swollen, with reduced mitochondrial cristae (Figure 10c). The mitochondria of thyroidectomized rats are compact, and many tiny vacuolar structures appear in their matrix (Figure 10b). Condensation of the endoplasmic reticulum is observed in the cytoplasm of the cells.

Differences in the level of thyroid hormone in the body are thus accompanied by changes in some of the cellular organelles of the liver tissue. The most constant changes in the conditions described above are a decrease or increase in the number of ribosomes with the granular endoplasmic reticulum more closely approximated to the mitochondria, and destruction of the mitochondrial cristae in the presence of thyrotoxic doses of the hormones. Our own investigations and data in the literature [90, 212, 259, 263] show that physiological doses (moderate hyperthyroidism) increase the

Table XV. Oxidative Phosphorylation of Liver Mitochondria of Rats Receiving Various Doses of Thyroxine

Rate of respiration, ng-atom O_2/min·mg protein	Normal (6)	Hyperthyroidism (6)	Thyrotoxicosis (11)	Thyroidectomy (15)
Before addition of ADP	44.3 ± 1.3	126.5 ± 7.2	271.5 ± 12.2	36.9 ± 1.8
In state 3	128.3 ± 8.5	229.9 ± 29.0	271.5 ± 12.2	115.8 ± 4.4
In state 4	38.2 ± 1.6	90.2 ± 10.8	271.5 ± 12.2	27.6 ± 2.1
Respiratory control	3.7 ± 0.2	3.4 ± 0.3	1	4.4 ± 0.3
ADP/O ratio	1.6 ± 0.07	1.6 ± 0.1	–	1.7 ± 0.1

Note: Number of experiments shown in parentheses.

basal metabolic rate and the rate of growth, but the coefficient of respiratory control of the isolated mitochondria shows no significant change under these circumstances.

The intensity of oxygen consumption by the liver mitochondria of normal rats during oxidation of succinate is 44.38 ± 1.35 mg-atom O_2/min·mg protein. ATP stimulates respiration to 128.33 ± 8.5; the coefficient of respiratory control under these circumstances is 3.78, and the ADP/O ratio is 1.63 (Table XV). After administration of small doses of thyroid hormone to animals (hyperthyroid rats), the intensity of oxidation of succinate in the mitochondria increased by 2.9 times above the normal level; the accelerated electron transport along the respiratory chain was not accompanied by any change in the respiratory control or the ADP/O ratio.

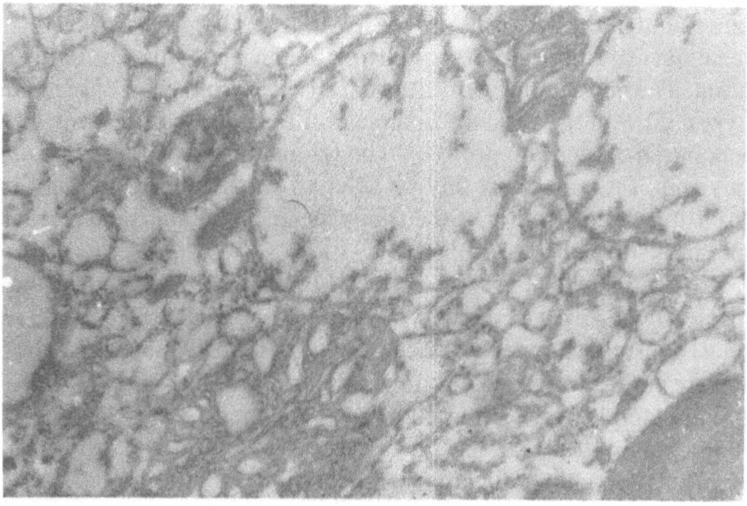

Fig. 11a

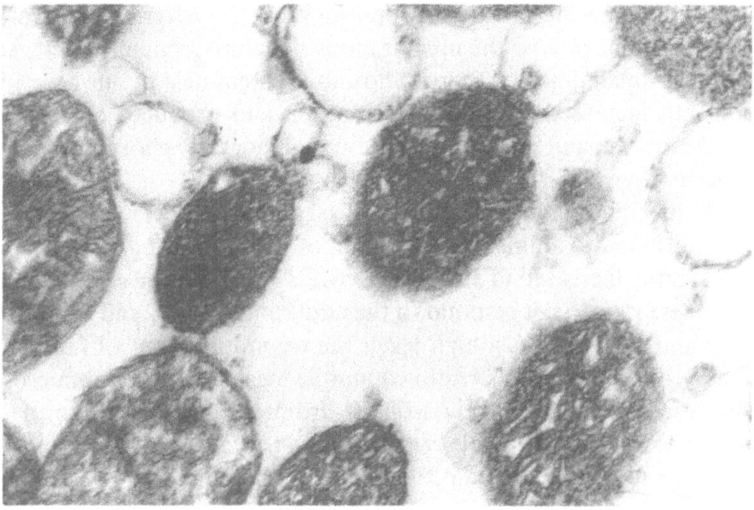

Fig. 11b

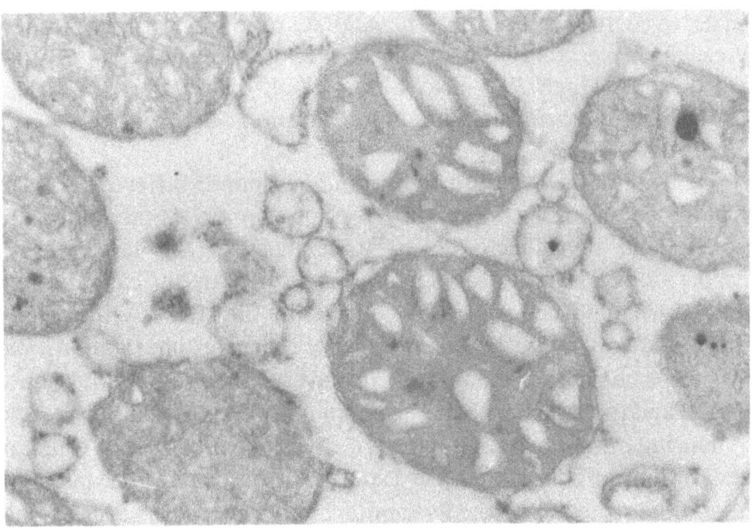

Fig. 11c

Fig. 11. Electron-microscopic structure of mitochondria of the rat liver: (a)–thyrotoxic, (b)–after thyroidectomy, (c)–normal.

Investigation of the morphology of the mitochondria of hyperthyroid rats shows that the isolated mitochondria are of large size and have a looser matrix with numerous intramitochondrial vacuoles. After administration of thyroid hormone *in vivo* the membranous structure remains intact. Administration of small doses of thyroid hormone to animals in our own investigation thus increased the rate of respiration and produced changes in the structure of the mitochondria, although oxidative phosphorylation remained unaffected.

A different picture is observed if large (toxic) doses of the hormone are administered to animals. Respiration of the mitochondria of thyrotoxic rats is sharply increased (Table XV) to 612.13% of normal. The mitochondria of these rats do not respond to the addition of ADP, and respiration in states 3 and 4 remains at a high level; the respiratory control falls to unity and, as a result, the ADP/O ratio cannot be measured. The submicroscopic organization of mitochondria isolated from the liver of thyrotoxic rats differs sharply from that observed in intact rats. The mitochondria are swollen, some of them contain fibrils and are bounded by a clearly defined membrane, and the matrix is electron-optically transparent (Figure 11a).

The liver mitochondria of thyroidectomized rats are smaller in size, and their matrix is less compact (Figure 11b). A slight decrease in the intensity of respiration was observed in mitochondria isolated from these animals, to 83.14% of normal. The ADP/O ratio was within normal limits, whereas the respiratory control was appreciably increased. In thyroidectomized animals Hoch [93] also observed an extremely high respiratory control which fell to normal after administration of thyroid hormone to the rats.

Depending on the dose of thyroid hormone, different effects were thus obtained on energy processes in the mitochondria. Stimulating doses of thyroxine and thyroidectomy led to changes in the level of electron transport along the respiratory chain, increasing it in one case and reducing it in the other, but the respiratory control and the ADP/O ratio, reflecting the degree of coupling of electron transport and phosphorylation, were not significantly changed. Toxic doses, however, led to rapid oxidation of the substrate and to disturbance of the coupling of oxidative phosphorylation.

During the study of the action of thyroxine *in vitro*, the effect of different concentrations (1×10^{-9} to 1×10^{-4} M) on respiration, phosphorylation, and the structure of the liver mitochondria were tested in normal rats and in rats receiving different doses of the hormone (stimulating and toxic). By contrast with higher concentrations (5×10^{-5} to 1×10^{-4} M), concentrations of 1×10^{-9} to 1×10^{-5} M of the hormone had no visible effect on biochemical processes in the mitochondria of these groups of rats. The results of an investigation into the effect of thyroxine (1×10^{-4} M) on respiration

Table XVI. Effect of Thyroxine (1×10^{-4} M) on Oxidative Phosphorylation of the Liver Mitochondria of Rats Receiving Different Doses of Thyroxine

Rate of respiration, ng-atom O_2min · mg protein	Normal (6)	Hyperthyroidism (6)	Thyrotoxicosis (6)	Thyroidectomy (6)
Before addition of ADP	51.6 ± 3.6	121.2 ± 11.5	260.8 ± 9.9	35.5 ± 2.1
Ditto + thyroxine	98.0 ± 7.3	290.8 ± 10.2	260.8 ± 9.9	54.5 ± 7.2
In state 3 + thyroxine	108.7 ± 20.2	290.8 ± 10.2	260.8 ± 9.9	177.5 ± 5.9
In state 4 + thyroxine	108.8 ± 20.2	122.7 ± 13.9	260.8 ± 9.9	92.3 ± 7.2
Respiratory control	1	2.47 ± 0.2	1	2.0 ± 0.2
ADP/O ratio	—	0.63 ± 0.025	—	1.1 ± 0.1

Note: The oxidation substrate was succinate. Number of experiments shown in parentheses.

and phosphorylation of the mitochondria of the rat liver are given in Table XVI.

In experiments with the mitochondria of normal rats, after the addition of thyroxine (1×10^{-4} M) the rate of respiration during oxidation of succinate increased, whereas the respiratory control fell to unity. In hyperthyroid animals this concentration of the hormone stimulated respiration by an even greater degree (by 2.4 times) than in normal rats; the respiratory control, however, was reduced by one-third and phosphorylation was also reduced. As a result, the ADP/O ratio fell to 0.69 ± 0.025 compared with 1.66 ± 0.10 before the addition of thyroxine. In this case, evidently, thyroxine led to incomplete uncoupling.

In experiments with the mitochondria of animals receiving a high dose of thyroxine, addition of the hormone (1×10^{-4} M) did not alter respiration, which remained at its previous high level in both the absence and the presence of phosphate acceptor. In the liver mitochondria of thyroidectomized animals, thyroxine led to a small increase (not statistically significant) in the rate of oxidation of the substrate to the level characteristic of normal mitochondria. The respiratory control was reduced by 2.2 times, and the ADP/O ratio also was low. It is important to note that Hoch [93] demonstrated a decrease in the respiratory control and an increase in the rate of respiration in state 4 by 2.01 and 1.76 times, respectively, after administration of an extremely low subcalorigenic dose of thyroxine (0.52 μg/100 g body weight) to hypothyroid animals. The phosphorylation coefficient in these animals, however, remained practically constant.

It will be clearly understood that the numerical values of the functional parameters of the state of the mitochondria given above are the averaged responses of mitochondria, which in general are extremely heterogeneous, to the preparation tested. As Hülsmann [99] reports, two types of mitochondria, described conventionally as M_1 and M_2, can be isolated from rat heart and skeletal muscles. The M_1 fraction, the yield of which increases with an increase in the dose of thyroid hormones administered, has a relatively high rate of respiration in the presence of added ATP and MG on account of spontaneous ATPase activity. The ADP/O ratio (for glutamate) is normally high (2.7), although the respiratory control is low (1.9). The mitochondria in the M_2 fraction have the typical properties of *firmly* coupled mitochondria, no spontaneous Mg^{++}-activated ATPase, high respiratory control, and high P/O ratio (5.1 and 2.8, respectively). These observations are explained by assuming that M_1 is the *aged* form of the M_2 fraction and that perhaps phospholipase participates in the mechanism of aging. Hülsmann considers that if the number of mitochondria of the M_1 type is also increased in other tissues in thyrotoxicosic animals, this could account for the increased basal metabolic rate.

Action of Thyroid Hormones on Mitochondrial Metabolic Responses and ATPase

When describing the uncoupling activity of the thyroid hormones, their effects on certain metabolic reactions and on the ATPase activity of isolated mitochondria must be examined. These processes have been widely investigated by many workers in order to obtain definite conclusions regarding the reaction of ATP synthesis as a whole.

The following metabolic reactions have most frequently been studied during attempts to analyze the mechanism of oxidative phosphorylation: P_{inorg}–ATP, H_2O–P_{inorg}, H_2O–ATP [142, 196]. According to one scheme proposed recently [103], these metabolic reactions are evidently interconnected within the framework of the following process:

$$HOPO_3^{2-} + ADP \overset{\sim}{\longleftrightarrow} ATP + HOH$$

where $\sim$ represents an intermediate high-energy compound (or state).

The metabolic reaction P_{inorg}–ATP does not require actual transport of electrons along the respiratory chain. It is depressed by many uncoupling agents, and its inhibition proceeds parallel with a decrease in oxidative phosphorylation [196]. As Lindberg et al. [150] and Bronk [23] point out, this reaction is effectively inhibited by thyroxine and its uncoupling analogs. The degree of inhibition depends on the concentration of hormonal products, the duration of the experiments, and the concentration of ATP and other controllable factors.

The metabolic reaction ADP–ATP evidently is also linked with oxidative phosphorylation [196]. The sensitivity of this reaction to DNP during aging of the mitochondria parallels the disturbance of oxidative phosphorylation [196]. More recently, weighty evidence has been obtained that this metabolic reaction is directly connected with the degree of integrity of the isolated mitochondria and inversely connected with the ATPase activity. It was therefore postulated that the metabolic system of ADP–ATP is a highly organized membrane complex, containing membrane ATPase among its other components.

Lindberg et al. [150] demonstrated inhibition of the metabolic reaction ADP–ATP by the use of deaminothyroxine and of submitochondrial particles obtained by mechanical disintegration of mitochondria in a high-speed blender. Inhibition of Mg^{++}-activated ATPase of the particles parallels the inhibition of the metabolic reaction. However, by contrast with intact mitochondria, the connection between the two effects noted above was unclear, for a metabolic reaction ADP–ATP sensitive to deaminothyroxine was found in fractions both with and without ATPase activity.

The ATPase activity of intact mitochondria reflects the reversal of the process of ATP synthesis. An enzyme catalyzing ATP hydrolysis has now been isolated from mitochondria in the purified form [128, 134, 196, 216]. Structurally the ATPase described by Racker et al. is the *head* of the mushroomlike structures on the inner surface of the internal membrane of the mitochondria, whereas the *stalk* of the mushroomlike formations contains the factor responsible for the sensitivity of ATPase to oligomycin. Purified ATPase is completely dependent on magnesium ions, and in the presence of magnesium it is activated by DNP. Many of the properties of this enzyme resemble those of the ATPase of submitochondrial particles [196].

In this connection it is instructive that thyroxine and its uncoupling analogs completely suppress ATPase activity in purified preparations of the enzyme and in the submitochondrial particles obtained from mitochondria after destruction by mechanical means and by ultrasound [23, 150]. On the other hand, thyroxine stimulates the ATPase activity of intact mitochondria, which increases parallel with their swelling [26, 68]. In the cases cited, the authors evidently were dealing with *magnesium-activated* ATPase, which is unmasked by damage to the structure of the mitochondria resulting from aging, swelling in a hypo-osmotic medium, in the presence of thyroxine, and so on. Using strontium ions, Caplan and Carafoli [29] showed that inhibition of magnesium-activated mitochondrial ATPase, after aging or swelling in the presence of thyroxine or phosphate, proceeds parallel with the stabilizing action of these agents on the structure of the mitochondria.

However, thyroxine, triiodothyronine, and deaminothyroxine effectively inhibit this ATPase activity in fragments of mechanically disintegrated mitochondira in which the level of magnesium-activated ATPase is sufficiently high [150]. The mechanism of inhibition is evidently the same as in purified preparations of the enzyme. Pentachlorophenol, chlorpromazine, atebrin, and so on had a similar action to thyroxine.

The ATPase activity of intact mitochondria rises sharply in the presence of classical uncouplers of oxidative phosphorylation, but with an increase in their concentration, stimulation of ATPase is replaced by inhibition. Characteristically, hydrolysis of ATP induced by uncouplers is observed when the structure of the mitochondria is intact, i.e., under unfavorable conditions for the detection of magnesium-activated ATPase. Hydrolysis of ATP stimulated by proton carriers probably reflects the energy expenditure of the mitochondria in restoring the ionic gradients and, in particular, the electrochemical H^+ gradient on the mitochondrial membrane, for the uncouplers discharge producing conductance along hydrogen ions. Activity of mitochondrial ATPase, acting as an H^+-translocator [171], in this case counteracts the shunting effect of the uncoupler, *pumping* protons into compartments of the mitochondria from which the uncoupler *expels* them.

According to the observations of Lindberg et al. [150], thyroid hormones inhibit DNP-activated ATPase of intact mitochondria. It is not clear, however, whether this inhibition is caused by an excess of uncouplers (if summation of the uncoupling action of DNP and thyroid hormones is accepted) or by thyroxine-induced structural damage to the mitochondria with parallel inhibition of DNP-activated ATPase and stimulation of Mg^{++}-activated ATPase. Partial removal of the inhibitory action of thyroxine in the presence of 4 mM magnesium may be evidence in support of this second hypothesis. On the other hand, the effect of magnesium can also be explained by the fact that it usually prevents swelling induced by thyroxine. The data on the action of thyroid hormones on DNP-activated mitochondrial ATPase are demonstrative also in that they reflect a characteristic feature of most of the effects of thyroid hormones that have been studied: the difficulty of choosing unambiguously between the *direct* uncoupling action of thyroxine and uncoupling taking place indirectly through structural disturbances induced by it in the mitochondria.

Action of Thyroid Hormones on the Transport of Energy in Submitochondrial Particles

After the discovery in Lehninger's laboratory and later elsewhere [142, 196] of methods of obtaining submitochondrial particles (by treating intact mitochondria with digitonin, Triton, alkali, ultrasound, mechanical fragmentation, and so on), it became possible to examine the relationship between the structural organization of the energy-transforming system and the action of thyroid hormones. In different types of submitochondrial particles (SMP), the possibility of oxidation of different substrates and the relative efficiency of phosphorylation at each of the three points vary considerably [196]. Considering the high efficiency of phosphorylation at the first coupling point in digitonin particles, it can be expected that the uncoupling action of the thyroid hormones in that case would be manifested more deeply than in ultrasonic SMP, for which the efficiency of phosphorylation at the first point is only 40% [196]. However, despite much evidence to show that the primary action of thyroxine is in fact localized at that phosphorylation point, possibly with the participation of the bound form of NAD [139, 144, 195], neither the coupling of respiration with phosphorylation nor the metabolic reactions P_{inorg}–ATP and ADP–ATP, nor ATPase activity was changed in digitonin fragments by the action of thyroxine or calcium [144]. Meanwhile, classical uncouplers such as DNP and dicoumarol affected all the processes mentioned above. The ineffectiveness of calcium ions is somewhat unexpected, for we know that calcium accumulates actively in digitonin SMP [272] and that is why it is potentially capable of influencing the intensity and direction of other alternative pathways of the transfer of energy. Possibly in order to demonstrate the effect of calcium ions in digitonin SMP, conditions somewhat different from those used by Lehninger et al. must be chosen.

On the other hand, the fact that thyroxine has no effect whatever on the metabolism of digitonin particles led to the hypothesis that the mechanism of disturbance of energy transfer in the presence of thyroid hormones is directly connected with changes in the structure of the intact mitochondrion, a highly organized system of great complexity. Consequently, maximal simplification of structural organization, as is achieved in the case of digitonin SMP, explains their resistance to the action of thyroid hormones. However, this conclusion evidently calls for some reexamination in view of a recent report that thyroid hormones disturb the mechanism of energy transfer in precisely this type of SMP [195].

By contrast with digitonin particles, ultrasonic SMP respond to the addition of thyroid hormones by a decrease in the P/O ratio during oxidation of both succinate and NAD-dependent substrates. Stimulation of respiration is observed in the absence of an acceptor system, and the activity of the metabolic reactions and of ATPase is inhibited [23]. Characteristically, an increase in the magnesium concentration in the medium does not reduce the inhibitory action of thyroxine on these processes. In Lehninger's opinion [139], the higher level of structural organization of the ultrasonic SMP explains their similarity with intact mitochondria and their difference from digitonin particles as regards functional responses to the addition of thyroid hormones.

In SMP obtained by mechanical disintegration of mitochondria in a high-speed blender [150], thyroid hormones and their uncoupling analog deaminothyroxine effectively inhibit Mg^{++}-activated ATPase and the metabolic reaction ADP–ATP as well as NAD-oxidase activity. A similar picture was observed when a classical uncoupler such as pentachlorophenol was used.

We must dwell for a while on the results obtained with the use of pigment granules, the volume of which is 0.1–0.0001 of the volume of the mitochondria of the liver. These granules from melanomas behave in their respiration and phosphorylation like mitochondria, except that, unlike mitochondria, they do not swell in a hypotonic medium or in the presence of Ca^{++} or detergents [90]. Thyroxine (5×10^{-5} M), like other uncouplers, completely disturbs the transfer of energy in preparations of these granules, stimulates their respiration, and inhibits the metabolic reaction P_{inorg}–ATP. Characteristically, the functional responses of melanoma granules to the addition of thyroxine were not accompanied by significant changes in their structure detectable turbidimetrically at 520 nm. However, the possibility cannot be ruled out that swelling of these granules nevertheless took place but could not be detected because the granules contain a pigment which also absorbs at a wavelength of 520 nm [90].

The action of thyroid hormones on the transformation of energy is thus manifested more or less constantly in systems that differ sharply from each other in the complexity of their structural organization. Meanwhile, the functional responses of mitochondria and of the various SMP are the same in most cases to both thyroid hormones and classical uncouplers such as DNP, dicoumarol, pentachlorophenol, and so on.

Effect of Thyroid Hormones on the Properties of Model Systems

A further assessment of the uncoupling properties of the thyroid hormones was carried out by the study of their activity on bimolecular phospholipid membranes (BPM) prepared from phospholipids of the brain [67, 266]. Thyroid hormones were found to reduce the resistance of BPM only a little (by 1.1–5 times, unlike the classical uncoupling agents, which reduce the resistance of these membranes by several orders of magnitude [8, 147, 228]. The same conclusion, namely, that thyroid hormones have no constant positive effect on artificial bimolecular membranes, was reached by Gruenstein and Wynn [80] at the same time as the present writer.

The low activity of thyroxine on bimolecular phospholipid membranes may be connected with its *atypical* lipid solubility. As Hillier [89] showed recently, the partition coefficient of thyroid hormones between the aqueous and lipid phases was comparatively high (1.7 in the case of a water–olive oil system) because of hydrophobic adsorption of the hormones on the phase boundary or in the juxtamembraneous layer. Only the undissociated aromatic part of the molecule penetrates into the lipid part of the membrane, and the dissociated *tail* of the molecule is in water. This fixed position evidently confers relatively low mobility on the hormone in the lipid layer, and this could explain its ineffectiveness on artificial membranes despite the fact that the *partition coefficient* is apparently very high.

Unlike thyroid hormones, the activity of DNP and other classical uncouplers on artificial bimolecular membranes is much greater. In particular, DNP (1×10^{-3} M) lowers the specific resistance of BPMs from 1.43×10^7 Ω/cm^2 to 6.1×10^4 Ω/cm^2, i.e., by more than 200 times [12].

The uncoupling of oxidative phosphorylation under the influence of thyroid hormones explains the reason for the more rapid oxidation of substrates in mitochondria. The reduced formation of ATP during each act of oxidation assumes the preservation of large quantities of phosphate acceptor (ADP) and of inorganic phosphorus in the system, where they act as physiological activators of tissue respiration. Such a mechanism of activation of respiration during the uncoupling of oxidative phosphorylation can be deduced, in particular, from the observations of Loomis and Lipmann [154] that the oxygen consumption under these conditions, during the oxidation of most substrates, increases by approximately the same degree as under the influence of phosphate-acceptor systems. If such systems are added to mitochondria, thyroid hormones do not exhibit their *calorigenic* effect [97, 130].

As was mentioned above, by reducing the liberation of ATP, uncoupling of oxidative phosphorylation can account for symptoms of thyrotoxicosis connected with energy deficiency and surplus heat production. The physiological role of uncoupling could lie in the utilization of reduced equivalents of the cell not for ATP production but for other (for example, biosynthetic) purposes.

Action of Thyroid Hormones on the Endergonic Reduction of NAD by Succinate and the Transhydrogenase Reaction

The endergonic reduction of NAD by succinate, discovered recently by Chance and Klingenberg [38, 118, 119], is regarded as the reversal of electron transport in the respiratory chain. On the addition of substrates oxidized through flavins (succinate, α-glycerophosphate) to mitochondria, the NAD is reduced, evidently through electron transport from flavins to NAD. Electron transport from FP_1 to NAD without the expenditure of energy is impossible, for the $NADH_2/NAD^+$ potential is 0.27 V more negative than the potential of FPH_2/FP, and if converted into free energy this is equivalent to 12 kcal. The energy of hydrolysis of intermediate high-energy compounds (HEC), according to the calculations of Klingenberg and Schollmeyer [119], lies within these same limits, i.e., energization of the mitochondria under favorable conditions can bring about the reversal of electron transport in the respiratory chain. The biological significance of reversed electron transport as a universal property of the mitochondria of most tissues studied may perhaps lie in the accumulation of a certain additional number of electron donors with negative potential in this way in the readily mobilized form of $NADH_2$ [226, 228]. Most of the mitochondrial NAD, it must be noted, is reduced through reversed electron transport from succinate.

Hess and Brand [88] showed that thyroxine and triiodothyronine in low concentrations inhibit the endergonic reduction of NAD by succinate in the presence of oligomycin. The inhibition of this reaction was discovered by these workers in mitochondria from the liver and also in sarcosomes, and the half-maximal effect was obtained with a concentration of 5×10^{-7} M T_3. Similar observations were made by Chance and Hollunger [39], in whose experiments thyroxine induced significant inhibition of reversed electron transport in a concentration of 1×10^{-7} M. On the other hand, Roche et al. [204] found no appreciable changes in the level of NAD oxidoreduction by the action of triiodothyronine or triiodothyronine acetate. Oxidation of $NADH_2$ was observed by these workers only when they used T_3 or T_3 acetate together with Ca^{++}, irrespective of the order in which these agents were added. The disagreement between the results obtained by different workers must evidently be attributed to the experimental conditions. Removal of Mg^{++} from mitochondria by the addition of EDTA to the medium, for instance, sharply increases the sensitivity of reversed electron transport to the action of thyroid hormones.

In the experiments cited below, a clear inhibition of reversed electron transport is demonstrated by thyroxine in a concentration of 6×10^{-5}. The addition of this hormone to a suspension of mitochondria oxidizing succinate leads to slow oxidation of $NAD(P)H_2$, while the subsequent addition of ADP does not induce any more cycles of NAD oxidoreduction, indicating inhibition of the reversed electron transport (Figure 12).

The inhibitory action of thyroid hormones on the endergonic reduction of NAD by succinate may be due, in particular, to suppression of electron transport in the $NADH_2 \rightarrow FP_1$ sector, as Chance and Hollunger [40] showed by the use of amytal and rotenone, by the inhibition of oxidation of succinate, or by de-energization of the mitochondria as a result of uncoupling. The mechanisms 1 and 3 are more realistic, for the addition of thyroid hormones to isolated liver mitochondria of euthyroid animals not only does not inhibit the oxidation of succinate but actually stimulates it, and on the

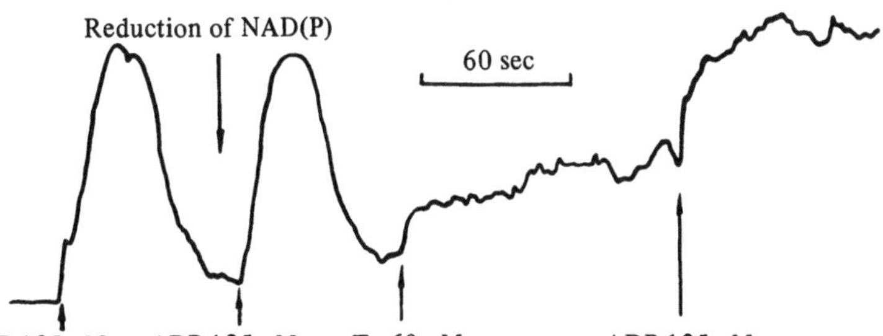

Fig. 12. Action of thyroxine and ADP on the level of reduction of endogenous NAD(P) in rat liver mitochondria (the level of reduction of NAD(P) was recorded fluorometrically; samples contained 120 mM KCl, 5 mM Tris-chloride, 2.5 mM KH_2PO_4, and 10 mM succinate; pH of the incubation medium 7.4).

other hand, thyroid hormones possess an uncoupling action with a simultaneous amytal-like effect on the electron transport chain [96].

Further details of the action of thyroid hormones on the energy transformation pathways in mitochondria can be obtained by examining the energy-dependent transhydrogenase reaction as a result of which NADP is reduced at the expense of $NADH_2$. This process, like reversed electron transport, depends on the presence of $\Delta\bar{\mu}_H$ on the membrane and is inhibited in the presence of the classical uncoupling agents [230]. The biological importance of the transhydrogenase reaction is examined by Vinogradov and Evtodienko [273] in their survey; it evidently lies in the generation of reducing equivalents essential for the synthesis of fatty acids, the 11-β-hydroxylation of steroids, the reduction of glutathione, and so on.

Estabrook et al. [58] found that half-maximal inhibition of the energy-dependent transhydrogenase reaction is attained in the presence of triiodothyronine in the incubation medium in a concentration of about 1.5×10^{-5} M. It is interesting to note that in the presence of triiodothyronine the analogous transhydrogenase in the chromatophores of *Rhodospirillum rubrum* is inhibited [112]. The influence of thyroid hormones on the transhydrogenase reaction is evidently connected with their uncoupling activity.

On the other hand, the inhibitory effect of thyroxine and triiodothyronine on the energy-independent transhydrogenase, catalyzing hydrogen transport between NAD and $NADPH_2$ [53], could also have important metabolic consequences and, in particular, the accumulation of $NADPH_2$ in the tissues. During acceleration of the oxidation of this pyridine nucleotide through $NADPH_2$-cytochrome c reductase, the activity of which is increased by thyroid hormones [188, 234, 256], the P/O ratio in the brain tissues could fall to 1, for electrons from $NADPH_2$ enter the respiratory chain bypassing both the first stages of phosphorylation. The oxidation of

$NADPH_2$ need not be coupled with phosphorylation but could take place through marked activation of tissue peroxidases by thyroxine [114]. Activation of $NADPH_2$-cytochrome c reductase could also lead to acceleration of the work of the pentose cycle and of the dehydrogenation of isocitrate in the hyaloplasm, as is in fact observed in thyrotoxicosis. Meanwhile, the fact that transhydrogenase is inhibited by thyroid hormones *in vivo* has not yet been proved. Stein et al. [243], for example, found no change in the activity of this enzyme in the tissues of hyperthyroid animals.

Calorigenic shunts of metabolism of the type described above could, as has already been mentioned, play an important role in the reduction of the energy efficiency of tissue respiration by the action of thyroid hormones. However, whether their action is of primary importance is a problem which has not yet been solved. Without mentioning the fact that each of these shunts separately cannot give rise to the whole picture of characteristic metabolic changes of hyperthyroidism, or that it is still doubtful whether they can actually function separately when thyroxine is administered *in vivo*, there are also other grounds for rejecting such a mechanism of the calorigenic effect of the thyroid hormones.

The functioning of each of the oxidation shunts described assumes a stable (although low) value of the P/O ratio in the tissues. Under the influence of thyroxine, however, this ratio changes depending on the dose of the hormone. It was mentioned earlier that during the action of physiological concentrations of thyroid hormones no decrease whatever in P/O can be found. Larger doses lower the P/O ratio for oxidation of α-ketoglutarate, but not of succinate. A further increase in the doses of hormones given reveals a decrease in the P/O ratio during the oxidation of succinate or of other substrate entering the respiratory chain at the flavoprotein level. Finally, in marked thyrotoxicosis the P/O ratio may be below 1 [97, 158, 159]. Complete uncoupling of oxidative phosphorylation can also be produced *in vitro* by the addition of appropriate quantities of thyroid hormones [116, 246, 285].

Variations in the P/O ratio through the action of thyroid hormones and the possibility of the complete uncoupling of oxidation and phosphorylation are thus evidence against a decisive role of calorigenic metabolic shunts in the mechanism of the effects of these hormones. The functioning of these shunts likewise does not explain the formation of carbon dioxide in the body. The respiratory quotient in thyrotoxicosis, however, is initially close to 1, and even in advanced stages of the disease it does not fall below 0.7.

Action of Thyroid Hormones on Ionic Transport in Mitochondria

Considerable energy is utilized in the mitochondria for active ionic transport. Several explanations of the mechanism of accumulation of ions in mitochondria have been put forward. They differ chiefly as regards the initial stages of ion accumulation or, more precisely, the motive forces responsible for this process.

According to one of the schemes, cations accumulate as a result of stoichiometric interaction between the cation and intermediate HECs generated on account of the work of the redox chain or of ATP hydrolysis [18, 35, 36]. Interaction of this type leads to the breakdown of the HEC with the liberation of H^+ into the extramitochondrial medium and to transfer of a cation inside the mitochondrion, where it is fixed on the negative charges of phospholipid or protein groups. If the medium contains anions able to pass through the mitochondrial membrane (phosphate, arsenate, acetate), translocation of cations can take place on a broader scale; eventually compounds of differing solubility, depending on the type of cation and anion, accumulate inside the mitochondria.

Alternatively Chappell and Crofts [47] suggested that the mitochondrial membrane contains a specific H^+-pump, the operation of which requires energy of the X∾Y component. The electrical neutrality of the membrane, disturbed because of the pumping out of H^+, is restored by the accumulation of cations (mainly potassium, calcium, strontium, and manganese ions). Anionic transport evidently takes place as an exchange-diffusion process in which the phosphate can be exchanged for $-OH$ and the undissociated molecules (CO_2, CH_3COOH) penetrate freely. According to these workers' observations, the mitochondrial membrane is impermeable to monovalent cations. However, antibiotics of polypeptide nature (valinomycin, gramicidin) render both mitochondrial membranes and artificial phospholipid membranes highly permeable to these cations [27, 46, 47, 83]. The flow of cations through the mitochondrial membrane induced by antibiotics stimulates the activity of the H^+ pump and requires a flow of ions inside the mitochondria to neutralize the alkaline medium, thus enabling further H^+ ions to be pumped out in exchange for cations. The expenditure of energy on ionic transport, according to Chappell's scheme, reflects the functioning of the energy-dependent H^+ pump, and uncoupling agents, by increasing the permeability of the mitochondrial membrane for H^+, cause the H^+ pump to *idle* [46].

The third mechanism, based on the chemo-osmotic concept of coupling [230], explains active ionic transport by assuming that it is directed and effected by the membrane potential. As Skulachev [230] points out, "in terms of the membrane potential concept the question of the energy supply for the transport of Ca^{++} ions is answered automatically: the accumulation of Ca^{++} against the concentration gradient is the simple result of electrophoresis of that ion, i.e., of movement along the electrical gradient." Accumulation of the cation is accompanied by movement of H^+ in the opposite direction. Fragmentation of the mitochondria by ultrasound leads to the formation of submitochondrial particles characterized by an opposite orientation of the membrane compared with intact mitochondria and a membrane potential of opposite sign [228]. Since the internal space of these particles is positively charged compared with the surrounding medium, active transport of cations becomes impossible; however, ability to accumulate anions is well marked [228–230, 290 291]. This fact is indisputable confirmation of Mitchell's mechanism. However, mention must be made of the latest communications from Racker's laboratory, where it has been shown that Ca^{++} ions can be transported, in principle, in ultrasonic mitochondrial fragments [197].

Further research is necessary, however, to determine the precise mechanism of ionic transport in mitochondria. Nevertheless, as a result of many investigations, the most important features and principles have been established, and the process of active ionic transport can now be described at least quantitatively [30, 32, 36, 43, 62, 141, 189, 208].

A series of papers published in the last few years have given information on the inhibitory action of thyroid hormones and their derivatives on the active transport of cations in mitochondria [67, 163, 164, 166, 204–206, 260–267]. The action of these hormones on the accumulation of bivalent cations has been studied in the greatest detail, and the following are the main results observed:

a. The sensitivity of the ion-transporting mechanism to the action of the hormones depends on the type of cation transported, and it increases in the order: manganese, strontium, calcium.
b. If inorganic phosphate is present in the incubation medium, higher concentrations of thyroid gland products are required to inhibit accumulation by 50%.
c. If the accumulation of Ca^{++} in the mitochondria is brought about by electron transport through the third coupling point (oxidation of ascorbate and TMPD), T_3 and T_3 acetate are virtually ineffective. T_3 has no inhibitory action on the accumulation of strontium even if it is energized by electron transport through coupling points I and II (with oxidation substrates β-hydroxybutyrate and succinate respectively).
d. Differences in the activity of thyroxine, triiodothyronine, and its derivatives when their effect is studied on ionic transport apply mainly to kinetic parameters: the velocity of the effects produced, the active concentrations, and so on, but not to the mechanism of action [205].

The addition of small quantities of Ca^{++} to a suspension of mitochondria leads to cyclic, temporary stimulation of respiration and oxidation of $NAD(P)H_2$, which stops after the accumulation of Ca^{++} is complete. It was shown by the use of thyroid hormones and Ca^{++} that, irrespective of the order of addition of these agents, a prolonged, steady, noncyclic stimulation of respiration and oxidation of $NAD(P)H_2$ takes place [166, 204]. It was postulated that this phenomenon was caused by the prevention of translocation of Ca^{++} if the T_3 or T_3 acetate was added before the Ca^{++}, or the outflow of the accumulated Ca^{++} from the mitochondria if the T_3 or T_3 acetate was added after Ca^{++}. In either case there is an increase in the content of free Ca^{++} in the extramitochondrial medium; however, the Ca^{++} ions interact with the ion-transporting mechanism but do not accumulate in the mitochondria, and they circulate between the intra- and extramitochondrial space.

The writers' experiments with ^{45}Ca showed [261] that thyroid hormones inhibit the accumulation of this cation whether taking place by oxidation of succinate or by dephosphorylation of ATP. Diiodotyrosine has practically no effect on the accumulation of this cation. Thyroxine inhibits active Ca^{++} transport in concentrations of 1×10^{-6} M and above. Analysis of the effect of thyroxine on Ca^{++} transport shows that the inhibitory effect develops with time; with an increase in the incubation time the mitochondria lose calcium which was accumulated in its initial stages.

A more detailed investigation of the action of thyroid hormones on Ca^{++} transport in mitochondria was carried out by the method of continuously recording small changes in the H^+ concentration in the medium accompanying the process of cation translocation. Certain other parameters of mitochondrial function were investigated at the same time. The experiment showed that during respiration of mitochondria after the addition of

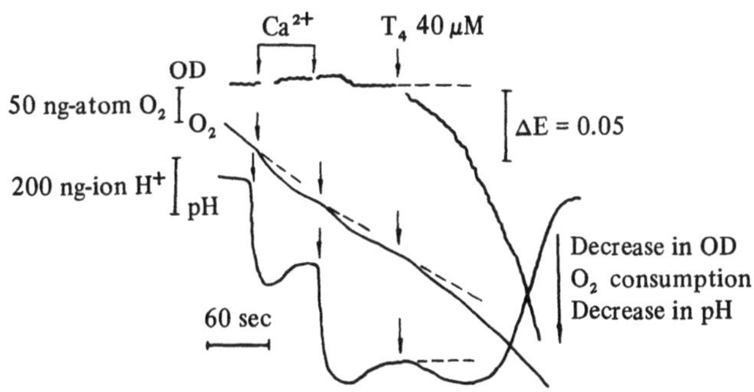

Fig. 13. Connection between changes in optical density (OD), rate of oxygen consumption, and H^+ concentration in the suspension during the action of thyroxine on mitochondria previously *loaded* with calcium (200 ng-ion added each time). Broken line indicates kinetics of processes in the absence of thyroxine. Incubation medium: 120 mM KCl, 5 mM Tris-chloride, 3 mM succinate; pH 7.4. Respiration recorded polarographically; decrease in optical density corresponds to swelling of mitochondria, decrease in pH to accumulation of Ca ions.

several doses of Ca^{++}, irrespectively of the presence of phosphate in the medium, the action of thyroxine and triiodothyronine returns the pH of the suspension to its initial level, pointing to the outflow of Ca^{++} from the mitochondria. Parallel with this, stimulation of respiration and swelling of the mitochondria are observed (Figure 13).

Changes in the parameters of mitochondrial function induced by thyroxine develop over a period of time whose duration is determined by the size of the *loading* of the mitochondria with calcium. For example, during the accumulation of 40, 80, and 120 ng-ion Ca^{++}/mg protein in the mitochondria, this shift in pH of the suspension to its initial value took place 390, 180, and 100 sec, respectively, after the addition of thyroxine (4×10^{-5} M). This latent period is perhaps essential for the hormone to penetrate to the centers of interaction inside the mitochondria where it exerts its effect. In this case the potentiating effect of Ca^{++} is evidently due to the increased permeability of the mitochondrial membranes for thyroxine as a result of swelling of the mitochondria, the rate of which is connected with the quantity of accumulated calcium [269]. This hypothesis also explains the great resistance of the transport of manganese and strontium ions to the action of thyroid hormones, because these cations sharply reduce the swelling of the mitochondria [29, 67].

Another possible explanation is that manganese and strontium ions, depending on their size and the density of their charge, interact electrostatically with the specific negatively charged groups of the mitochondrial membrane and, unlike calcium, they cause *blocking* of the membrane and stabilization of the structure of the mitochondria. This, in turn, may lead to a change in the conformation of the membrane proteins so that the centers of interaction with thyroid hormones become less accessible. During the inhibition of Ca^{++} transport by thyroid hormones, no significant change in the initial rate of accumulation or in its stoichiometric parameters takes place. However, thyroid hormones reduce the Ca^{++}-accumulating capacity of the mitochondria almost by half [67, 264, 265].

Unlike Ca^{++}, endogenous K^{+} leaves the mitochondria only in the presence of comparatively high concentrations of thyroid hormone: Even 1×10^{-4} M triiodothyronine is practically without action on this process [166]. It is also interesting to note that almost half the endogenous Mg^{++} leaves the mitochondria during incubation with T_3 acetate for 20 min [163]. Raising the temperature from 20 to 30°C more than doubles the rate of this process. This fact must certainly be examined in connection with the important role of Mg^{++} in the regulation of metabolism and the membrane permeability of the mitochondria [7, 56, 142]. On the other hand, addition of Mg^{++} to the incubation medium, where it evidently prevents the *leakage* of this cation from the mitochondria in the presence of thyroid hormones, considerably and, in some cases, completely abolishes the characteristic effect of these hormones on mitochondrial processes [90, 120, 195]. Conversely, a decrease in the magnesium concentration in the incubation medium provides a clearer demonstration of the uncoupling effect of thyroid hormones [90, 195].

The physiological mechanism regulating the permeability of mitochondrial membranes with the participation of magnesium ions has recently attracted particular attention in connection with the discovery of cytoplasmic metabolic factor (CMF)—an acid cyclic polypeptide with a molecular weight of 2200 (20 amino acid residues), present in the cells of different tissues and active in an extremely low concentration, of the order of 1×10^{-8} M [13, 14, 136, 152]. The mechanism of action of CMF *in vitro* and *in vivo* consists of preventing the leak of membrane-bound magnesium. Allowing for the well-known antagonism between the effects of Mg^{++} and thyroxine on oxidative phosphorylation and the other parameters of the state of the mitochondria, it would evidently be of great interest to study the activity of this factor in the presence of thyroid hormones and also their effect on its biosynthesis and its subcellular distribution.

Magnesium acts as an antagonist of thyroid hormones in experiments *in vivo* also. Administration of this cation to experimental animals prevents the uncoupling action of thyroid hormones on oxidative phosphorylation. Keeping animals on a magnesium-deficient diet leads to the appearance of uncoupling [90, 195, 274]. However, there is evidence that mitochondria of normal and thyrotoxic animals contain equal amounts of Mg^{++} [156] and that magnesium is ineffective in various types of disturbances of the thyroid gland. Injections of magnesium into such patients caused neither changes in the basal metabolic rate nor blocked the calorigenic effects of triiodothyronine (cited by [259]).

Unlike magnesium, calcium ions act as synergists of thyroid hormones [41, 132, 269]. The addition of small quantities of calcium before and after thyroid hormones leads to changes in the mitochondria compa-

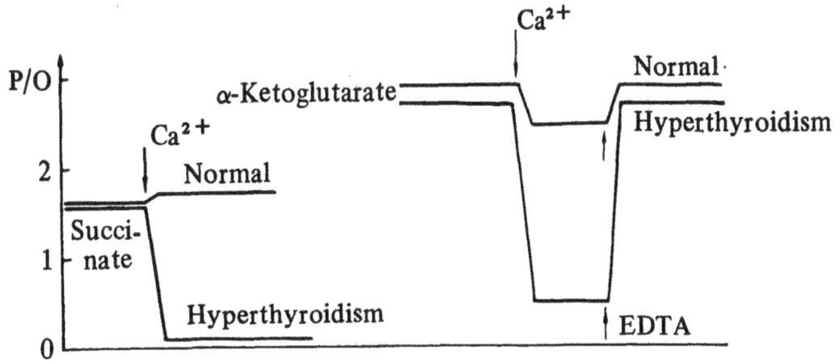

Fig. 14. Detection of uncoupling of oxidative phosphorylation in mitochondria in hyperthyroidism by addition of calcium ions to the incubation medium (from data of various workers [224]).

tible with the action of large doses of calcium or of an uncoupling agent [67, 166, 204]. Severin and Yang Fu-yü [217], as well as other workers [90, 224], showed that the addition of very small quantities of Ca^{++} to the incubation medium *unmasks* the uncoupling in hyperthyroidism, but the subsequent binding of this cation by the addition of a chelating agent (EDTA) to the medium *masks* the hyperthyroid uncoupling once again (Figure 14). In this connection Staehelin postulated that thyroid hormones exert their action through changes in the concentration of free calcium (cited by [90]). However, the validity of this conclusion can be questioned if only because thyroid hormones cause uncoupling in ultrasonic mitochondrial fragments in which the effect of calcium ions on the pathways of energy transfer is absent [23, 90, 272].

Calcium ions not only potentiate, strengthen, and unmask the action of thyroid hormones but, by themselves, also induce changes in the structure and functions of mitochondria which correspond to the similar effects of thyroid hormones [67, 205, 266]. In particular, the process of swelling of the mitochondria induced both by thyroxine and by calcium is characterized by equal sensitivity to inhibitors of electron and energy transport [205].

Under special conditions the addition of thyroxine to a suspension of mitochondria in a forced metabolic state has virtually no effect on the rate of respiration. However, the ability of the mitochondria to accumulate Ca^{++} is altered. The addition of thyroxine, as already mentioned, causes prolonged stimulation and not cyclic stimulation of respiration, and there is a failure to return to the initial metabolic state of rest. The same increase in respiration is found if the order of the additions is varied, i.e., if thyroxine acts on mitochondria previously loaded with calcium. A similar action is shown by triiodothyronine and by doses of calcium greater than the accumulating capacity of the mitochondria (Figure 15).

The stimulation of respiration observed is accompanied by loss of sensitivity of the mitochondria to ADP (coefficient of respiratory control = 1). Consequently, an excess of Ca^{++}, like the combination of hormone + calcium, gives rise to a qualitatively uniform picture of change in mitochondrial functions: stimulation of respiration and abolition of respiratory control. In experiments with calcium and thyroxine, however, no summation effect is observed. In particular, Roche et al. [205] observed that the activity of thyroxine is 200 times higher than that of calcium, so that any question of additivity is ruled out.

Intact mitochondria can accumulate considerable quantities of calcium, although only up to a certain limit, without causing significant disturbances in the state of oxidative phosphorylation. The accumulation beyond this limit leads to high-amplitude swelling of the mitochondria accompanying uncoupling [44, 45, 269]. There is indirect evidence in the literature to

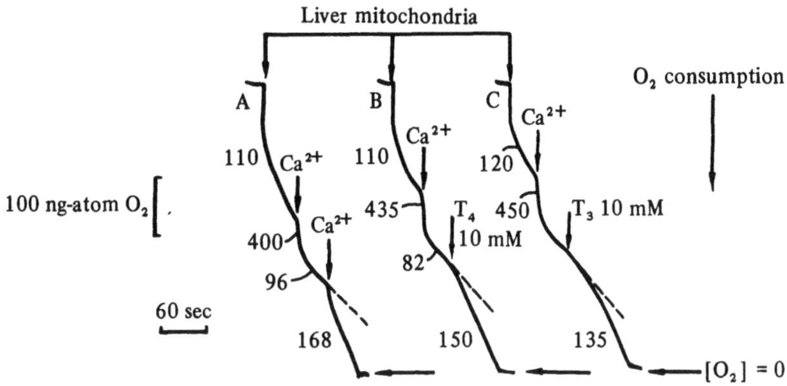

Fig. 15. Action of calcium, thyroxine, and triiodothyronine on respiration of mitochondria after accumulating 200 ng-ion Ca^{++}. Respiration recorded polarographically; incubation medium contained 120 mM NaCl, 10 mM Tris-chloride (pH 7.4), 5 mM succinate, and 2.5 mM KH_2PO_4. The rate of oxygen utilization in ng-atom O_2/min is shown on the polarographic records.

suggest a decrease in the Ca^{++}-accumulating activity of the mitochondria in hyperthyroidism, as a result of which much lower concentrations of Ca^{++} are required for the uncoupling of oxidative phosphorylation than in the mitochondria of normal animals; i.e., the Ca^{++}-accumulating *capacity* of mitochondrial preparations from normal animals is higher than that observed in the presence of an excess of thyroid hormones. To verify this hypothesis, direct measurements were made of the Ca^{++}-accumulating activity of mitochondria isolated from the liver of normal, thyrotoxic, and thyroidectomized rats [67]. The results showed that thyroidectomy of the animals, unlike thyrotoxicosis, produces no significant changes in the individual parameters of Ca^{++} transport. The Ca^{++}-accumulating capacity of the mitochondria was increased by 10% after thyroidectomy and reduced by 40% in thyrotoxicosis, as compared with normal. Consequently, the same amount of Ca^{++} can give rise to uncoupling in the case of mitochondria from thyrotoxic animals or it can be completely accumulated without any consequent changes in function in the mitochondria of normal and thyroidectomized animals. This fact may be the reason why some workers observed a potentiating, unmasking action of calcium ions when investigating certain effects of thyroid hormones. The results described are evidently interesting also as an aid to the understanding of the physiological mechanisms controlling mitochondrial ionic transport.

Investigations of the sensitivity of calcium ion transport to exogenous thyroxine showed that the inhibitory action of the hormone is strongest in mitochondrial preparations from the liver of thyroidectomized rats. Differences in the responses of mitochondria from normal, thyroidectomized, and thyrotoxic animals to exogenous thyroxine could be explained by differences in the initial content of thyroid hormones in the corresponding mitochondrial preparations. Inhibition of calcium accumulation by endogenous amounts of thyroid hormones is evidently another cause of the variation in the Ca^{++}-accumulating capacity of the mitochondria of these groups of animals.

Further research in this direction will possibly show that antagonism between magnesium ions and thyroxine, as established by many workers, is connected with the ability of magnesium to increase the Ca^{++}-accumulating capacity of the mitochondria many times [269, 271, 272] and, consequently, to prevent the indirect action of thyroid hormones on the structure and function of the mitochondria through their effect on Ca^{++} transport.

Like their action on mitochondria, *in vivo*, thyroid hormones also reduce the Ca^{++}-binding capacity of fragments of sarcoplasmic reticulum (FSR), without affecting ATPase activity [6]. The difference in the absorption of Ca^{++} by FSR from the muscles of control animals and animals receiving thyroxine was 57%. This effect may be the result either of delayed accumulation of Ca^{++} or its more rapid liberation. Careful analysis of these alternatives showed that the rate of accumulation of Ca^{++} is reduced in the FSR of animals treated with thyroxine. Meanwhile, an increased initial rate of Ca^{++} liberation by itself is unconnected with the decrease in the Ca^{++}-binding capacity of the reticulum, for the overall rate of liberation is only very slightly altered.

Two possibilities emerge from the analysis of the mechanism of the inhibitory action of thyroid hormones on ionic transport in the mitochondria: (a) interaction between thyroid hormones and carriers of bivalent cations and (b) their effect on the permeability of the mitochondrial membrane and, as a result, on the transmembrane potential. Interaction between thyroid hormones and intermediate HEC, to which the role of carriers of bivalent cations is ascribed in Chance's well-known scheme [36], was first suggested by Roche et al. [203–205] to explain the inhibitory action of T_3 and T_3 acetate on the transport of calcium, strontium, and manganese ions in the mitochondria of the liver. According to their hypothesis, these compounds form a complex with $X{\sim}Y$, which later breaks up into its components. Rupture of the high-energy bond prevents interaction of the bivalent cations with the ion-transporting mechanism. A special type of competition is thus observed between the thyroid hormones and cations for $X{\sim}Y$, with an evident weighting in favor of the former. It can be deduced from this hypothesis that the initial rate of accumulation of bivalent cations is reduced in the presence of increasing doses of thyroid hormones, for there must be a corresponding decrease in the stationary concentration of the carrier. However, the rapid recording methods used in the present writer's experiments were able to show that there is no change in the initial rate of

Ca^{++} accumulation when thyroxine is added to isolated mitochondria [67, 265, 266]. Unlike thyroid hormones, the titer of the carrier of bivalent cations can be modified with the aid of lanthanides, with a resulting definite decrease in the initial rate of Ca^{++} accumulation [32, 162].

On the other hand, the possibility cannot be ruled out that thyroid hormones could lead to a decrease in the stationary concentration of the carrier simultaneously with an increase in its *number of cycles* or with a decrease in its affinity for bivalent cations. The overall rate of translocation of the cation under these circumstances need not be substantially changed. However, special kinetic investigations are required to study this possibility, and the situation is complicated at the present by the absence of reliable information on the nature of the carrier.

It can be postulated, on the basis of the recently suggested mechanism of action of thyroid hormones in a manner unlike the proton carriers, that the effect of these hormones on ionic transport in mitochondria is determined by a change in the electrical properties of the membrane. The transmembrane potential, the motive force in the mechanism of accumulation of cations in the mitochondria, is evidently lowered when the properties of the membrane structures are modified by metabolic products of the thyroid hormones, as Gruenstein and Wynn [80] suggested.

Recent experiments in the laboratory of biophysics, Institute of Biochemistry, Academy of Sciences of the Uzbek SSR, have shown that the electrical component of the membrane potential of the mitochondria recorded by Mitchell's method [175] is in fact significantly reduced in the presence of thyroid hormones and that this effect has a certain latent period.

It can be concluded from the facts relating to the action of thyroid hormones on the function of isolated mitochondria and submitochondrial particles described above and also from the study of their activity in model systems that the comparatively weak degree to which the properties of classical uncouplers are exhibited by these hormones indicates that the activity of these iodinated compounds must be effected in other ways. One such way would be for the thyroid hormones to function as carriers of *activated* iodine in membrane structures [80, 176, 195]. The biologically active form of iodine in this view is I^+ and the free radical I^- which are

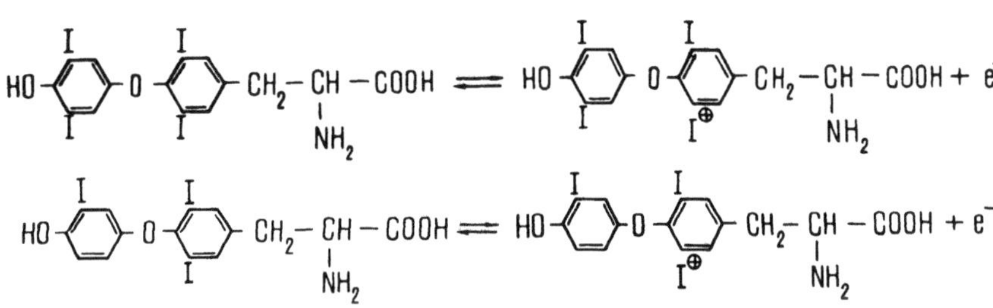

formed by deiodination of the β-ring of the molecule of the thyroid hormones [80] or by the giving up of an electron by the molecules of these hormones with the conversion of the iodine atom in position 5 into the I^+ form or into something close to it [176].

As was mentioned earlier, many functional responses of the mitochondria to the addition of thyroid hormones have been simulated by means of ICN and molecular iodine [80, 168, 205]. According to Rachev [193], the action of molecular iodine differs from the effects of thyroxine in that thyroxine affects the functional state of both chains—respiratory (stimulation) and phosphorylating (inhibition)—whereas I_2 acts chiefly on the rate of oxygen utilization. However, these views are to some extent in conflict with those of other workers who consider that the active principle is the same for both I_2 and thyroid hormones, and also for ICN and that it is connected with the presence of I^+ in these substances [176, 205] or with its liberation from them [80]. On the other hand, the reduced form of iodine (I^-) has no activity on mitochondria, although it can diffuse through the membrane in the presence of I_2, which acts as an iodide carrier and lowers the resistance of bimolecular phospholipid membranes [133, 149]. If uncoupling in the presence of thyroid hormones is in fact due to the action of the active form of iodine I^+, it is to be expected that similar uncoupling will be produced in the presence of molecular iodine and bromine, which, as Mokhnach [176] showed spectroscopically, contain the form of the element with a valence of +1 or near to it. Other workers have expressed similar views [195, 204].

In this connection a series of experiments was carried out in Turakulov's laboratory [67, 267] to study the effect of various forms of iodine and also of molecular bromine on oxidative phosphorylation of isolated mitochondria. It can be concluded from the results of these experiments, illustrated in Figure 16, that KI has practically no effect on the transforma-

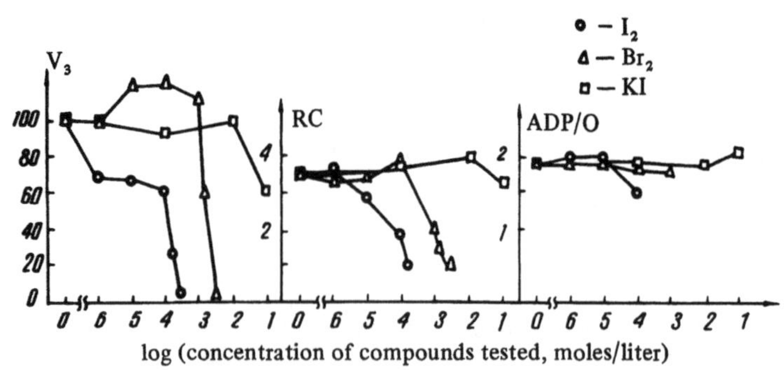

Fig. 16. Action of molecular iodine and bromine and also of potassium iodide on the rate of respiration in state 3 (V3) (ng-atom O_2/min·mg protein), coefficients of respiratory control (RC), and ADP/O ratio for rat liver mitochondria. (Oxidation substrate was succinate.)

tion of energy and that molecular iodine has almost ten times the uncoupling activity of molecular bromine. The action of I_2 and Br_2 on this function of the mitochondria outwardly resembles the action of low concentrations of uncoupling agents: The value of RC is sharply reduced, but ADP/O is more stable. Unfortunately, the coupling of oxidative phosphorylation cannot be followed by experimental polarographic methods (from ADP/O) after equality of the rates of oxygen consumption has been reached in metabolic states 3 and 4 (when RC = 1), and only a preliminary analysis of the analogy with uncouplers is therefore possible.

Relatively high concentrations of molecular iodine and bromine (0.5 and 5 mM, respectively) inhibit mitochondrial respiration practically completely; the inhibition observed is not steady in character but sudden and abrupt, as if some specific component of the membrane regulating the operation of the respiratory chain by the "all or nothing" principle is being titrated. In both cases, however, the change in respiratory control is smoother in character.

Thus, the results of these experiments agree with the view that the action of halogen-containing compounds, including the thyroid hormones, is connected with the character of the valence of the halogens in these compounds [176]. Consideration of the form of the iodine valence is evidently useful when the mechanism of action of the thyroid hormones is examined, for this approach has recently enabled some workers [80] to postulate a single principle for materialization of the effect of these hormones at the cellular and subcellular level, namely, by a universal change in individual parameters (such as permeability) of biological membranes.

Effect of Thyroid Hormones on the Permeability of the Mitochondrial Membranes

Accessibility of the substrate for the enzyme in the cell is controlled by the spatial separation of the stocks of substrate and enzyme. The role of barrier is performed usually by membranes of the mitochondria, nucleus, endoplasmic reticulum, lysosomes, and so on. According to this regulatory principle, known as *compartmentalization*, the regulator induces transitions between two states of the membrane in which it blocks or, conversely, opens the substrate's access to the enzyme [228].

Action of Thyroid Hormones on the Structure of the Mitochondria

Aebi and Abelin [2] demonstrated photometrically in 1953 that mitochondria isolated from the liver of hyperthyroid rats are swolen. The ability of thyroid hormones and other agents to modify the structure of the mitochondria and, consequently, the state of permeability of the mitochondrial membranes has subsequently been extensively investigated in several laboratories.

Analysis of the changes in volume of the mitochondria shows that they are of two principal types:

a. the passive and comparatively rapid swelling or contraction of the mitochondria, depending on the osmotic concentration of impermeable substances in the incubation medium;
b. the relatively slow, *active* swelling, dependent on respiration or the presence of HEC, which is induced or considerably accelerated by agents such as calcium ions, thyroxine, phosphate, free fatty acids, and so on [141, 142].

The first type of changes in volume has been investigated by many workers [139]. It reflects the behavior of the mitochondrion as an osmometer, and it evidently cannot play an important role under the conditions of the cell, where the osmotic pressure of the medium is kept more or less constant.

Packer [185], who studied the second type of swelling, described two phases of the changes in volume taking place in mitochondria of the heart. Phase I, or low-amplitude swelling or contraction (about 20–40% of the change in volume of the mitochondria) is relatively rapid and reversible. This phase of swelling has been shown to depend on the mechanisms of coupling and/or respiration; the possibility of reversal of the low-amplitude changes in volume is also connected with the activity of these mechanisms. Low-amplitude swelling and contraction of the mitochondria is observed during the transition from the resting state (state 4) into the active state (state 3) in the presence of ADP [184], and it also corresponds to changes in the volume of the mitochondria caused by the accumulation of small quantities of Ca^{++} in them in the presence of phosphate [269]. As Lehninger observes, Packer's experiments demonstrated integration of the electron flux, phosphorylation, and the structural state of the mitochondria provided that the changes were reversible, i.e., such as take place in the intact cell [142]. The low-amplitude changes in volume of the mitochondria are evidently the physiological mechanism for the regulation of functions connected with the state of permeability of mitochondrial membrane. This follows, in particular, from the experiments of Packer and Golder, who showed that changes in the dispersion of light, relatable to changes in the volume of the mitochondria, are observed in a suspension of Ehrlich's ascites cells during variations in their respiratory activity [139].

Phase II in the active swelling of the mitochondria (two- to threefold change in volume) is observed as a high-amplitude swelling and is only partially under the control of respiration and the energy transformation system

[140, 185]: The mitochondrial functions disappear step by step, and the volume of the mitochondria increases proportionally. The high-amplitude cycle of swelling is more marked, and it leads to profound and irreversible disturbances in mitochondrial structure [140, 142, 143].

Mitochondria in a state of high-amplitude swelling can be restored to their initial volume in a medium containing factors such as ATP, Mg^{++}, serum albumin, chelating agents, and so on, but under these circumstances the normal coupling of oxidation with phosphorylation and the original structure of the mitochondria are not restored [9, 140, 142]. This type of swelling of the mitochondria is evidently a process which is outside normal cell control [140].

According to much evidence obtained in various laboratories [7, 100, 139, 140, 142, 155, 184, 185, 269], the active change in volume of the mitochondria is an energy-dependent process. Some workers consider that the energy requirement reflected in the process of swelling is most probably satisfied passively by the endergonic accumulation of ions in the mitochondria [46, 49, 155, 180, 209]. The connection between ionic transport and swelling is demonstrated particularly clearly in experiments involving the direct comparison between the degree of swelling and the number of monovalent and bivalent cations accumulated by mitochondria in the presence of penetrating anions [46, 83, 180, 209, 269]. In that case the two processes exhibit quantitatively equal sensitivity to specific inhibitors of respiration and of energy conversion.

After a thorough analysis of the causes leading to changes in the structure of mitochondria, Yasaitis [291] concluded that these changes can be largely explained in terms of the osmotic properties of the internal mitochondrial membrane and the energy-dependent distribution of ions between the space of the matrix and the surrounding medium. In the presence of sources of energy the mitochondria can maintain a high level of endogenous osmotically active ions for a long time. This evidently determines the degree of hydration of the matrix and the size of the space bounded by the osmotic barrier of the internal membrane. Interruption of the process of energy-dependent absorption of cations by the addition of appropriate inhibitors to the incubation medium can possibly lead to the disappearance of ionic gradients between the matrix and environment and, consequently, to contraction of the mitochondria under conditions of de-energization. This can also occur after the addition of ADP, which is capable of competing with the ionic transport system for energy.

Another extremely attractive possibility, examined by Skulachev [230], is that structural changes in the mitochondria are the result of gradations of rigidity of the framework of the internal membrane. The decrease in rigidity essential for maintenance of a high hydrostatic pressure (about 3 atm) in the matrix prevents osmotic swelling of the mitochondria. It exists after breakdown of the protein–phospholipid–protein complex which takes place with the participation of the endogenous phospholipase of the mitochondria. As a result of hydrolysis of the phospholipid, the rigidity of the membrane must be reduced, and its elasticity must increase. This permits the mitochondrial membrane to swell instead of becoming ruptured. Conversely, resynthesis of the cross-linking phospholipid molecules leads to restoration of the original (high) rigidity of the membrane skeleton and to contraction of the swollen organelles. In Skulachev's opinion, reversibility of the changes described above is "evidence that interconversions between rigid and elastic states of the mitochondrial membrane may lie at the basis of regulatory acts acompanied by changes in the degree of coupling of oxidation and phosphorylation."

Some workers have postulated that swelling is due to the transport of cations and anions inside the mitochondria and to the subsequent gel–sol conversions of the intramitochondrial lipoprotein gel along the lines of myosin transformations [155]. On the other hand, it is postulated that swelling is connected with reconstruction of the internal membrane of the mitochondria as the result of a change in the geometry of the *repeating units* built into the membrane. These changes, in turn, are caused by cation-induced coiling or uncoiling of the specific proteins of the repeating unit [16]. Thus, absorption of water by the mitochondria depends directly or indirectly on energization which evidently does not require the whole assortment of processes of oxidative phosphorylation [140].

For mitochondria to contract during low-amplitude cycles of changes in volume, it is sufficient for energy production to be blocked. This can be done in various ways. Reversal of high-amplitude swelling of mitochondria calls for the more complex procedure described above. Depending on the method of reversal, either the chain of energy transfer or the respiratory chain must be in good working order; in either case, however, the discharge of water from the mitochondria is accompanied by expenditure of energy. Low-amplitude changes in volume are observed only in strongly contracted preparations of mitochondria, and for that reason the presence or absence of an energy requirement for the swelling of the mitochondria to be reversed may reflect the amplitude of the changes in volume.

The changes observed in the structure of the mitochondria are principally changes in the configuration of the internal membrane bounding the intramitochondrial space or matrix, impermeable to sucrose, and regulating the passage of various substances inside or outside the mitochondria [11, 139, 290]. An increase in permeability of the mitochondrial membranes produced by the action of thyroid hormones leads to the outflow of NAD, cytochrome c, substrates of the tricarboxylic acid cycle, and so on from the mitochondria [139, 143, 212, 217, 218]. Thyroid hormones induce an increase in the volume of the mitochondria not only *in vivo*, but also *in vitro* in preparations of these particles isolated from parenchymatous tissues and heart and skeletal muscles [90, 139]. For thyroid hormones to exert their effect on mitochondrial structure, electron transport, coupled with phosphorylation, must be present through any of the three energy transformation points [215], or, at least, through the second point [168].

A similar increase in volume of the mitochondria is produced by I_2 or ICN but not by KI [168, 205]. It is interesting to note that inhibitors of respiration and uncouplers prevent the action of thyroid hormones on mitochondrial structure, whereas guanidine, oligomycin, and rutamycin are ineffective [165, 168, 205]. Conversely, ATP-induced contraction of mitochondria swollen in the presence of thyroxine is inhibited by oligomycin, by atractylate, and, in some cases, by DNP, but it is insensitive to inhibitors of electron transport [139]. If swelling of the particles is maintained by the energy of ATP, like contraction it is inhibited by oligomycin. The clear interconnection between thyroxin-induced swelling of the mitochondria and their energization may perhaps reflect the passive dependence of volume changes on the endergonic accumulation of ions and may characterize the osmotic nature of the swelling process. It has recently been shown [54] that thyroxine analogs under certain conditions (energization of the mitochondria by ATP), like valinomycin, induce selective permeability of the mitochondrial membranes to K^+ ions. It is more likely that this phenomenon is the cause of the swelling.

Changes in volume produced, on the one hand, by calcium ions and, on the other hand, by thyroxine have much in common both kinetically and in their sensitivity to inhibitors [139, 205]. On the basis of their investigations into Ca^{++}-induced swelling of mitochondria, Chappell and Crofts postulated the *physical* uncoupling of oxidative phosphorylation as the result of spatial separation of the electron transport chain from components of the energy transfer chain in swollen mitochondria [45]. Similarly the study of mitochondrial swelling produced by thyroxine led Lehninger et al. [143] to conclude that thyroid hormones disorganize the process of oxidative phosphorylation as the result of the structural disturbance of coordinated interaction between the mitochondrial enzyme systems.

The action of thyroxine on mitochondrial structure can be observed with the hormone in *physiological* concentrations [90, 139], and peripheral antithyroid preparations inhibit the volume changes mentioned above. It must also be added that digitonin submitochondrial particles, in which the role of the structural integrity factor is reduced to the minimum, are not sensitive to thyroxine in relation to various functional parameters [90, 144]. However, Rachev's experiments on particles of this type suggest the opposite—this factor evidently has no role to play in the manifestation of the uncoupling action of thyroid hormones [195].

State of Mitochondrial Permeability and Regulation of Oxidative Metabolism

In the case of intact mitochondria, it is recognized that under physiological conditions thyroid hormones can modify the permeability of mitochondria and increase the outflow of substrates of the tricarboxylic acid cycle from them into the hyaloplasm. Their oxidation in the hyaloplasm is stimulated by the appropriate dehydrogenases with the participation of extramitochondrial NAD [212, 218]. As a result, the relationship between oxidation in the mitochondria accompanied by ATP production and nonphosphorylating oxidation, with the participation of cytochrome b_5, can be regulated. A possible mechanism for the regulation of the two oxidation pathways in the mitochondria of the liver is shown in Figure 17. The outer nonphosphorylating pathway must be activated by the loss of some of the cytochrome c from the inner membrane into the intermembranous space. As Severin and Yang Fu-yü have suggested, such a situation can arise in thyrotoxicosis [217]. Cytochrome c could shuttle to and fro from the outer membrane to the inner, carrying electrons between cytochrome b_5 and cytochrome oxidase [228]. Nonphosphorylating oxidation may also take place with the participation of cytochrome P-450, bound with the endoplasmic reticulum [182]. The content of cytochromes b_5 and P-450 in the liver, it is worth noting, is controlled by thyroid hormones [200]. According to Skulachev [228], the role of free oxidation may amount to removing the excess of

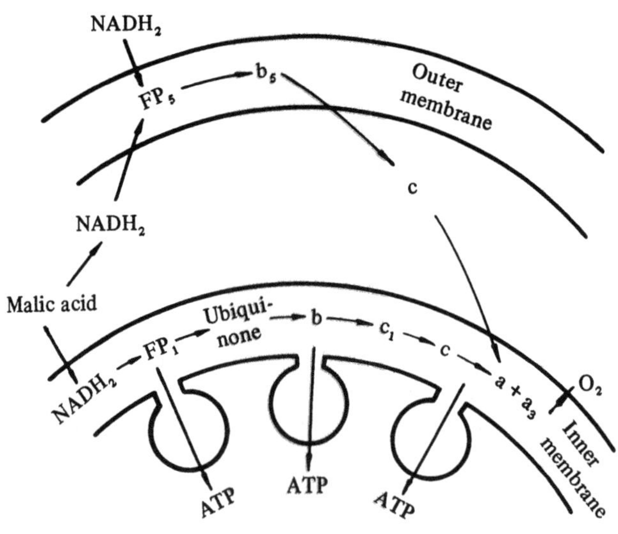

Fig. 17. Spatial separation of two electron transport pathways in the liver mitochondria (after Skulachev [228]).

substrate independently of phosphorylation or, no less important, the regulation of the $NADH_2/NAD$ ratio in the hyaloplasm independently of the value of the other ratio $[ADP] \cdot [P_{inorg}]/[ADP]$ controlling the work of the inner respiratory pathway.

Maslova, Raikhman, and Skulachev [160] have summarized the data on the role of the free hydroxylation system located in the endoplasmic membranes of liver cells and including $NADPH_2$, flavoprotein, a nonheme ferroprotein, and cytochrome P-450. This system participates in the detoxication of aromatic compounds but cannot receive electrons from fatty acid hydroxylase. As a result, fatty acids undergo omega-oxidation. Considering the increase in the free fatty acid level occurring under the influence of thyroid hormones, and also the fact that, not being linked with the production of high-energy compounds, this system functions at a rate limited only by the availability of the substrates, it can be presumed to play a special role in the mechanism of reduction of the P/O ratio by thyroxine. There is other evidence to show that thyroidectomy inhibits the activity of this system (in the same way as it is inhibited by catecholamines).

The increase in the contribution of free oxidation to the total oxygen consumption of the body can explain only the increased basal metabolism and heat production, whereas the other aspect of the thyrotoxicosis syndrome—the reduced energy capacity of the body—cannot be so explained. In addition, the system including cytochrome P-450 is found in some tissues (liver, adrenals), whereas the decrease in the P/O ratio under the influence of thyroid hormones occurs in other organs besides. Finally, during activation of $NADPH_2$–cytochrome c reductase, which was mentioned above, it is difficult to accept any considerable acceleration of the $NADPH_2$-dependent hydroxylation of fatty acids.

Another important consequence of the increase in permeability of the mitochondrial membrane is the redistribution of Ca^{++}, Mg^{++}, and other ions between the mitochondria and the surrounding medium [90, 151]. Under these circumstances changes in the activity of several enzymes of the mitochondria and hyaloplasm activated by these cations may be observed (ATPase, adenylate-kinase, ATP-creatine transphosphorylase, phospholipase A, glutamate dehydrogenase, and so on). Characteristically, the activating effect of thyroxine on lipase is achieved entirely through regulation of the availability of Ca^{++} for the enzyme [90, 145].

Metabolic Shunts of the Mitochondria

Intact mitochondria are impermeable to $NADH_2$ and $NADPH_2$ and also, in some cases, to the oxidized forms of these coenzymes [142]. This phenomenon is regarded by Racker [196] as "a safety measure designed by nature to preserve the important and multiple function of intramitochondrial reduced pyridine nucleotides in fatty acid synthesis, glutathione reduction, detoxication mechanisms, and so on." However, changes in the structure of the mitochondria produced by Ca^{++} or of thyroxine-induced swelling increase the permeability of the mitochondrial membrane for pyridine nucleotides. In intact, unswollen mitochondria the permeability barrier for pyridine nucleotides is overcome by *bypasses*—the so-called metabolic shunts that function like shuttling systems [124, 142, 223, 228, 276]. The principle of action of metabolic shunts is that both components of the redox system, in which oxidoreduction is carried out by appropriate forms of NAD or NADP, penetrate freely through the mitochondrial membrane and thereby regulate the level of reduction of these systems so that it is the same inside the mitochondria and in the extramitochondrial medium, and also in different organs with the aid of the vascular system. The metabolic shunt of this type consists of the transport of hydrogen from the mitochondria to the hyaloplasm and vice versa, depending on the functional needs of the different compartments of the cell for reducing equivalents for use in glyconeogenesis, fatty acid synthesis, reductive amylation of α-ketoglutarate, the 11β-hydroxylation of steroids, and so on [223, 272].

A characteristic feature of the action of thyroid hormones is that they reduce the content of mitochondrial NAD and NADP [90, 104, 143, 248]. Kadenbach [104] showed that the NAD/cytochrome c ratio is 8–10 under normal conditions but falls to 3 in hyperthyroidism despite the fact that NAD-bound substrates continue to be oxidized at a fast rate. The NAD and NADP concentration in the tissues falls significantly in thyrotoxicosis as a result of disturbances of the biosynthesis of these coenzymes. The rate of conversion of nicotinamide into the coenzyme is evidently reduced because of a deficiency of ATP but not on account of any enzymic defects [90].

A constant effect of the thyroid hormones is stimulation of the oxidation of $NADH_2$ and $NADPH_2$ parallel with the inhibition of endergonic processes of NAD reduction by succinate and hydrogen transport from $NADH_2$ to NADP [58, 88, 90, 248]. Thyroid hormones also regulate the relative quantities of reducing equivalents used in the two compartments separated by the mitochondrial membrane. For example, in rats fed with thyroid preparations there is a 22-fold increase in the activity of mitochondrial α-glycerophosphate dehydrogenase [90]. This evidently leads to sharp disproportion in the *limbs* of the α-glycerophosphate shunt, for the cytoplasmic α-glycerophosphate dehydrogenase activity remains virtually unchanged. One result of this disproportion could be the *leaking* of reducing equivalents from the cytoplasm into the mitochondria and the stimulation of extramitochondrial processes leading to NAD reduction (for example, aerobic glycolysis).

The dependence of mitochondrial α-glycerophosphate dehydrogenase activity on the thyroid hormone level in the body described by Lardy et al. [131, 137, 138] can also lead to many other characteristic metabolic changes. The increased activity of this enzyme produced by thyroid hormones takes place only in tissues that react to thyroxine by increased oxygen consumption [137]. This reaction is highly specific with respect to thyroid hormones [210] and correlates with their dose. An increase in mitochondrial α-glycerophosphate dehydrogenase activity ought to accelerate the function of the α-glycerophosphate–dihydroxyacetone phosphate cycle, thereby not only reducing the value of the P/O ratio to 2 (since α-glycerophosphate is oxidized in the respiratory chain, bypassing NAD and the first phosphorylation point), but also enabling constant regeneration of the oxidized NAD in the cytoplasm. The latter is evidently an important condition enabling a speeding up of the breakdown of carbohydrates, including the endogenous tissue glycogen. This possibility, as is well known, can be converted into a reality in the presence of an excess of thyroid hormones in the body. Working with the isolated perfused rat heart, Isaacs et al. [101] also found a considerable increase in the rate of lactate utilization in thyrotoxicosis. Since lactate dehydrogenase activity in the myocardium is always high and cannot limit the conversion of lactate into pyruvate [211, 282] and since thyroid hormones, at least in the liver, do not affect the activity of this enzyme [179], the rate of lactate utilization can evidently only be limited by the availability of oxidized NAD. With an increase in the rate of operation of the α-glycerophosphate shunt, the supply of this pyridine nucleotide is increased, and this explains the faster rate of lactate oxidation. However, the mechanism just described cannot explain why there is no decrease in the utilization of lactate by the heart of hypothyroid animals, in which mitochondrial α-glycerophosphate dehydrogenase activity is sharply reduced [101].

There is no evidence of the participation of the β-hydroxybutyrate–acetoacetate shunt in the modified metabolic processes induced by thyroid hormones. The activity of mitochondrial β-hydroxybutyrate dehydrogenase in most organs is slightly lower than normal in hyperthyroidism and hypothyroidism [104].

It is also worth noting that activity of mitochondrial NAD-specific isocitrate dehydrogenase is increased in hyperthyroidism, whereas activity of the NADP-specific enzyme is actually below normal [104]. The oxidation of isocitrate in the mitochondria evidently takes place according to the scheme proposed by Chappell (see [228]) with the participation of the malate–oxaloacetate shunt. The possibility cannot be ruled out that the ratio between the activities of these two forms of isocitrate dehydrogenase in hyperthyroidism controls the rate of oxidation of $NADH_2$ in the mitochondria and of $NADPH_2$ in the microsomes. If this shunt works in the opposite direction, oxaloacetate can be removed from the mitochondria, an extremely important matter in connection with the observed inhibitory effect of oxaloacetate on the oxidation of succinate.

The materialization of the regulatory effect of thyroid hormones on the pathways of utilization of reducing equivalents in the intra- and extramitochondrial compartments of the cell is evidently linked with their effect on the permeability of the mitochondrial membranes, which controls the accessibility of oxidation and phosphorylation substrates to the corresponding mitochondrial systems, the supply of ATP and hydrogen to the hyaloplasm, and the distribution of key metabolites between the mitochondria and other parts of the cell.

Protein Synthesis and Regulation of the Enzyme Content by Thyroid Hormones

An important stage in the elucidation of the mechanism of action of thyroid hormones was the discovery of their regulatory action on the early stages of biosynthesis of enzymes and other proteins [56, 181, 248–258, 260, 282]. Investigations by Tata et al. led to the conclusion that the general anabolic action of thyroid hormones on cell processes is due, not to the uncoupling of oxidative phosphorylation, but to the synthesis of new respiratory enzymes. It must be emphasized that the addition of inhibitors of RNA or protein synthesis (actinomycin D, 5-fluorouracil, puromycin, cycloheximide) caused 70–100% inhibition of the stimulatory action of thyroxine and triiodothyronine on the basal metabolism and on the rate of growth in both normal and thyroidectomized animals [248]. Thyroid hormones were found to increase the rate of incorporation of amino acids not only in the microsomal fraction, but also in isolated mitochondria [81, 82, 207, 248–258].

It thus becomes necessary to examine the problem of the action of thyroxine on the biosynthesis of mitochondrial respiratory enzymes, for the chief physiological effect of thyroid hormones, manifested at all levels, is the stimulation of respiration. It is now generally accepted that respiration is stimulated by thyroid hormones, not as a result of their direct activating action on the corresponding enzymes, but as a result of increased synthesis of respiratory enzymes in the tissues. This view of the mechanism of action of thyroid hormones provides a better understanding of the reason for the latent period in the action of these hormones, for the synthesis *de novo* of the amount of enzyme required to modify the action velocity clearly requires a certain time.

Analysis of the relevant literature showed that the administration of thyroxine or triiodothyronine *in vivo* in fact leads to an increase in the concentration of certain oxidation enzymes. The most striking example is the increased concentration of mitochondrial α-glycerophosphate dehydrogenase mentioned above in some organs of rats receiving thyroid preparations [131, 138]. The addition of dried thyroid gland to the diet of rats for 10 days increased the rate of oxidation of α-glycerophosphate by the tissue mitochondria of these animals sixfold. Thyroidectomy led to the virtually total disappearance of the enzyme from mitochondria of the liver and kidneys. Replacement therapy restored the content of this dehydrogenase back to or above normal. The content of enzyme also varied, although by a lesser degree, in the myocardium and skeletal muscle. However, no change in the content of α-glycerophosphate dehydrogenase could be found in organs not responding to thyroxine by an increase in their oxygen consumption (the brain, spleen, lungs, ovaries, and testes). The fact that in such cases it is a true formation of enzyme protein *de novo* is confirmed by blocking the effect of thyroxine with ethionine.

However, the mechanism of action of thyroid hormones cannot be reduced simply to their effect on mitochondrial α-glycerophosphate dehydrogenase, first, because under the influence of these hormones the oxidation of substrates that must pass through a stage of glycerophosphate formation is accelerated and, second, because in tissues that utilize glycerophosphate much more actively than the liver (muscles, for instance) its content is altered less by thyroid hormones than in the liver.

So far as the synthesis of other oxidative enzymes *de novo* is concerned, Phillips and Langdon [188] describe the induction by thyroxine of $NADPH_2$–cytochrome c reductase. This enzyme system also catalyzes the calorigenic metabolic shunt, but the mechanism of action of thyroid hormones likewise cannot be reduced simply to this effect, for they activate not only NADP-, but also NAD-dependent dehydrogenation in mitochondria.

It is often stated in the literature that the number of electron-transport chains in the mitochondria or even the number of mitochondria in the cell is increased by the action of certain doses of thyroid hormones. In fact, if small concentrations of thyroxine or triiodothyronine are injected into animals for a short time, the number of mitochondria in the liver or muscle cells increases considerably. This could bring about an increase in the overall oxidative potential of the cell and could thus explain the increase in the oxygen consumption arising under the influence of thyroid hormones. Under those conditions, however, there is an increase in respiration not only of the whole cell, but also of the mitochondria themselves, calculated per unit mass of protein or nitrogen in them. Consequently, thyroxine primarily increases the specific respiratory activity of the mitochondria. Further, while the synthesis of mitochondrial proteins is stimulated by relatively small doses of thyroid *in vivo*, prolonged administration of the hormones or treatment with high doses reduces mitochondrial protein synthesis, whereas tissue respiration continues to rise. This has been shown in Golber's laboratory for mitochondria of the rabbit myocardium by Kandror and Svyatkina. Increased activity of cytochrome c in the mitochondria of animals receiving thyroid hormones could play an important role in this problem. The actual technique of determining this electron carrier is evidence that the increased activity obtained in hyperthyroidism [156, 259] is actually connected with a change in the content of enzyme protein. An increase in its concentration is observed in the liver, kidneys, myocardium, and skeletal muscle, i.e., in tissues that respond to thyroxine by an increased oxygen consumption. The close connection between the increased respiration and the cytochrome c content of the tissues is illustrated by the findings of Whaley et al. [279]. They point out that the time taken for the calorigenic effect to arise after a single injection of thyroxine in different tissues is inversely proportional to the content of cytochrome c in those tissues. For instance, increased respiration is observed soonest in homogenates of heart muscle, in which the cytochrome c content is twice as high as in the diaphragm; increased respiration in the diaphragm, however, develops much sooner than in skeletal muscles, with the smallest cytochrome c content. Tata et al. [256] administered physiological concentrations of thyroid hormones to thyroidectomized rats and also observed an increase in the content of certain other cytochromes in the mitochondria.

The increased synthesis of specific respiratory enzymes under the influence of thyroid hormones makes it necessary to analyze the possibility that these hormones may exert their primary effect on the protein-synthetic apparatus in the cell. In the last decade the regulation of protein synthesis by thyroid hormones has been studied intensively in Tata's laboratory.

In experiments on thyroidectomized animals (usually rats) receiving single very small doses of thyroid hormones (of the order of 2–25 μg/100 g body weight), Tata, like many other workers, observed that the incorporation of amino acids into proteins was stimulated in the organs taken from these animals (the experiments were usually carried out on liver tissue). Assuming the role of RNA in the synthesis of protein molecules, Tata concentrated his attention on the effect of thyroid hormones on the metabolism of these compounds. He found an increase in the RNA content in the microsomal fraction isolated from the liver of the experimental rats. This increase occurred before the increase in RNA-polymerase activity in the nuclei of the liver cells. However, the earliest of all the observed effects of triiodothyronine was an increase in the rate of synthesis and metabolism of the fast-labeled fraction of nuclear RNA (to judge from the incorporation of ^{14}C-orotic acid into it). Evidently under the impression of the work of Karlson [111], who postulated the hormonal regulation of transcription, these findings were interpreted as evidence of a change in messenger RNA synthesis produced by thyroid hormones. However, it was shown later that the regulation of protein synthesis in the cells of higher animals can take place at various levels: at the stage of RNA transport from nucleus to cytoplasm, at the stage of the structural organization of the ribosomes, their translation activity, and so on. This work led to a revision of the earlier views.

On the basis of their experiments, Tata and co-workers were able to review the changes recorded in the protein-synthetic apparatus of the cell from the time of administration of triiodothyronine to the animals. They found that an increase in the synthesis of fast-labeled nuclear RNA was detectable within 4–6 h in rats. RNA-polymerase activity increased later, but characteristically this was preceded by a change in activity of the enzyme forming ribosomal RNA. Later, after an increase in the synthesis of phospholipids in the microsomes and simultaneously with activation of the incorporation of amino acids into mitochondrial and microsomal proteins, there was an increase in the activity of the polymerase participating in the synthesis of DNA-like mRNA. At the same time an increase in the oxygen consumption of the animals was noted. The increase in RNA-polymerase activity in isolated cell nuclei described by Tata and Widnell [257] is often cited as proof of the direct action of thyroid hormones on the protein-synthetic apparatus. However, it is sometimes forgotten that these workers administered the hormone *in vivo* and only later extracted the liver and isolated the nuclear fraction; they did not incubate this fraction with thyroxine. The addition of thyroid hormones *in vitro* to isolated cell nuclei does not stimulate RNA metabolism [239, 257].

Whatever the true state of affairs, careful analysis of nuclear RNAse whose synthesis is stimulated by thyroid hormones showed that the clearest changes taking place in the protein-synthetic apparatus in the early stages of action of the hormone are changes in the rate of synthesis of ribosomal RNA [252]. This effect of thyroid hormones is not manifested after administration of small doses of actinomycin D, to which the synthesis of ribosomal RNA is more sensitive than the synthesis of messenger RNA [201].

It has also been shown by the use of labeled orotic acid and ^{32}P that thyroid hormone accelerates the synthesis of mitochondrial and soluble RNA as well as of ribosomal RNA [257]. The stimulation of protein and phospholipid synthesis is coordinated with that of RNA synthesis, suggesting simultaneous control over the rate of formation of RNA and of cell membranes [251]; meanwhile, an increase in both the mean size and the number of polysomes is also observed [257]. Characteristically, the hormonal effect on incorporation of amino acids is also manifested in the ribosomes, but the hormonal action is most marked if the ribosomes are bound to the cytoplasmic membranes formed concomitantly with the additional ribosomes [249, 257, 258]. This situation as a whole leads to changes in the cell architecture that are an important and proved stage in the anabolic action of thyroid and other hormones of growth and development [248, 258]. Having demonstrated the effect of triiodothyronine on the synthesis of ribosomal RNA and, later, on the redislocation of the ribosomes in the cell, on their aggregation, their binding with phospholipid cytoplasmic membranes, and so on (other anabolic hormones, of course, affect these processes also), Tata felt that his multiplicity of mechanisms of action, of thyroid hormones does not give them the necessary specificity of action. A way out of this difficulty is provided by the hypothesis of simultaneous acceleration of the synthesis of messenger and ribosomal RNA with a disproportionately large yield of the latter [252]; this hypothesis has received some experimental confirmation.

By fractionating a preparation of nuclear DNA-dependent RNA-polymerase on a column with DEAE-Sephadex, Smuckler and Tata [235] obtained three fractions each with enzymic activity. By administering triiodothyronine or growth hormone to experimental animals they showed that these two hormones act differently on the yield and specific activity of the three fractions. In particular, triiodothyronine stimulated both the amount and the specific activity of the enzyme participating in the synthesis of ribosomal RNA. At the same time, this hormone increased sensivitivity to α-amanitine, an inhibitor of RNA synthesis of nonribosomal type.

Most hormonal effects described by Tata and co-workers [248]—stimulation of the synthesis of fast-labeled RNA and of DNA-dependent RNA-polymerase, the mitochondrial and microsomal incorporation of amino acids into proteins, the synthesis of mitochondrial cytochrome oxidase and microsomal $NADPH_2$–cytochrome c reductase, stimulation of the basal metabolism, increase in the weight of organs, and so on—take place within a time range of several hours to several days. However, the activity of other enzymes, such as nuclear NAD-phosphorylase, mitochondrial ATPase, isocitrate dehydrogenase, creatine phosphokinase, the system of amino acid activation, D-glucan phosphorylase, and UDP-glucosaglycogen-glucosyl transferase, was unchanged even after prolonged treatment of the animal with the hormone [248]. On the other hand, the increase in the activity of many enzymic processes induced by thyroid hormones is undoubtedly brought about by an increase in the quantity of the enzyme and not by changes in its catalytic activity or in the accessibility of the substrate to the enzyme. This has been demonstrated most clearly for succinate dehydrogenase, cytochromes c, b, and a, ubiquinone, (NAD)-isocitrate dehydrogenase, α-glycerophosphate oxidase, etc. [104, 115, 213, 248]. In order to separate the effects of thyroid hormones on the catalytic activity of the enzyme and on the quantity of enzyme, the latter can be determined directly, as with the cytochromes [104], or inhibitors of protein synthesis can be used [17]. In particular, it has been shown by the use of the last method that stimulation of the activity of several enzymes concerned with glucose metabolism by thyroid hormones is the result of increased enzyme protein synthesis, whereas the activity of phosphoenolpyruvate carboxykinase is controlled by different channels. This differentiation of the hormonal effects is useful in any case, for there is evidence of the effect of diet and of avitaminoses on the stimulation of enzyme activity accompanying development or caused by administration of thyroid hormone [153, 286]. In particular, the activity of *malic*-enzyme is controlled both by diet and by hormonal changes.

The stimulation of protein synthesis is induced not only by thyroid hormones, but also by corticosteroids, insulin, growth hormone, glucagon, and so on [121, 253, 281]. However, not all hormones act in the same way or even produce the same effect. For instance, corticosteroids, insulin, and glucagon induce tyrosine transaminase synthesis in rat liver, but the mechanism is different in each case [121].

Developmental hormones stimulate the synthesis of proteins not hitherto synthesized in the body. In these cases derepression of part of the genome is perhaps observed, so that new types of mRNA can be synthesized [121]; the most likely explanation is that the hormone does not act directly to derepress the gene but at intervals with the compound which is the actual repressor (Figure 18). The hormone can play its role in the regulation of protein biosynthesis according to the Jacob and Monod scheme not only by indirectly regulating RNA transcription or formation, but also by coordinating translation (the transfer of information from RNA to the protein molecule) or RNA function [253, 260]. There are as yet insufficient grounds for considering that repressors are proteins, but if such should prove to be the case, their inhibition could be reduced to changes in quaternary structure (disaggregation with a change in activity and substrate specificity) similar to those produced by thyroid hormones in the structure of glutamate dehydrogenase [66, 287].

Many new facts were discovered in the 1960s concerning the role of cyclic 3′,5′-AMP (c-AMP) in the response of cell metabolism to hormonal stimulation [84]. One interpretation of the mechanism of action of c-AMP assumes that it may regulate the translation of mRNA in polysomes. This point of view explains, in particular, most of the early effects of TSH on thyroid tissue, for in that case c-AMP evidently acts as an intracellular mediator of the hormone [121]. It was also shown that c-AMP accelerates protein synthesis in the case of ACTH. In most other cases (insulin, growth hormone), however, the results suggest that c-AMP plays no part in the anabolic action of hormones on protein synthesis [121].

According to some reports the synthesis and steady-state concentration of adenyl cyclase from the myocardium are increased in thyrotoxicosis [19]. However, results obtained by other workers show that the activity of

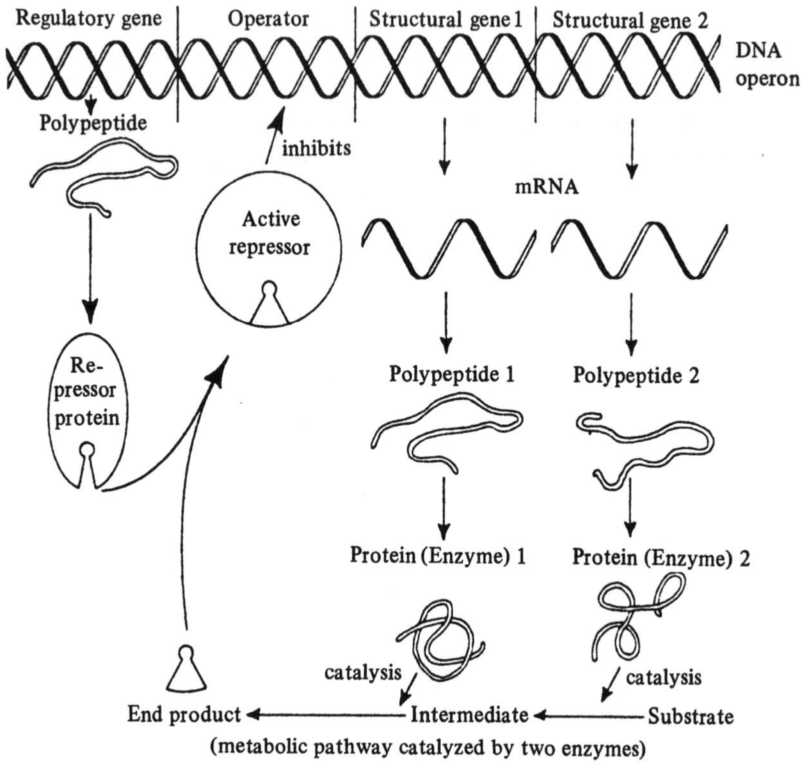

Fig. 18. Possible mechanism of action of some depressor hormones in Jacob and Monod's scheme of the regulation of protein biosynthesis (scheme taken from Green and Goldberger [77]).

enzymes participating in both the synthesis (adenyl cyclase) and the degradation (phosphoesterase) of c-AMP is about equal in the myocardium of hyperthyroid and euthyroid animals [236]. On the other hand, experiments *in vitro* demonstrated an increase in adenyl cyclase activity in the presence of thyroid hormones [146], although the same workers found no such increase in experiments *in vivo* [236]. These differences of opinion can evidently be explained on the basis of the well-known difference in the effects of thyroid hormones on enzyme activity *in vivo* and *in vitro*. It has also been shown that maximal accumulation of c-AMP in the myocardium is significantly below normal in hypothyroidism [146]. The stimulant action of thyroid hormones on the conversion of ATP into c-AMP has also been demonstrated in macaque spermatozoa [33]. What is equally important is that compounds structurally related to thyroxine had no effect on the accumulation of c-AMP.

The stimulant effect of thyroid hormones on the cell level of c-AMP can be attributed, according to the workers cited, to their direct action on adenyl cyclase. Anaerobic fructolysis in spermatozoa responds to different concentrations of triiodothyronine in the same way as adenyl cyclase activity, i.e., in two phases with a maximum to correspond to a triiodothyronine concentration of about 7.5 μM.

Krishna et al. [126] obtained evidence that adenyl cyclase participates in the thyroid hormones. According to this mechanism, thyroxine potentiates the action of catecholamines on the lipolytic system as follows:

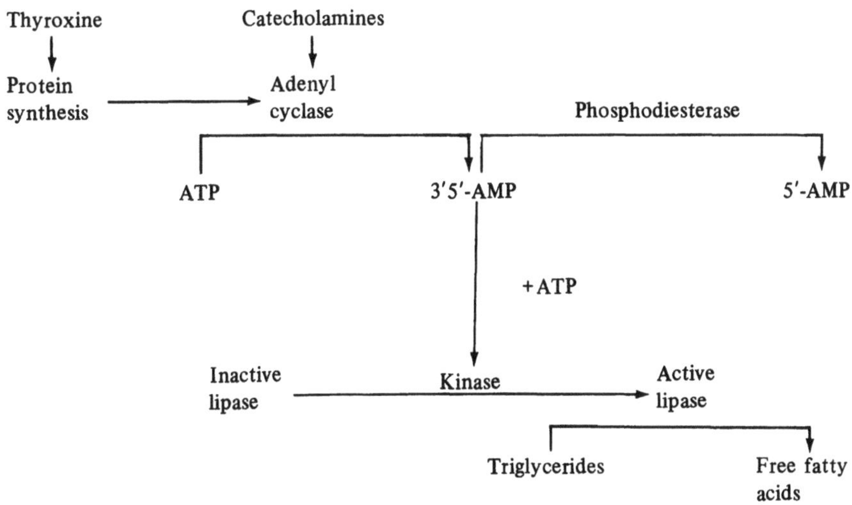

It must be stated in connection with this scheme that the more than twofold increase in adenyl cyclase activity in hyperthyroid rats compared with normal is unaccompanied by any changes in phosphodiesterase activity. Such a situation must undoubtedly be favorable for the accumulation of c-AMP in the cell.

On the other hand, comparison of the effects of thyroid hormones and of dibutyryl-c-AMP on the absorption and incorporation of amino acids and also of inorganic substrate into the intact pelvic bone of a 10-day chick embryo indicates a fundamental difference between the mechanisms of action on these agents [3]. Further support is given by the impossibility of replacing thyroxine by c-AMP in order to obtain the selective stimulant effect on carbamoyl phosphate synthetase of the tadpole liver. On the whole, however, considering all the facts described above, it is a difficult problem at the present time to give any reliable and unambiguous assessment of the role of c-AMP in the anabolic activity of thyroid hormones.

Mitochondria and the Action of Thyroid Hormones on Intracellular Protein Synthesis

The study of the connection between the effects of thyroid hormones on the intracellular system for protein synthesis and the state of metabolism in the mitochondria is a particularly interesting problem. In the simplest case this connection is seen in the fact that thyroid hormones primarily activate the processes of intracellular protein synthesis, with the result that cell respiration is stimulated as a secondary effect, through triggering of the respiratory control mechanism. The difficulty facing the analysis of this connection is that large doses of thyroxine and triiodothyronine, with a general catabolic rather than anabolic effect *in vivo*, inhibit RNA and protein synthesis in the organs, whereas the absorption of oxygen by the tissues continues to rise. Evidence of the phasic effect of thyroid hormones on protein synthesis in various organs was given above. It will suffice to recall, for example, that in the experiments of Gol'ber, Kandror, and co-workers [70–75, 106–109] activation of phosphate incorporation into the various fractions of RNA and of amino acids into proteins of the myocardial cells occurred in the early stages of the experiment in rabbits receiving increasing doses of thyroid for one month, whereas in the later stages these processes were definitely inhibited. As a result of special precautions taken by these workers when analyzing their data, it could be stated that the changes found in fact reflected the rate of RNA and protein synthesis and were not due, for example, to changes in dilution of the label in the tissues, and so on. These results agree with those obtained by other workers who found an inhibitory effect of *toxic* doses of thyroid hormones on protein synthesis in the cells of various organs.

Depending on the dose of thyroid hormones given to the animals, the effect on the intracellular protein-synthetic system could be in opposite directions (activating and inhibitory). This was shown by results obtained in Turakulov's laboratory by Khalikov and Seitmuratova on cross-reconstruction of the ribosomes and polysomes of normal and experimental animals receiving *stimulating* and *toxic* doses of thyroxine with the cell sap of normal and experimental animals (Table XVII). It is important to emphasize that activation or inhibition of tyrosine-^{14}C incorporation in this system is observed in the presence of R_e and P_e as well as of CS_e and that the direction of the effect depends entirely on the dose of thyroxine. Further, within the range studied, it increases 1–7 days after administration of thyroxine. Meanwhile, another group of workers in the same laboratory [263] found that the administration of stimulating (200 μg/100 g body weight) and toxic doses of the hormone (4 mg/100 g body weight) results in a uniform type of response of the respiratory chain of liver mitochondria (see the rate of respiration of mitochondria in state 4 in Table XVI).

Table XVII. Incorporation of Tyrosine-^{14}C (pulses/min) into Acid-Insoluble Material of Cell Systems Containing Ribosomes, Polysomes, and Cell Sap from the Liver of Normal and Experimental Rats

Time after administration of thyroxine, days	Ribosomes				Polysomes			
	$R_n + CS_n$	$R_e + CS_e$	$R_n + CS_e$	$R_e + CS_n$	$R_n + CS_n$	$R_e + CS_e$	$R_n + CS_e$	$R_e + CS_n$
Thyroxine, 25 mg/100 g body weight								
1	444 ± 30	546 ± 44	510 ± 38	503 ± 40	674 ± 48	787 ± 48	708 ± 38	705 ± 34
3		603 ± 38	519 ± 46	554 ± 34		827 ± 36	746 ± 43	764 ± 53
5		714 ± 48	584 ± 51	587 ± 29		986 ± 63	794 ± 56	904 ± 46
7		764 ± 63	618 ± 46	660 ± 40		1176 ± 72	838 ± 52	1084 ± 57
Thyroxine, 4 mg/100 g body weight								
1	380 ± 21	694 ± 33	462 ± 13	674 ± 58	689 ± 56	1280 ± 84	726 ± 19	1204 ± 80
3	510 ± 31	475 ± 28	430 ± 27	530 ± 39	635 ± 33	720 ± 54	685 ± 33	830 ± 49
5	410 ± 36	174 ± 13	364 ± 19	230 ± 17	744 ± 64	314 ± 27	614 ± 52	480 ± 27
7	465 ± 40	82 ± 6	254 ± 21	134 ± 12	780 ± 65	146 ± 9	460 ± 29	190 ± 17

Note: R_n, R_e = ribosomes of normal and experimental rats respectively, P_n, P_e = polysomes of normal and experimental rats, CS_e C_eS = cell sap of normal and experimental rats.

Since the changes in one process take place in different directions (depending on the dose of the hormone), whereas changes in the other process (tissue respiration) are all in one direction, the second process cannot be regarded as a derivative of the first. In other words, cell respiration cannot be considered to increase as a result of an increase in the consumption of high-energy compounds for protein synthesis.

This contradiction was eliminated by Tata [248] by assuming different mechanisms of action of physiological and pharmacological doses of the hormone. "It is often not realized," Tata writes, "that large doses of the hormone act on cell structures on which it does not act in much smaller concentrations." He further states that "the effect of large doses can be reduced to direct action on structures which, under normal, physiological conditions, do not react to thyroid hormones." This means that an effect of thyroid hormones which is in the same direction whatever the dose, such as the increased oxygen consumption, must differ in its origin depending on whether the hormone acts in physiological or in pharmacological doses. In the first case it is compensation for the increased consumption of ATP for protein biosynthesis, whereas in the second case it reflects certain direct changes in the tissue respiration system. Such a possibility must be accepted in principle. However, this concept is no more than a hypothesis, and as the subsequent account will show, it is possible to resolve this contradiction in another way.

This other way was revealed, in particular, by work carried out in Sokoloff's laboratory [238, 242]. In 1959, Sokoloff and Kaufman confirmed the observations of Dutoit [55] that the rate of incorporation of amino acids into protein of liver slices of thyroidectomized rats is slowed and that this process can be restored to normal by replacement thyroid treatment. These workers extended Dutoit's conclusion to cell-free preparations of the liver from control rats and rats receiving thyroxine. They found that the reduced rate of protein synthesis in chronic thyroid insufficiency is not just restored to normal by administration of thyroxine to the rats. Even if given to control animals (with an intact thyroid gland), thyroxine stimulated the incorporation of amino acids into cell-free liver preparations. Acceleration of protein synthesis was also found in the myocardium and kidneys, whereas no such effect was observed in brain tissue, the testis, or the spleen. In other words, this effect of thyroxine (100 μg per rat daily for 10 days) had the same distribution among the organs and tissues as the calorigenic action of this hormone.

Unlike Tata, Sokoloff and Kaufman [240, 241] also investigated the effect of thyroxine, added *in vitro*, on protein synthesis in individual fractions of a cell-free liver homogenate. They found that, starting with a concentration of 1×10^{-7} M of thyroxine, the rate of protein synthesis in the microsomal fractions of the homogenate increased. With an increase in the concentration of the hormone, the percentage rise in radioactivity of the protein also increased. However, on the addition of thyroxine in concentrations exceeding 4×10^{-4} M, the effect of the hormone changed sharply in direction; stimulation changed into inhibition of protein synthesis:

Thyroxine concentration	Change in specific activity of protein, %
1.3×10^{-7} M	+4
6.6×10^{-7} M	+5
1.3×10^{-6} M	+9
1.3×10^{-5} M	+17
6.5×10^{-5} M	+42
1.3×10^{-4} M	+61
3.9×10^{-4} M	+77
6.5×10^{-4} M	+62
1.3×10^{-3} M	−85

Apart from D-thyroxine, only physiologically active analogs or derivatives of the hormone gave a similar effect [28].

The results obtained by this group of workers concerning the role of mitochondria in the mechanism of the effect of thyroid hormones on intracellular protein synthesis are of the greatest interest. The liver was removed from three groups of rats: control, thyroidectomized, and those receiving thyroxine. Mitochondrial, microsomal, and *cell sap* fractions were then obtained from a homogenate of the organ by differential centrifugation. The rate of protein synthesis was investigated in the reconstituted homogenate obtained by adding together these subcellular fractions of control and experimental animals in all possible combinations. They found that the acceleration of protein synthesis (chiefly microsomal) was observed only in homogenates containing mitochondria obtained from the liver tissue of hyperthyroid rats. The origin of the other fractions of the reconstituted homogenate was unimportant.

Investigations with the addition of thyroxine *in vitro* fully confirmed the role of the mitochondria in the mechanism of stimulation of microsomal protein synthesis. If these organelles were left out of the homogenate, thyroxine had no effect whatsoever on the incorporation of amino acids into protein. These experiments showed conclusively that contact between the thyroid hormone molecule and the energy-producing organelles of the cell is an essential condition for the increase in translation activity of the cell ribosomes [242].

It is important to emphasize that, by contrast with Tata's findings, the increase in the translation acitivity of the ribosomes in these experiments was independent of the effect of thyroxine on the synthesis of all types of RNA. It remained completely intact in the presence of substances inhibiting the synthesis of these compounds (deoxyribonuclease, actinomycin D) and even in the presence of synthetic polyribonucleotide in the homogenate [242]. Experiments on lysates of reticulocytes, in which thyroxine (in the presence of mitochondria) stimulated the synthesis of the α- and β-chains of hemoglobin, also showed that this was connected with activation of the translation stage of protein synthesis, for under these conditions only lengthening of the polypeptide chain or the completion of its formation took place [123].

Yet another difference from the results of the experiments of Tata et al. was that in the experiments of Sokoloff et al. activation of microsomal protein synthesis appeared after 5–7 min, and not after 27–30 h, i.e., after an immeasurably shorter time than was required for even the earliest effect to be manifested in Tata's system—exchange of fast-labeled nuclear RNA.

The analysis of this short latent period in the action of thyroxine on protein-synthesizing activity of the ribosomes showed that preincubation of the reaction mixture (before addition of the labeled amino acid) for a short time with the hormone caused disappearance of the lag period. This effect was observed only when mitochondria and oxidation substrates were present in the reaction mixture during preincubation with the hormone. The presence of microsomes, cell sap, and other components of the medium (except adenine nucleotides, buffer solution, and magnesium ions) in the system during preincubation with thyroxine was not necessary for disappearance of the latent period in the action of the hormone. These results show that during the lag period some form of interaction takes place between hormone and mitochondria, as a result of which a compound with a direct activating action on protein synthesis in the ribosomes passes into the supernatant. In fact, the addition of this supernatant to a system containing ribosomes increases the protein-stimulating activity of these organelles even in the absence of thyroxine.

The main problem is now reduced to the identification of the product (or products) of interaction between thyroxine and mitochondria which pass into the supernatant and activate the translation activity of the ribosomes. The attempts of Sokoloff et al. to define this product have not yet proved successful. All that has been shown is that the desired factor is dialyzable, thermostable, and destroyed by acid. On the basis of these investigations Sokoloff [237] rules out the possibility that the factor is of nucleic acid or protein nature. Likewise it is not cyclic AMP.

The known role of the mitochondria as *power stations* of the cell in the modern view permits only one possible form of their participation in the processes taking place in other cell organelles—that of supplying these processes with the energy of phosphate bonds. Meanwhile Sokoloff rejects the possibility that the product of interaction between thyroxine and mitochondria, stimulating the protein-synthesizing activity of the ribosomes, is ATP or any other nucleoside phosphate. For example, replacing mitochondria in the reaction mixture by another ATP-generating system (phosphocreatine + creatine kinase) does not permit the stimulating effect of thyroxine on protein synthesis in microsomes to be exhibited. Furthermore, the addition of ATP to the system not only did not stimulate, but it actually depressed the initial rate of synthesis of microsomal protein, whereas under the same conditions the effect of thyroxine was fully preserved.

Protein synthesis in ribosomes is known to consist of two energy-dependent stages: first, the activation of the free amino acid by the energy of ATP and the formation of an amino acid—transfer RNA complex, and second, the addition of the amino acid contained in this complex to the growing polypeptide chain through the energy of GTP. Ono et al. [183] calculated that during the incorporation of each amino acid into the growing peptide chain at least two molecules of GTP are hydrolyzed. By careful experiments Sokoloff et al. [242] showed that thyroxine, in the presence of mitochondria and oxidation substrate, stimulates the second stage of protein synthesis. Thyroxine stimulation, moreover, was most marked when a-ketoglutarate was used as the oxidation substrate, and GTP is generated in the course of its oxidation. Further evidence of the role of generation of GTP as the factor mediating the stimulating effect of thyroxine on protein synthesis in the microsomes is given by the fact that the GTP-dependent stage of protein synthesis limits the rate of the process as a whole. The addition of GTP to the system accelerates the incorporation of amino acids, both free and bound with transfer RNA, into microsomal proteins. However, Sokoloff et al. [242] showed that, even in a reaction mixture with optimal GTP concentrations, thyroxine (in the presence of mitochondria and oxidation substrate) continues to stimulate protein synthesis. These results question the role of GTP as the product of interaction between the hormone and oxidative phosphorylation looked for in the mitochondria.

It is difficult at present to answer the question whether by adding a standard dose of GTP to the system the effect of a variable yield of this compound in the course of oxidative phosphorylation can be completely replaced. It would therefore, in the writer's view, be premature to deny the role of GTP as a mediator of the hormonal effect on protein synthesis on the basis of these observations. Moreover, as will be shown later, the character of the change produced by thyroid hormones in the energy supply for intracellular processes explains the phasic nature of their action on protein synthesis. Kremer [125], after an analysis of the literature, concludes that "although the mechanisms through which the hormone manifests its action are not yet completely clear, it is most probably connected with the regulation of energy metabolism and the supply of energy for anabolic processes."

Some important evidence in support of this view of the mechanism of action of thyroid hormones was described by Cohen et al. [50]. In experiments on contracting rat atria these workers showed that protein synthesis taking place in a tissue when incubated *in vitro* for 2–3 h does not require the formation of new molecules of messenger RNA. The rate of incorporation of leucine-^{14}C into protein in fact was unchanged after the addition of actinomycin D to the incubation medium. On this basis they concluded that the availability of mRNA does not play the role of the rate-limiting factor for tissue protein synthesis. On the other hand, a decrease in the availability of energy (caused by a decrease in the partial pressure of oxygen in the system or by specific concentrations of DNP or oligomycin) sharply reduced the rate of protein synthesis in the tissue. It is interesting to note that no loading of the contractile structures of the muscle was used in these experiments, and for that reason the expenditure of energy on atrial contraction was minimal.

The linear relationship between energy production and the rate of incorporation of an amino acid into protein is evidence of the close link between these processes. Similar observations were made by Schreiber et al. [214] on the isolated perfused heart. In the opinion of Cohen et al., the stimulus for increased energy production in the mitochondria could be a very early, if not the earliest, reaction in the chain of events leading to the acceleration of protein synthesis. Finally, the possibility of an energy-dependent effect of hormones on protein synthesis is also confirmed by the fact that agents whose action is known to be exerted on oxidative phosphorylation (for example, DNP, salicylates) in small doses can stimulate growth and protein synthesis *in vitro* [130, 241, 278], increase the tissue glycogen reserves [65, 177], and so on. Large doses of these agents, like high concentrations of thyroid hormones, have the opposite effects.

Comparison of the effects of thyroxine as described, on the one hand, by Sokoloff's group and, on the other hand, by Tata is extremely interesting. As was pointed out above, Tata et al. observed activation of the synthesis of nuclear RNA hours, not minutes, after administration of the hormone *in vivo*. Attempts to find similar effects after the addition of thyroxine to the system *in vitro* were unsuccessful [25, 256]. Activation of protein synthesis by relatively small doses of thyroid hormones can thus be regarded as taking place in two successive stages. The first, appearing after a very short lag period (5–7 min), as already stated is absolutely dependent on interaction between the hormone and the oxidative phosphorylation system in the cell mitochondria and totally independent of the effect of the hormone on the synthesis of any form of RNA. This stage did not come to light in Tata's experiments because his system did not contain mitochondria. The second stage begins not earlier than 30 h after the administration of thyroxine, it is independent of the presence of mitochondria, and it is preceded by the activation of synthesis of nuclear (chiefly ribosomal) RNA. This was the stage responsible for the *primary* effect of thyroid hormones in the system of

Tata et al. This time sequence of the events developing in the protein-synthetic system of the cell suggests that the second stage of the changes in this system, involving the presumed participation of the nuclear-ribosomal complex, is not the result of the direct action of the hormone but merely reflects the adaptive response of the cell to its direct action [237]. The second stage in fact has the characteristic features of an adaptive reaction of the cell to the *primary* action of the hormones: It has a long lag period, it appears only after administration of the hormone *in vivo*, and it depends on several factors determining the general condition of the organism. For example, it does not appear during starvation [256, 257], which would not affect the specific primary action of hormones. In its general form this reaction is evidently a manifestation of the rule that an increase in the function of any structure (in this case the intracellular ribosomes) involves an increase in mass of the functioning structures [161].

Meanwhile, the activation of the protein-synthesizing function of the ribosomes by thyroid hormones can evidently be regarded as the primary effect of these hormones only with respect to the activation of new ribosome formation. The facts described above are evidence that the primacy of this effect is not absolute. In turn, it is a product of earlier changes arising under the influence of thyroxine in the mitochondria, the power stations of the cell.

Consequently, the facts now available provide an answer to the first of the questions raised at the beginning of this section: The most acceptable view is that thyroid hormones act *primarily* on the mitochondrial processes of electron transport and energy transformation. However, the view that mitochondrial metabolism is connected with the influence of hormones on the cytoplasmic protein-synthesizing system would be incomplete without any consideration of the role of the mitochondrial system of protein sysnthesis in the overall regulatory effect of thyroid hormones at the cell level.

Comparison of the system for protein synthesis in the cytoplasm and mitochondria reveals certain special features of the latter. As in the case of microsomal protein synthesis the source of energy is ATP but not its high-energy precursors [78, 207]. Protein synthesis in the mitochondria is independent and includes the same basic stages as cytoplasmic protein synthesis (Figure 19). However, there are differences between mitochondrial and microsomal systems for protein synthesis, affecting the size of the ribosomes, the structure of the RNA and DNA, sensitivity to specific inhibitors, and so on [192, 207]. On the other hand, there is convincing evidence of the similarity between the process of protein synthesis in bacteria and mitochondria [1, 207]. The rate of protein synthesis in the mitochondria rises to a maximum before cell division; synthesis is preceded by the rapid, energy-dependent transport of amino acids inside the mitochondria [280]. It is interesting to note that the synthesis of mitochondrial proteins is accompanied

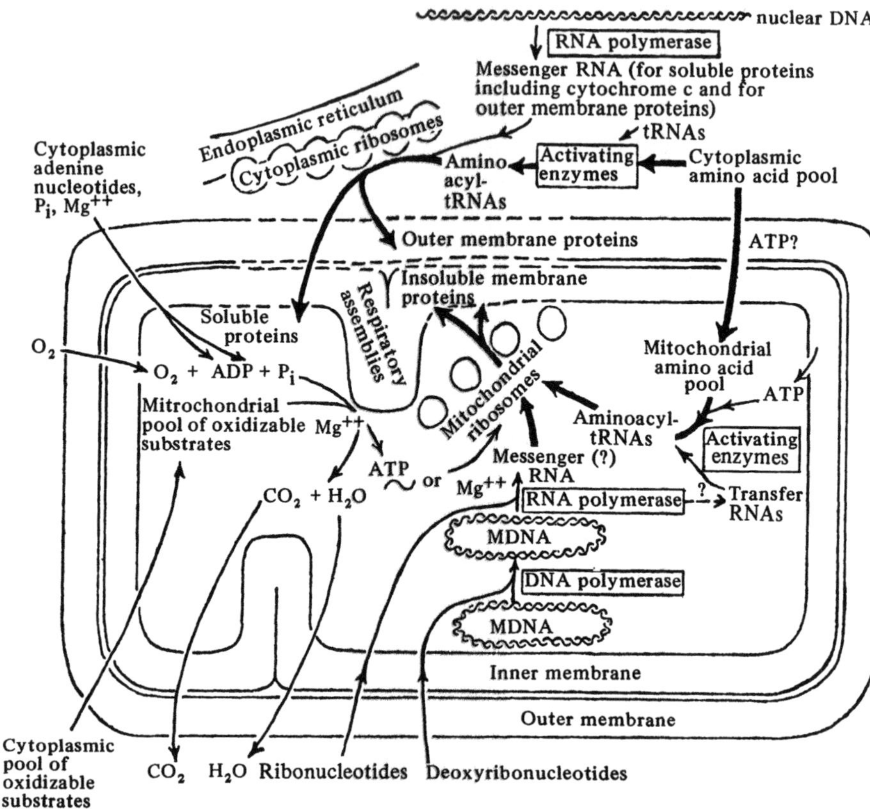

Fig. 19. Scheme of protein biosynthesis in the mitochondria (after Roodyn and Wilkie [207]). Bold arrows indicate amino acid incorporation, the other arrows related processes. Dashed lines denote the sites of membrane formation.

by corresponding synthesis of phospholipids. This could be the basis for the coordinated formation of a thermodynamically stable structure—the membrane [142, 255].

Mitochondrial protein synthesis is evidently a controlled and integrated process. Most workers nowadays consider that soluble enzymic mitochondrial proteins are synthesized on the cytoplasmic ribosomes and then transported inside the mitochondria [207]. Most probably protein synthesis in the mitochondria leads to the formation of structural protein only [82, 142, 207, 289]; this structural protein possibly plays the role in the membrane of a *stand* ensuring the correct interaction between the fixed mitochondrial components in the organized membrane. Work in Green's laboratory has shown that the structural protein can bind certain mitochondrial proteins and phospholipids and that it has specific sites for the attachment of cytochrome of the respiratory chain [76, 77, 207].

Consequently it is only through the combined action of thyroid hormones on protein synthesis in the microsomes and mitochondria that the necessary regulatory effect can be produced on the energy-transformation system in the cell that is ultimately revealed and assessed as morphological and functional manifestations, and as the composition of populations and the rate of *turnover* of the mitochondria themselves or of their more important components [79, 192].

Clear proof has now been obtained of the existence of two populations of mitochondrial DNA and protein, *cycled* at different rates after the administration of thyroid hormones to hypothyroid or euthyroid animals [79, 192]. The differences in the rate of turnover indicate that a new, active population of mitochondria, synthesizing at a higher level of thyroid hormones, has accumulated in the cell, whereas the previous mitochondrial population has undergone rapid degradation. According to this view, qualitative changes arising in the mitochondria after administration of thyroid hormones are not due to modification of the previous population but are embodied in the nature of the new population. Physiological concentrations of thyroid hormones evidently establish optimal proportions in each organ between the enzymes (*constant proportions*). Nonphysiological doses of the hormones change these proportions and thereby reduce the potential of the organism as a whole [104, 213].

Recent investigations [26, 190, 191] in which rats were treated with thyroxine confirmed the activation of mitochondrial protein synthesis. It is important to emphasize that this activation occurred sooner than any detectable stimulation of amino acid incorporation into the proteins of ribosomes isolated from the same animals. These experiments thus demonstrate the independent and primary effect of thyroxine on the mitochondria and thus rule out the stimulation of microsomal protein synthesis as the cause of the calorigenic action of the hormone on the cell. It is evidently a more difficult matter to exclude the role of stimulation of the synthesis of the mitochondrial proteins themselves, although it has been shown that there are none of the known dehydrogenases among these thyroxine-induced proteins.

Kaplay and Sanadi [110] reported recently that one of the fractions of water-soluble mitochondrial proteins of thyroidectomized animals to which thyroxine was given 1–3 h before sacrifice increases respiration in the liver mitochondria from thyroidectomized rats in state 4 by about the same degree as a single injection of the hormone. Meanwhile the rate of respiration in state 3 was practically unchanged. On the other hand, the analogous fraction obtained from the liver mitochondria of euthyroid animals did not have the above-mentioned effect when added to the mitochondria from thyroidectomized rats. Since, of all the fractions tested, only one specifically affects the rate of respiration in state 4 and since the stimulation of respiration is not abolished by bovine serum albumin, it is unlikely that the effect is due to the presence of protein-bound thyroxine. These workers' experiments with thyroxine-^{14}C gave further evidence in support of this view.

On the basis of these results, a clear line can be drawn between the direct action of thyroxine on the mitochondria and its action effective through the synthesis of specific mitochondrial proteins. The many effects of thyroxine on rat liver mitochondria *in vivo* are represented in the following scheme [110]:

	Thyroidectomy $+T_4$	
Direct effect	60–180 min	36 h
Increased mitochondrial respiration in state 4. Reversed by bovine serum albumin (BSA).	Rapid extramitochondrial selective synthesis of protein and its incorporation into the mitochondrion. Increased mitochondrial respiration in state 4. Not reversed by BSA.	Synthesis of new respiratory groups. Increased basal metabolic rate.

The direct effect of thyroxine is an increase in the rate of respiration of mitochondria in state 4, which is insensitive to cyclohexamide and reversed by the addition of BSA to the isolated mitochondria *in vitro*. The next effect, manifested in the course of 1 h after administration of T_4, is the rapid synthesis of specific protein (or proteins) by the extramitochondrial protein-synthesizing system. This protein is incorporated into the mitochondria where it evidently maintains the stimulant effect during the intermediate period. This stimulation is not reversed by the addition of BSA *in vitro*. The third response to administration of T_4, observed only after a lag phase of about 36 h, is expressed as the synthesis of new respiratory groups.

Modern Views of the Mechanism of Action of Thyroid Hormones at the Subcellular Level

Modern ideas of the mechanism of action of the hormones are based on the assumption that their manifold biological effects arise through interaction of the hormone with a single site or *target*. However, there are no weighty theoretical or practical objections to the assumption that these sites are double or multiple in nature, at least for the hormones of growth and development [254]. Possible models of manifestations of multiple biological effects as the result of interaction between the hormone and a single site (models 1 and 2) or with several sites (model 3) are illustrated in Figure 20. In Tata's opinion [254], the last model overcomes many of the difficulties arising through the acceptance of mutually exclusive mechanisms based

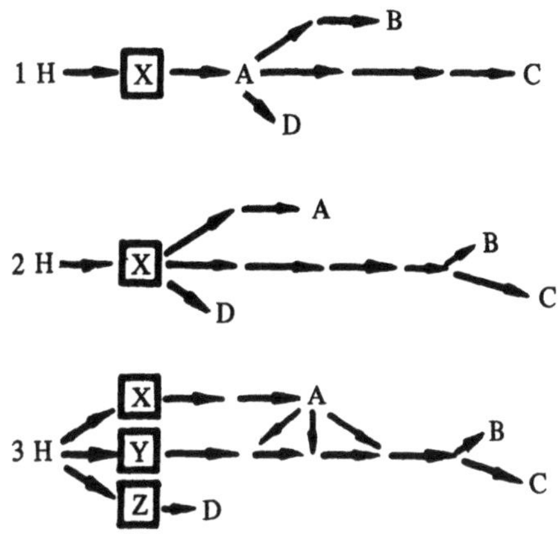

Fig. 20. Three hypothetical models explaining how multiple biological effects (A, B, C, D) of the hormone (H) can arise from a single primary site of interaction (X) in models 1 and 2, or from multiple sites (X, Y, Z) in model 3. In the last model the effect of interaction between the hormone and one of the sites (X) facilitates the course of the slower processes dependent on its action on another site (Y). The number and length of the arrows are intended to reflect the fact that the lag period and the degree of remoteness of the various effects from the action of the hormone on the primary sites are different (after Tata [254]).

only on the regulation of membrane permeability (for example, the site X) or only on intereaction with the gene or repressor controlling the synthesis of specific protein (for example, through the site Y). In particular, model 3 envisages the reconstruction of the permeability barrier as one of the earliest hormonal effects. However, this hormonal regulation by itself does not characterize the specificity of action, but it may facilitate the course of processes regulating the synthesis of compounds specific for that given hormone (processes B and C). As a result the slowest process C is controlled through interaction between the hormone and different sites or targets.

In Hoch's opinion [94], the criteria of the selective primary action of a hormone must include the correlation of the observed effects *in vivo* and *in vitro*, the rate of action, the effectiveness of small doses of the hormone, and the localization of the hormone in the target site where the functional changes are manifested. Observations made as early as in 1954 by Lee and Williams [135] show that about 8% of the radioactivity of thyroxine-^{131}I injected into an animal is concentrated within 5 min in the liver and that 40% of this radioactivity is localized in the mitochondria. Shimada [221] found that 10–25% of labeled thyroxine accumulating in the liver was in the nuclei, 20–30% in the mitochondria, and 30–40% in the microsomal fraction. Hoch has recently shown that the injection of small doses of thyroxine (5.2 μg/g body weight) into hypothyroid animals increases the content of this hormone by 550 times in the liver mitochondria in the course of 3 h after injection.

Thyroxine accumulates in the mitochondria not only when it is injected into experimental animals, but also if it is incubated directly with isolated mitochondria, which assimilate from 1/3 to 4/5 of the total quantity of hormone present in the reaction mixture [97, 245]. However, numerous attempts to establish correlation between the metabolic effect and intensity of binding of the hormone in the mitochondria proved unsuccessful [97, 116, 245]. There is evidence in the literature that the assimilation of thyroid hormones by isolated mitochondria is passive in character and is independent of metabolism [116, 245]. Thyroxine binding was observed equally at 0°C and at 20°C, while thermal denaturation of the mitochondria actually increased it twofold [116]. The assimilation of thyroxine in the mitochondria takes place very quickly and is virtually complete in 1 min [245].

Intact mitochondria are divided into several structurally and functionally separate compartments (Figure 21). To discover in which compartment most of the thyroxine accumulates, different workers have disintegrated mitochondria with ultrasound or detergents and then fractionated the components of the mitochondrial membranes [5, 221]. Very weighty evidence of the localization of thyroxine in fragments of the membranes, especially the inner membranes housing the oxidation and coupling systems, has thus been obtained. The highest content of thyroxine, expressed per milligram protein, was found in the fraction of *elementary particles*, with rather less in the fraction of structural protein of the inner mitochondrial membranes [221]. Recent investigations in Turakulov's laboratory have shown that the role of phospholipids in the mechanism of thyroxine and tri-

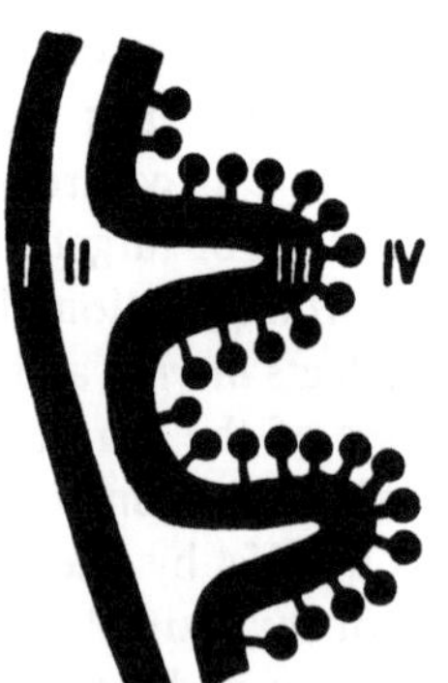

Fig. 21. Scheme showing different *compartments* of the mitochondria (after Ernster and Kuylenstierna [57]): I–outer membrane, II–intermembraneous space, III–inner membrane with characteristic *mushroom-like* projections, IV–mitochondrial matrix.

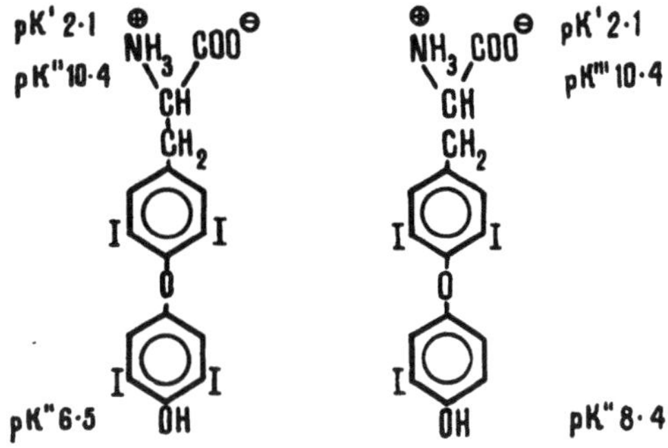

Thyroxine Triiodothyronine

iodothyronine binding by the mitochondria is of secondary importance: Removal of about 80% of the phospholipids by acetone extraction by the method of S. and B. Fleischer [64], for instance, had virtually no effect on the binding process [262, 266]. Presumably the binding of thyroxine with the protein components of the mitochondrial membranes, as also with other proteins (of the albumin type, for example), takes place with the participation of free lysyl-ε-amino groups of the proteins [244]. The bond between the anionic part of the hormone molecule and the cationic groups of the protein has the character of electrostatic forces of attraction, and interaction with the enzyme proteins of the subcellular particles evidently takes place through the OH-group of the hormone [195, 244].

Hillier [89] investigated the binding of thyroxine and triiodothyronine on natural and model systems and concluded that the hydrophobic adsorption of hormones by the lipid part of the membrane plays an important role. Interaction of this type is due to loss of the charge of the phenolic group in the juxtamembranous layer as a result of the fact that its pH is close to the pK value of the phenolic group. Under these conditions the undissociated aromatic part of the hormone molecule penetrates into the hydrophobic layer of the lipids, whereas the hydrophilic *tail* lies in the outer aqueous layer.

However, this method of penetration of the hormone into the lipid phase evidently does not give it the necessary mobility in the lipid layer in order to create effective conductance for H^+, i.e., uncoupling within the framework of the schemes examined earlier (Figure 9). The stability of thyroxine when adsorbed hydrophobically on the water–lipid phase boundary, according to Hillier, is the main source during interaction of the hormone with the membranes. This mechanism of thyroxine accumulation in the membrane evidently also takes place *in vivo*. At any rate, Hillier was able to demonstrate correlation between the phospholipid content in the tissues and their ability to bind thyroxine *in vivo*. However, it is difficult to say how universal this principle is; as was stated above, no decrease in the binding of thyroxine with the mitochondria was found when 80% of their phospholipids had been removed [262, 266]. Possibly not only phospholipids, but also other components of the membranes, including certain types of proteins such as structural protein with hydrophobic properties and lipoproteins, may also have a hydrophobic mechanism of hormone binding.

The intensive accumulation of thyroid hormones in parts of the mitochondria where the energy transformation mechanism is located, and its accumulation in quantities comparable with the number of respiratory ensembles [95], is evidently by no means accidental. According to Hoch [95], a single injection of thyroxine into hypothyroid animals (5.2 μg/g body weight) restores functional parameters of the isolated mitochondria such as P/O, the respiratory control, the rate of respiration in state 4, and sensitivity to DNP to normal within 2 min. As much thyroxine as is usually given in experiments *in vitro* to demonstrate particular functional responses of the mitochondria in the presence of that hormone accumulates in the mitochondria under these circumstances.

Thyroid hormones can accumulate on the surface of the membrane, where they create a much higher local concentration than in the surrounding solution. This more nonspecific type of concentrating effect may play the role of the initial stage in transporting the hormone to the centers of its action or metabolism. Assuming that the *thyroxine receptor* is bound with the membrane, the amount of hormone accessible to it will be determined not by the level of free thyroxine in the solution, but by the local concentration of the hormone on the membrane surface [89].

However, it must be recognized that the elucidation of the actual mechanism of interaction between thyroxine localized in the membranes and the components of the electron and energy transfer chains is a matter for further investigation. Meanwhile certain facts already available emphasize the main differences between the mechanism of action of thyroid hormones and of classical uncouplers of the DNP type. The following, in particular, may be mentioned:

a. Thyroid hormones do not significantly affect the conductance of bimolecular phospholipid membranes [67, 80, 266].
b. The multiple effects of thyroid hormones in experiments *in vivo* cannot be simulated by other uncouplers.
c. Unlike DNP, in some cases a certain latent period is required for the effects of thyroid hormones to take place; this latent period is perhaps required to enable the hormone to penetrate to the target areas where it is converted into the *active* form [90, 248, 259].
d. The classical uncouplers prevent the swelling of the mitochondria induced by thyroid hormones [90, 139]. These facts, as well as the discovery of the regulating action of thyroid hormones on the early

stages of enzyme biosynthesis [254], have led one group of workers to criticise the *uncoupling* mechanism vigorously and to relegate it to the sphere of the *toxic* effects of the hormone; in exchange they have formulated the view that thyroid hormones, by controlling the activity of protein-synthesizing systems in the cell, have a multiple effect on the enzymes and organized groups of enzymes, including the system for mitochondrial oxidative phosphorylation [56, 104, 248–254, 257, 258].

However, this concept also, shifting the center of gravity from the mitochondria to the genetic system of the cell, is not without its faults. For example, changes in the activity of many enzymes, including α-glycerophosphate dehydrogenase, observable in the liver, are not found in the brain or spleen [90, 104]. Furthermore, the increases in the basal metabolic rate and in heat production after administration of thyroxine to guinea pigs are not accompanied by significant changes in α-glycerophosphate dehydrogenase or succinate dehydrogenase activity in the mitochondria of the liver, heart, and muscles of these animals, unlike in rats. The α-glycerophosphate dehydrogenase of the mitochondria of hyperthyroid dogs is actually a little less active than normally [85]. Several other facts also are difficult to reconcile with the above concept:

a. the abnormally high respiratory control in the liver mitochondria of hypothyroid rats,
b. the fact that mitochondria are necessary for thyroxine-induced protein synthesis in the microsomes,
c. the ability of thyroxine to modify the reactivity of mitochondria [for example, to DNP *in vivo* and to amobarbital *in vitro*) in concentrations of the hormone which have no action either on calorigenesis or on the synthesis of new respiratory ensembles,
d. the normalizing action of thyroxine on the functions of the liver mitochondria of hypothyroid rats if injected as little as 2 min before death of the animal, i.e., many hundreds of times faster than the increase in protein synthesis taking place in the mitochondria and microsomes or of RNA synthesis in the nucleus [92–96].

According to Hoch's most recent findings, changes in the mitochondrial functions after administration of thyroid hormones to animals must be classed as an effect on the mechanism of energy transformation preceding activation of the genetic system of the cell as observed by Tata and other workers. The decrease in respiratory control of the mitochondria after injection of subcalorigenic doses of thyroid hormones leads to an increase in the rate of ATP synthesis, for respiration in state 4 can be coupled with phosphorylation or with ionic transport and, consequently, this phenomenon can be regarded as an anabolic effect of the thyroid hormones, leading to an increase in potential for intracellular biosynthesis [95, 96].

In these experiments the decrease in respiratory control characteristically took place on account of the activation of mitochondrial respiration in state 4 (i.e., after complete exhaustion of the reserves of ADP, the phosphate acceptor), whereas the assimilation of oxygen by the mitochondria in state 3 was unchanged by these low doses of thyroxine. On the other hand, in a series of investigations by Kimata and Tarjan [113, 247], who used mitochondria from the ventricular myocardium of rabbits treated with a comparatively large dose of thyroxine (20 μg/100 g) for a long period of time, no changes whatsoever in the indices reflecting the coupling of oxidation with phosphorylation were found. In their opinion, changes observed in the experiments by other workers are due to the fact that respiratory control by adenine nucleotides (which is itself unchanged) becomes extremely sensitive to substrates of the Krebs cycle.

The metabolic changes described above are the earliest known effect of thyroid hormones. This effect is in agreement with observations made in Sokoloff's and Hoch's laboratories on the *primacy* of interaction between thyroxine and the mitochondria. Considering the practically complete absence of a latent period of the effect (it appeared simultaneously with the entrance of the hormone into the mitochondria) and also its appearance after doses of the hormone so small that they cannot be placed in either the *pharmacological* or the *toxic* category, it is reasonable to suppose that this effect is most closely linked with the *molecular* mechanism of action of physiological concentrations of thyroxine. Whatever the mechanism of attenuation or abolition of respiratory control, it leads to an increase, and not a decrease, in the output of high-energy compounds per unit time. Analysis of the data given in Table XIV shows, for instance, that during weakening of coupling, ATP formation per unit time must be increased by 50%. A similar situation was observed by Slater and Hülsmann [232] when investigating the oxidation of *a*-ketoglutarate by the sarcosomes of the pectoral muscles of the fly in the presence of 2,4-DNP. After the uncoupling of free phosphorylation in the electron transport chain and the preservation of only one substrate phosphorylation, the acceleration of oxidation more than compensated for the complete inhibition of phosphorylation in the respiratory chain. The end result was that DNP increased the rate of phosphorylation although the efficiency of the conversion of the energy of oxidation into ATP was of course reduced.

Skulachev [224] has summarized the results of much research to show that the rate of oxidation and the degree of its coupling with phosphorylation are inversely proportional to each other and that some degree of uncoupling sharply accelerates the flow of electrons along the respiratory chain. According to Lardy and Maley [130], in such cases phosphorylation is uncoupled at points where it limits the rate of the whole process of oxidation. As a result of the considerable increase in the overall rate of respiration arising under these circumstances, the initial level of ATP production is exceeded. As Skulachev [228] points out, the concept of thermodynamic and biological efficiency of energy accumulation do not coincide, but "for living systems the total amount of energy is not so important as the rate of its liberation" [60]. When coupling is *weakened*, and no decrease in the P/O ratio can be found, there is naturally a far greater increase in the rate of phosphorylation and in the output of ATP per unit time.

The ability of low concentrations of thyroid hormones to raise the P/O ratio without any change in the rate of oxidation has also been described [52], although Bronk [20, 21] found an increase both in the P/O ratio and in the oxygen consumption in the mitochondria and even in submitochondrial particles under the influence of these minimal concentrations of the hormone. Whatever the case, just as during the weakening of coupling, the ATP output evidently rises.

All these observations show that low concentrations of thyroid hormones can change the coupled processes in the mitochondria so that the output of ATP is increased; larger doses of these hormones, however, by their effect on the efficiency of phosphorylation, can reduce the output of this product of tissue respiration. In that case two distinct processes have to be taken into account—oxidative phosphorylation in the mitochondria and the synthesis of RNA and protein in the nucleo-ribosomal apparatus of the cell by targets of physiological and toxic doses of the thyroid hormones. All doses of these compounds can act on the same process, the difference being only in the extent to which they change its course.

The mechanism of abolition of respiratory control is evidently identical in nature with the true uncoupling of oxidative phosphorylation, and it usually precedes it. The decrease in P/O arising with low concentrations of uncouplers may be so small that it cannot be detected, whereas the consequences of this uncoupling—the decrease in the respiratory control, the increase in the rate of respiration in state 4, and the increase in the output of ATP per unit time—appear clearly enough.

The above hypothesis is not supported by the observed normal value of the P/O ratio in the mitochondria of hypothyroid animals [22, 157]. However, as Skulachev [228] rightly points out, further improvements in the methods of measuring P/O may permit values of this ratio greater than 3 to be obtained. Maley and Lardy have already observed changes in the sensitivity of the mitochondria of thyroidectomized rats to 2,4-DNP, and they have concluded on this basis that even *normal* concentrations of thyroid hormones can uncouple oxidative phosphorylation. Evidence in support of this view is given by Heninger et al. [87]. They investigated the thyroxine and triiodothyronine content in the liver mitochondria of totally and partially thyroidectomized animals (by the isotope equilibrium method) and the P/O ratio in the mitochondria during the oxidation of glutamate. They found that the P/O ratio in thyroidectomized animals was much higher than the characteristic values for mitochondria of the control rats. Moreover, with a decrease in the concentration of thyroid hormones in the mitochondria (from 0.35 to 0.00 ng/mg nitrogen) the P/O ratio increased from 2.4 to 3. The negative correlation observed between the hormone level in the mitochondria of thyroidectomized animals and the value of P/O means that thyroxine, even in concentrations below those present in the mitochondria of normal rats, can dissociate oxidative phosphorylation.

Largely through the delicate experiments of Hoch and other investigators it can be firmly accepted that the mitochondria satisfy criteria of selectivity of hormonal action such as the correlation between effects observed *in vivo* and *in vitro*, rate of action, effectiveness of small doses of hormone, and localization of the hormone in the target area where the functional changes are manifested.

The fact that the increased oxygen consumption by the tissues under the influence of thyroid hormones *in vivo* and *in vitro* is based on the same mechanism is illustrated, in particular, by the observations of Goh Kong-oo and Dallam [69]. These workers showed that the addition of thyroid extract to the diet of rats leads to an increase in the oxygen assimilation of myocardial slices. A similar effect was observed when thyroxine was added *in vitro* to slices of heart muscle from control animals. However, the addition of the hormone *in vitro* to myocardial slices from hyperthyroid rats was not followed by any further increase in the oxygen consumption of this tissue. Experiments by Khusainova (in Turakulov's laboratory) in which thyroxine was added to preparations of thyroid gland mitochondria also gave the same result: Thyroxine increased respiration of the thyroid mitochondria from normal and hyperplastic tissue but, in a concentration of 1×10^{-5} M, it did not stimulate the absorption of oxygen by mitochondria isolated from the tissue of thyrotoxic glands.

When the ways by which thyroid hormones affect the mechanism of energy transformation in the mitochondria are examined, attention must be paid to a recent paper by Gruenstein and Wynn [80] in which the molecular mechanism of action of thyroxine is represented as the result of modification of the membrane phospholipids by iodine (Figure 22). The universal criterion by which, in these workers' opinion, both the physiological and toxic effects of thyroid hormones can be estimated is the degree of decrease in the electrical resistance of the membrane or increase in its ionic conductance as a result of a free-radical mechanism of thyroxine degradation with the liberation of iodine from its molecule as $I^{\bullet}$ (or I^{+}). A decrease in the resistance of biological membranes is thus postulated as the primary mechanism of action of thyroxine. The process of thyroxine degradation is accompanied

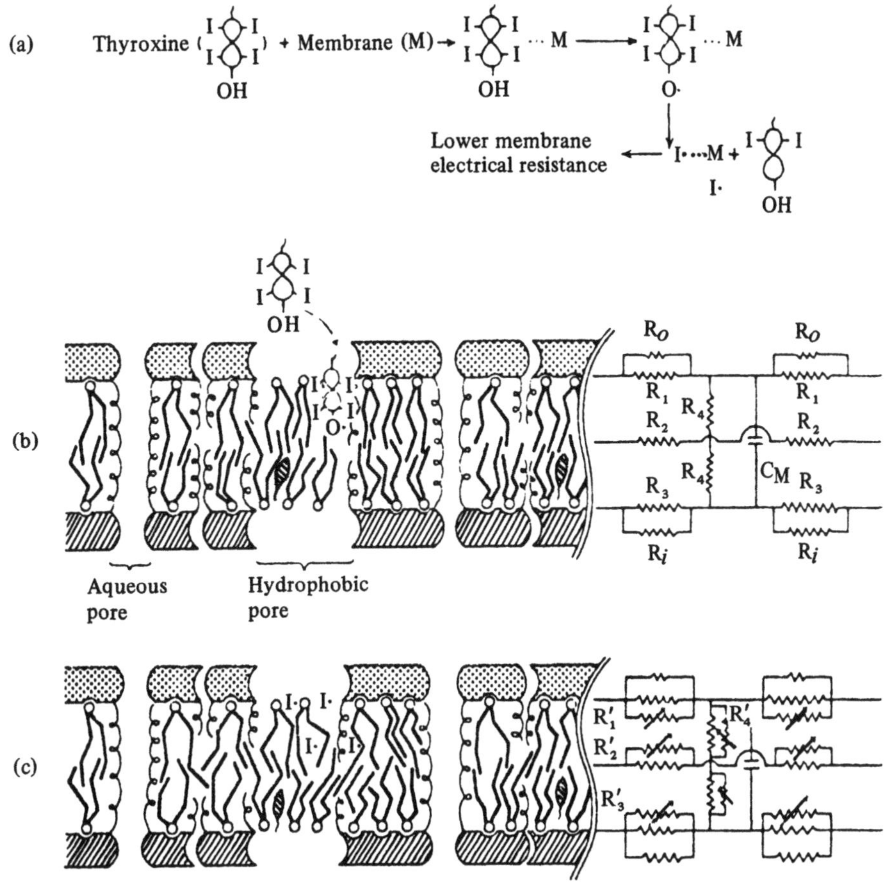

Fig. 22. Scheme showing the general theoretical proposals for the mechanism of action of thyroxine put forward by Gruenstein and Wynn [80]. (a) This summarizes the general theoretical proposal for the mechanism of thyroxine action. Thyroxine plus membrane yields a membrane-thyroxine complex. This complex in turn gives rise to a membrane-thyroxine free radical, which decomposes leaving some or all of the iodine from the thyroxine associated with the phospholipid portion of the membrane. (b) *Left*. This is a diagrammatic representation of the membrane before and during the initial association with thyroxine. Although the phospholipid is seen closely associated with the membrane protein, some phospholipid bilayer nature remains. *Right*. Shows a simple equivalent electrical circuit for the membrane on the left, including longitudinal resistances along the inner and outer surfaces (R_1, R_3) and through the center (R_2) of the bilayer, as well as transverse (R_4) to the membrane. R_o and R_i are resistances of the outer and inner solutions respectively, and C_m is the membrane capacitance. (c) *Left*. This shows the membrane following the degradation of the thyroxine-free radical. Although no major structural alterations of the phospholipids are depicted. such changes may be important aspects of the I^- (or I^+) in the membrane. *Right*. The longitudinal and transverse membrane resistances are now modified, as a result of the presence of the I^- (or I^+), by the schematic insertion of parallel resistances (R'_1, R'_2, R'_3, and R'_4). These parallel resistors are shown as variables since the decrease in membrane resistance may change as a function of such factors as membrane voltage.

by manifestation of the protective antioxidant function of the hormone which, in this respect, is much more active than ascorbic acid, vitamin E, and cysteine [80, 288].

It may be that this mechanism, incorporating a decrease in membrane potential through the action of thyroxine, can explain the inhibition of the endergonic functions of the mitochondria and the similarity of their individual responses to the addition of thyroid hormones and of the classical uncouplers. However, by contrast with the latter, which function as H^+ carriers into the hydrophobic parts of the membranes, thyroxine evidently acts as donor of *active* iodine in the membrane structures [80, 195]. Changes in individual physical and physicochemical characteristics of the membranes evidently arise through interaction between iodine liberated from the thyroxine molecule and unsaturated fatty acids in the side chain of the phospholipids.

Evidence has been obtained to show, however, that there is no appreciable deiodination of the thyroid hormones while they induce specific effects at the mitochondrial level, suggesting that metabolism of the hormones does not occur in the course of their action [191, 259]. In the light of the above hypothesis it is difficult to explain some other aspects of the action of thyroid hormones. In particular, it is not clear by what mechanism the classical uncouplers and inhibitors of respiration prevent the action of thyroxine, ICN, and I_2 on mitochondrial structure. It is also questionable whether the interaction between thyroxine and cytochrome oxidase is important, in principle, as Gruenstein and Wynn [80] emphasize, for according to Arbogast and Hoch [5] there is one molecule of thyroxine in the mitochondria for every 200 respiratory chains, or at least for every 66 if the distribution of thyroxine in ultrasonic fragments of the mitochondria is considered.

Nevertheless, the conclusion which follows from this hypothesis can be accepted, namely, that the mechanism of action of thyroxine is universal despite the multiplicity of the effects observed both on isolated mitochondria and in experiments *in vivo.* The reason is evidently that the *target* proposed by Gruenstein and Wynn—the biological membrane—can respond in many different ways, with many variations of each, for the functions of membranous structures are also diverse. However, the hypotheses we have examined still provide no criterion for correlating changes observed in cell structures under the influence of thyroid hormones and their physiological effects.

The most difficult task is evidently to explain the abrupt morphological and chemical changes arising in tadpoles during metamorphosis, that are known to be linked with the effects of thyroid hormones, from the standpoint of this hypothesis. During the metamorphosis of amphibians, new enzyme proteins connected with urea synthesis (carbamoyl phosphate synthetase) and with digestion, and also a new structure of hemoglobin, are formed in these animals [66]. These changes correspond more with the view that thyroxine influences the synthesis of messenger RNAs in the nuclei than with their primary action on the supply of energy for the processes of protein synthesis.

Nor must the possibility of species specificity in the mechanism of action of the hormones be forgotten. This specificity could determine the direction in which the increased output of ATP, taking place under the influence of physiological concentrations of thyroxine through activation of cell respiration, is utilized. In other words, in amphibians thyroid hormones could also have oxidative phosphorylation processes as their target, and the species specificity could be manifested as the use of the surplus energy for the formation of new specific proteins. This, however, is nothing more than a hypothesis, although the experiments of Cutting and Tainter [51] using 2,4-DNP led to the earlier appearance of some morphological features of metamorphosis in tadpoles. The possibility cannot be ruled out that metamorphosis could not be completely reproduced by DNP because of the toxicity of this compound and the consequent rapid death of the tadpoles.

According to Wilt [284] and to Paik and Cohen [186] the acceleration of protein biosynthesis during metamorphosis may be produced by the catabolic action of thyroid hormones.

Another group of observations, on the basis of which metamorphosis in amphibians can be regarded as a special manifestation of activation of the thyroid gland, is connected with the insufficient specificity of thyroid hormones in this respect. For example, in thyroidectomized larval forms of amphibians metamorphosis can be induced by acetylated thyroxine, by diiodotyrosine, by inorganic salts of iodine, or even by iodine itself [4], none of which affect metabolism quantitatively. In some species of fish, moreover, thyroid hormones lead to changes in the rate of growth and shape of the body but do not affect the oxygen consumption [59, 233]. Lardy and Lee [132] found no activation of mitochondrial α-glycerophosphate dehydrogenase in tadpoles under the influence of thyroid hormones. Experiments with *Rana pipiens* showed that, although injection of thyroid hormone into the tadpoles stimulated metamorphosis, it did not cause changes in their oxygen consumption; in the adult frogs this hormone increased metabolism although, of course, its action was no longer accompanied by the characteristic changes of metamorphosis, and at certain temperatures (greater than 13°C) it lowered the body temperature [86, 277]. These results point to differences in the mechanisms of action of thyroid hormones on amphibians at different age periods.

The results of the investigations described above reveal the great difficulties that beset all attempts at the present time to identify the process modified primarily by thyroid hormones. Nevertheless it can be concluded that, except for the role of these hormones in metamorphosis, most of the evidence points to mitochondrial processes of oxidative phosphorylation as the cellular target for thyroxine and triiodothyronine. The adoption of this *monistic* view enables the rejection of suggestions that different doses of the hormone have different mechanisms of action or, at least, that physiological and pharmacological concentrations of the hormone in the cell act on spatially different sites.

REFERENCES FOR PART III

1. Aay, C., and Kroon, A. M. In: *Abstracts of the 5th Meeting of FEBS, Prague,* 1968, p. 51.
2. Aebi, H., and Abelin, I. *Biochem. Z. 324*:364, 1953.
3. Adamson, L. E. *Biochim. Biophys. Acta 201*:446, 1970.
4. Allen, B. M. (1963), cited by Prosser and Brown, 1967.
5. Arbogast, B., and Hoch, F. L. *FEBS Lett. 1*:315, 1968.
6. Ash, A. S. F., Besch, H. R., Jr., Harigaya, S., and Zaimis, E. *J. Physiol. (London) 224*:1, 1972.
7. Azzi, A., Rossi, E., and Azzone, G. *IEG No. 1, Sci. Memo,* 529, 1966.
8. Babakov, A. V., Liberman, E. A., Skulachev, V. P., Topaly, V. P., Sharaf, A. A., and Yaguzhinskii, L. S. In: *Mitochondria. Enzymic Processes and Their Regulation* (in Russian), Nauka, Moscow, 1968, p. 137.
9. Bartley, W., and Enser, N. B. *Biochem. J. 93*:332, 1964.
10. Beechey, R. B. *Biochem. J. 98*:284, 1966.
11. Bentzel, C. J., and Solomon, A. K. *J. Gen. Physiol. 50*:1547, 1967.
12. Bielawski, J., Thompson, T. E., and Lehninger, A. L. *Biochem. Biophys. Res. Commun. 24*:948, 1966.
13. Binet, A., Gros, C., and Volfin, P. *FEBS Lett. 17*:193, 1971.
14. Binet, A., and Volfin, P. *FEBS Lett. 17*:197, 1971.
15. Blair, P. V., and Wee Chong Tan. *Biochim. Biophys. Acta 143*:630, 1967.
16. Blondin, G. A., and Green, D. E. *Proc. Nat. Acad. Sci. (Washington) 58*:612, 1967.
17. Böttger, I., Kriegel, H., and Wieland, O. *Eur. J. Biochem. 13*:253, 1970.
18. Brierley, G. P. In: *Energy-Linked Functions of Mitochondria,* Academic Press, New York, 1963, p. 237.
19. Brodie, B. B., et al. *Pharmacol. Rev. 18*:273, 1966.
20. Bronk, J. R. *Biochim. Biophys. Acta 27*:667, 1958.
21. Bronk, J. R. *Biochim. Biophys. Acta 35*:562, 1959.
22. Bronk, J. R., and Bronk, M. S. *J. Biol. Chem. 237*:897, 1962.
23. Bronk, J. R. *Biochim. Biophys. Acta 69*:375, 1963.
24. Bronk, J. R. *Biochim. Biophys. Acta 97*:9, 1965.
25. Brown, D. M. *Endocrinology 78*:1252, 1966.
26. Buchanan, J. L., Primack, M. P., and Tapley, D. F. *Endocrinology 89*:534, 1971.
27. Buzhinskii, E. P., Gotlib, V. A., and Lev, A. A. In: *Mitochondria. Enzymic Processes and Their Regulation* (in Russian), Nauka, Moscow, 1968, p. 141.
28. Campbell, P. L., Deibler, G. E., Gelber, S., and Sokoloff, L. *Endocrinology 75*:304, 1964.
29. Caplan, A. I., and Carafoli, E. *Biochim. Biophys. Acta 104*:317, 1965.
30. Carafoli, E., Weiland, S., and Lehninger, A. L. *Biochim. Biophys. Acta 97*:88, 1965.

31. Carafoli, E. *J. Gen. Physiol. 50*:1849, 1967.
32. Carafoli, E. *Biochem. J. 116*:2P, 1970.
33. Casillas, E. R., and Hoskins, D. D. *Biochem. Biophys. Res. Commun. 40*:255, 1970.
34. Chance, B. In: *Regulation of Cell Metabolism* (Russian translation), IL, Moscow, 1962, p. 111.
35. Chance, B. In: *Energy-Linked Functions of Mitochondria,* Academic Press, New York, 1963, p. 253.
36. Chance, B. *J. Biol. Chem. 240*:2729, 1965.
37. Chance, B. In: *Control of Energy Metabolism,* Academic Press, New York, 1965, p. 415.
38. Chance, B., and Hajihara, B., *Proceedings of the 5th International Biochemical Congress* (in Russian), 1962, vol. 5, p. 10.
39. Chance, B., and Hollunger, G. *J. Biol. Chem. 238*:445, 1963.
40. Chance, B., and Hollunger, G. *J. Biol. Chem. 238*:418, 1963.
41. Chance, B., Parsons, D., Rasmussen, H., and Williamson, J. R. *Abh. Dtsch. Akad. Wiss. Berlin Kl. Med. 1966*(4):1.
42. Chance, B., and Williams, G. R. *Adv. Enzymol. 17*:65, 1956.
43. Chappell, J. B., Cohn, M., and Greville, G. D. In: *Energy-Linked Functions of Mitochondria,* Academic Press, New York, 1963, p. 219.
44. Chappell, J. B., Crofts, A. R. *Biochem. J. 95*:378, 1965.
45. Chappell, J. B., and Crofts, A. R. *Biochem. J. 95*:387, 1965.
46. Chappell, J. B., and Crofts, A. R. *Biochem. J. 95*;393, 1965.
47. Chappell, J. B., and Crofts, A. R. In: *Regulation of Metabolic Processes in Mitochondria,* Elsevier, Amsterdam/London/New York, 1966, p. 293.
48. Cockrell, R. S. *Fed. Proc. 27*:528, 1968.
49. Cockrell, R. S., Harris, E. J., and Pressman, B. C. *Nature 215*:1487, 1967.
50. Cohen, J., Felman, R. E., and Whitbeck, A. A. *Am. J. Physiol. 216*:76, 1969.
51. Cutting, W. S., and Tainter, M. L. *Proc. Soc. Exp. Biol. Med. 31*:97, 1933–34.
52. Dallam, R. D., and Howard, R. B. *Biochim. Biophys. Acta 37*:188, 1960.
53. Devlin, T. M. *J. Biol. Chem. 234*:962, 1959.
54. Dow, D. S. *J. Bioenerg. 1*:423, 1970.
55. Dutoit, C. H. In: *Phosphorus Metabolism, 1*:597, 1951.
56. Ernster, L. *Fed. Proc. 24*:1222, 1965.
57. Ernster, L., and Kuylenstierna, B. In: *Mitochondrial Structure and Function,* Academic press, New York, 1969, vol. 17, p. 5.
58. Estabrook, R. W., Hommes, F., and Gonze, G. In: *Energy-Linked Functions of Mitochondria*, Academic Press, New York, 1963, p. 143.
59. Etkin, W. N., Root, R. W., and Mofskin, B. P. *Physiol. Zool. 13*:415, 1940.
60. Evlhejm, C. A. In: *Respiratory Enzymes* (Russian translation), IL, Moscow, 1952, p. 7.
61. Evtodienko, Yu. V. *The Study of the Cytochrome System of Mitochondria by Differential Spectrophotometry*. Author's abstracts of candidate's dissertation, Moscow, 1967.
62. Evtodienko, Yu. V., and Kudzina, L. Yu. In: *Mitochondria. Biochemistry and Morphology* (in Russian), Nauka, Moscow, 1967, p. 18.
63. Evtodienko, Yu. V., and Mokhova, E. N. In: *Mechanisms of Respiration, Photosynthesis, and Nitrogen Fixation* (in Russian), Nauka, Moscow, 1967, p. 35.
64. Fleischer, S., and Fleischer, B. *Methods Enzymol. 10*:406, 1967.
65. Fonnesu, A., and Severi, C. *Br. J. Exp. Pathol. 10*:35, 1951.
66. Frieden, C. *Enzymes 7*:3, 1963.
67. Gagel'gans, A. I. *Ionic Transport in Mitochondria and the Action of Thyroid Hormones.* Candidate's dissertation, Tashkent, 1970.
68. Glick, J. L., and Bronk, J. R. *Biochim. Biophys. Acta 97*:16, 1965.
69. Goh Kong-oo, and Dallam, R. D. *Am. J. Physiol. 188*:514, 1957.

70. Gol'ber, L. M., and Kandror, V. I. In: *Problems in Pathological Physiology* (in Russian), Erevan, 1966, p. 32.
71. Gol'ber, L. M., and Kandror, V. I. In: *Textbook of Pathological Physiology in Several Volumes* (in Russian), vol. 4, 1966, p. 219.
72. Gol'ber, L. M., and Kandror, V. I. *Kardiologiya 7*:53, 1967.
73. Gol'ber, L. M., and Kandror, V. I. In: *Abstracts of Proceedings of Symposia at the Second All-Union Biochemical Congress* (in Russian), Tashkent, 1969, p. 142.
74. Gol'ber, L. M., Kandror, V. I., and Dagaeva, L. N. *Patol. Fiziol. Éksp. Ter. 10*:16, 1966.
75. Gol'ber, L. M., Kandror, V. I., and Salakhova, N. S. In: *Mechanisms of Regulation of Vital Activities under Pathological Conditions. Proceedings of the 1st All-Union Congress of Pathophysiologists* (in Russian), Baku, 1970, p. 216.
76. Green, D. E., and Fleischer, S. In: *Horizons in Biochemistry* (Transl. from Russian), Mir, Moscow, 1964, p. 293.
77. Green, D. E., and Goldberger, R. *Insights into the Living Process,* Academic Press, New York, 1967.
78. Grivell, L. A., and Roodyn, D. B. *Biochem. J. 116*:26P, 1970.
79. Gross, N. Y. *J. Cell Biol. 48*:29, 1971.
80. Gruenstein, E., and Wynn, J. *Theor. Exp. Biol. 26*:343, 1970.
81. Gustafson, R., Tata, J. R., Lindberg, O., and Ernster, L. *J. Cell. Biol. 26*:555, 1965.
82. Haldar, D., Freeman, K., and Work, T. S. *Nature 211*:9, 1966.
83. Harris, E. J., Cockrell, R., and Pressman, B. C. *Biochem. J. 99*:200, 1966.
84. Haynes, R. C., Jr., Sutherland, E. W., and Rall, T. W. *Recent Prog. Horm. Res. 16*:121, 1960.
85. Heier, G., and Wollenberger, A. In: *Abstracts of the 3rd Meeting of FEBS,* Warsaw, 1967, p. 94.
86. Helft, O. M. *J. Exp. Zool. 45*:69, 1926.
87. Heninger, R. W., Mong, F. N., and Albright, E. C. *Proc. Soc. Exp. Biol. Med. 133*:110, 1970.
88. Hess, B., and Brand, K. *Biochem. Z. 338*:376, 1963.
89. Hillier, A. P. *J. Physiol. 211*:585, 1970.
90. Hoch, F. L. *Physiol. Rev. 42*:605, 1962.
91. Hoch, F. L. *Endocrinology 77*:991, 1965.
92. Hoch, F. L. *IEG No. 1 Sci. Memo*, 457, 1965.
93. Hoch, F. L. *J. Biol. Chem. 241*:524, 1966.
94. Hoch, F. L. *IEG No. 1 Sci. Memo*, 605, 1966.
95. Hoch, F. L. *Proc. Nat. Acad. Sci. 58*:506, 1967.
96. Hoch, F. L. *Arch. Biochem. Biophys. 124*:238, 1968.
97. Hoch, F. L., and Lipmann, F. *Proc. Nat. Acad. Sci. 40*:909, 1954.
98. Howland, J. L. *Biochim. Biophys. Acta 153*:309, 1968.
99. Hülsmann, W. C. *Biochem. J. 116*:32P, 1970.
100. Hunter, F. E. *Proceedings of the 5th International Biochemical Congress* (in Russian), vol. 5, Moscow, 1962, p. 301.
101. Isaacs, G. H., Sactor, B., and Murphy, T. A. *Biochim. Biophys. Acta 177*:196, 1969.
102. Jagendorf, A. T., and Uribe, E. G. *Proc. Nat. Acad. Sci. 55*:170, 1966.
103. Jones, D. H., and Boyer, P. D. *J. Biol. Chem. 244*:5767, 1969.
104. Kadenbach, B. *Biochem. Z. 344*:4, 1966.
105. Kagawa, Y., and Racker, E. *J. Biol. Chem. 246*:5477, 1971.
106. Kandror, V. I. *Probl. Endokrinol. 11*:88, 1965.
107. Kandror, V. I. In: *Molecular Bases of Disease* (in Russian), Meditsina, Moscow, 1965,
108. Kandror, V. I. *Mechanisms of Cardiovascular Disorders in Thyrotoxicosis* (*Experimental Investigation*). Doctoral dissertation, Moscow, 1968.

109. Kandror, V. I., and Shakhnarovich, V. M. *Dokl. Akad. Nauk SSSR 192*:218, 1970.
110. Kaplay, S. S., and Sanadi, D. R. *Arch. Biochem. Biophys. 144*:440, 1971.
111. Karlson, P. *Prospect. Biol. Med. 6*:203, 1963.
112. Keiser, D. L., and Yike, N. *J. Biochem. 6*:3847, 1967.
113. Kimata, S. L., and Tarjan, E. M. *Endocrinology 89*:378, 1971.
114. Klebanoff, S. J. *J. Biol. Chem. 234*:2480, 1959.
115. Kleitke, B., and Wollenberger, A. In: *Abstracts of the 5th Meeting of FEBS,* Prague, 1968, p. 83.
116. Klemperer, H. G. *Biochem. J. 60*:122, 1955.
117. Klemperer, H. G. *Biochem. J. 60*:128, 1955.
118. Klingenberg, M., and Schollmeyer, P. *Biochem. Z. 333*:335, 1960.
119. Klingenberg, M., and Schollmeyer, P. *Proceedings of the 5th International Biochemical Congress* (in Russian), vol. 5, Moscow, 1962, p. 55.
120. Kolotilova, A. I., and Rachev, R. R. In: *Chemistry in the Natural Sciences* (in Russian), Leningrad, 1965, p. 65.
121. Korner, A. *Biochem. J. 115*:30P, 1969.
122. Kotel'nikova, A. I. In: *Mechanisms of Respiration, Photosynthesis, and Nitrogen Fixation* (in Russian), Nauka, Moscow, 1967, p. 74.
123. Krause, R. L., and Sokoloff, L. *J. Biol. Chem. 242*:1431, 1967.
124. Krebs, H. A., Gascoyne, T., and Natton, B. M. *Biochem. J. 102*:275, 1967.
125. Kremer, Yu. N. *The Biochemistry of Protein Feeding* (in Russian), Zinatne, Riga, 1965.
126. Krishna, G., Hynie, S., and Brodie, B. B. *Proc. Nat. Acad. Sci. 59*:884, 1968.
127. Laber, L. J., and Black, C. C. *J. Biol. Chem. 244*:3463, 1969.
128. Lambeth, D. O., Lardy, H. A., Senior, A. E., and Brooks, J. C. *FEBS Lett. 17*:330, 1971.
129. Lardy, H. A., and Feldott, G. *Ann. N. Y. Acad. Sci. 54*:636, 1951.
130. Lardy, H. A., and Maley, J. G. *Rec. Prog. Horm. Res. 10*:129, 1954.
131. Lardy, H. A., Lee, Y. P., and Takemori, A. *Proc. N. Y. Acad. Sci. 86*:506, 1960.
132. Lardy, H. A., and Lee, Y. P. (1961), cited by: Lee, Y. P., and Hsu, H. H. T. *Endocrinology, 85*:251, 1969.
133. Läuger, P., Richter, J., and Lesslauer, W. *Ber. Bunsenges. Phys. Chem. 71*:906, 1967.
134. Le Deaut, J. Y., Ledig, M., and Mendel, P. *FEBS Lett. 20*:153, 1972.
135. Lee, N. D., and Williams, R. H. *Endocrinology 54*:5, 1954.
136. Lee, N. M., Wiedmann, I., and Kun, E. *FEBS Lett. 18*:81, 1971.
137. Lee, Y. P., and Lardy, H. A. *J. Biol. Chem. 240*:1427, 1965.
138. Lee, Y. P., Takemori, A., and Lardy, H. A. *J. Biol. Chem. 234*:3051, 1959.
139. Lehninger, A. L. *Physiol. Rev. 42*:467, 1962.
140. Lehninger, A. L. In: *Horizons in Biochemistry* (Russian translation), Mir, Moscow, 1964, p. 326.
141. Lehninger, A. L. *Ann. N. Y. Acad. Sci. 137*:700, 1966.
142. Lehninger, A. L. *The Mitochondrion. The Molecular Basis of Structure and Function* (Russian translation), Mir, Moscow, 1966.
143. Lehninger, A. L., Ray, B. L., and Schneider, M. *J. Biophys. Biochem. Cytol. 5*:97, 1959.
144. Lehninger, A., Watkins, C. L., and Remmert, F. *Regulation of Cell Metabolism* (Russian translation), IL, Moscow, 1962, p. 154.
145. LeJohn, H. B., Jackson, S. C., and Klassen, G. R. *J. Biol. Chem. 244*:5346, 1969.
146. Levey, G. S., Skelton, C. L., and Epstein, S. E. *J. Clin. Invest. 48*:2244, 1969.
147. Liberman, E. A., Mokhova, E. N., Skulachev, V. P., and Topaly, V. P. *Biofizika 13*:188. 1968.
148. Liberman, E. A., and Topaly, V. P. *Biofizika 13*:1025, 1968.
149. Liberman, E. A., Topaly, V. P., Tsofina, L. M., and Shkrob, A. M. *Biofizika 14*:56, 1969.

150. Lindberg, O., Low, H., Conover, T. E., and Ernster, L. In: *Biological Structure and Function,* Academic Press, New York, 1961, p. 3.
151. Litwack, G. In: *Actions of Hormones on Molecular Processes,* New York/London/Sydney, 1964, p. 132.
152. Loh, H. H., Volfin, P., and E. Kun, E. *Biochemistry 7*:726, 1968.
153. Lockwood, E. A., Balley, E., and Taylor, C. B. *Biochem. J. 115*:40P, 1969.
154. Loomis, W. F., and Lipmann, F. *J. Biol. Chem. 173*:807, 1948.
155. Lynn, W. S., and Brown, R. H. *Biochim. Biophys. Acta 110*:445, 1965.
156. Maley, G. F. *Am. J. Physiol. 188*:35, 1957.
157. Maley, G. F., and Lardy, H. A. *J. Biol. Chem. 215*:377, 1955.
158. Martius, C., Bielling, H., and Nitzlitzow, D. *Biochem. Z. 327*:163, 1955.
159. Martius, C., and Hess, B. *Arch. Biochem. Biophys. 33*:486, 1951.
160. Maslova, G. M., Raikhman, L. M., and Skulachev, V. P. *Usp. Sovr. Biol. 67*:400, 1969.
161. Meerson, F. Z. *The Myocardium in Hyperfunction, Hypertrophy, and Failure of the Heart* (in Russian), Meditsina, Moscow, 1965.
162. Mela, L. *Biochemistry 8*:2481, 1969.
163. Michel, R., Autissier, N., and Dumas, P. *C. R. Soc. Biol. 161*:1515, 1967.
164. Michel, R. *C. R. Soc. Biol. 161*:1887, 1967.
165. Michel, R., Michel, O., Huet, P., Huet, M., and Roche, J. *C. R. Soc. Biol. 158*:1034, 1964.
166. Michel, R., Michel, O., and Huet, P. In: *Third Meeting of FEBS, Abstracts,* Warsaw. 1966, p. 96.
167. Michel, R., Michel, O., and Raoul, B. *C. R. Acad. Sci. 267*:969, 1968.
168. Michel, R., Roche, J., Michel, O., Girard, M., and Rall, J. E. *J. Biol. Chem. 239*:3062, 1964.
169. Michel, R., Truchot, R., Tron-Loisel, H., and Quignard, A. M. *C. R. Soc. Biol. 161*:1512, 1967.
170. Mitchell, P. *Nature 191*:144, 1961.
171. Mitchell, P. *Chemoosmotic Coupling in Oxidative and Photosynthetic Phosphorylation,* Bodmin, Cornwall, 1966.
172. Mitchell, P. *Biol. Rev. 41*:455, 1966.
173. Mitchell, P. *Biochem. J. 116*:5P, 1970.
174. Mitchell, P., and Moyle, J. *Biochem. J. 104*:588, 1967.
175. Mitchell, P., and Moyle, J. *Eur. J. Biochem. 7*:471, 1969.
176. Mokhnach, V. O. *The Theoretical Basis of the Biological Action of Halogen Compounds* (in Russian), Nauka, Leningrad, 1968.
177. Murano, T., Yasuda, S., Rhee, T. I., Uenshi, T., and Ueda, J. *Chem. Abstr. 55*:19015h, 1961.
178. Niemeyer, H., Crane, R. K., Kennedy, E. P., and Lipmann, F. *Fed. Proc. 10*:229, 1951.
179. Nikkilä, E. A., and Pitkänen, E. *Acta Endocrinol. 31*:573, 1959.
180. Ogata, E., and Rasmussen, H. *Biochemistry 5*:57, 1966.
181. O'Malley, B. W. *Trans. N. Y. Acad. Sci. 31*:478, 1969.
182. Omura, T., Cammer, W., Cooper, D., Rosental, O., and Estabrook, R. W. *Abh. Dtsch. Acad. Wiss. Berl. Kl. Med., 1966*(4):25.
183. Ono, Y., Skoultchi, A., Waterson, J., and Lengyel, P. *Nature 222*:645, 1969.
184. Packer, L. *J. Biol. Chem. 235*:242, 1960.
185. Packer, L. *J. Cell Biol. 18*:487, 1963.
186. Paik, W. K., and Cohen, P. P. *J. Gen. Physiol. 43*:683, 1960.
187. Patriarca, P., and Carafoli, E. *J. Cell Physiol. 72*:29, 1969.
188. Phillips, A. H., and Langdon, R. G. *Biochim. Biophys. Acta 19*:380, 1956.
189. Pressman, B. C. *Proc. Nat. Acad. Sci. 53*:1076, 1965.

190. Primack, M. P., Buchanan, J. Z., and Tapley, D. F. *Endocrinology 87*:1355, 1970.
191. Primack, M. P., Tapley, D. F., and Buchanan, J. L. *Biochim. Biophys. Acta 244*:349, 1971.
192. Rabinowitz, M., and Swift, H. *Physiol. Rev. 50*:376, 1970.
193. Rachev, R. R. *Uncoupling of Oxidative Phosphorylation in the Mitochondria and Its Reversibility.* Author's abstract of candidate's dissertation, Leningrad, 1964.
194. Rachev, R. R. *Oxidative Phosphorylation in the Mitochondria and Thyroid Hormones.* Author's abstract of doctoral dissertation, Leningrad University, Leningrad, 1969.
195. Rachev, R. R. *The Mitochondria and the Thyroid Hormones* (in Russian), Meditsina, Leningrad, 1969.
196. Racker, E. *Bioenergetic Mechanisms* (Russian translation), Mir, Moscow, 1967.
197. Racker, E. *Umsch. Wiss. und Tech. 1969*(1):25.
198. Racker, E., and Kandrach, A. *J. Biol. Chem. 246*:7069, 1971.
199. Ramakrishna, C. K., and Sanadi, D. R. *Arch. Biochem. Biophys. 126*:722, 1968.
200. Raw, I., and da Silva, A. S. A. *IEG No. 1 Sci. Memo,* 428, 1965.
201. Reich, E., and Goldberg, I. H. *Prog. Nucleic Acid Res. Mol. Biol. 3*:184, 1964.
202. Reid, R. A., Moyle, J., and Mitchell, P. *Nature 212*:257, 1966.
203. Roche, J., Michel, R., and Huet, P. *C. R. Soc. Biol. 159*:1891, 1965.
204. Roche, J., Michel, R., and Huet, P. *C. R. Soc. Biol. 159*:1935, 1965.
205. Roche, J., Michel, R., Michel, O., and Huet, P. *Ann. Endocrinol. 26*:705, 1965.
206. Roche, J., Michel, R., and Michel, O. *C. R. Soc. Biol. 160*:64, 1966.
207. Roodyn, D. B., and Wilkie, D. *The Biogenesis of Mitochondria,* Methuen, London, 1963.
208. Rossi, E., and Azzone, G. F. *Eur. J. Biochem. 7*:418, 1969.
209. Rossi, C., Scarpa, A., and Azzone, G. F. *Biochemistry 6*:3902, 1967.
210. Ruegamer, W. R., Newman, G. H., Richert, D. A., and Westerfield, W. W. *Endocrinology 77*:707, 1965.
211. Sacktor, B., and Dick, A. R. *Science 145*:606, 1964.
212. Samoilov, P. M. *Vopr. Med. Khim. 11*:3, 1965.
213. Schäfer, G., and Nägel, L. *Biochim. Biophys. Acta 162*:617, 1968.
214. Schreiber, S. S., Oratz, M., and Rothschild, M. A. *Am. J. Physiol. 213*:1552, 1967.
215. Scott, A., and Hunter, E. F., Jr. *J. Biol. Chem. 241.*:1060, 1966.
216. Senior, A. E., and Brooks, J. C. *FEBS Lett. 17*:327, 1971.
217. Severin, S. E., and Yang Fu-yü *Biokhimiya 25*:855, 1960.
218. Severin, S. E., and Samoilov, P. N. In: *Abstracts of Proceedings of the 1st All-Union Biochemical Congress* (in Russian), No. 1, 1963, p. 184.
219. Shambaugh, G. E., Balinsky, J. B., and Cohen, P. P. *J. Biol. Chem. 244* :5295, 1969.
220. Shafar, A. A. *A Study of the Mechanism of Action of Uncouplers of Oxidative Phosphorylation.* Author's abstract of candidate's dissertation, Moscow, 1968.
221. Shimada, H. *Sci. Pap. Coll. Gen. Educ. Univ. Tokyo 13*:231, 1963.
222. Short, S. H., and Riegamer, W. R. *Endocrinology 79*:90, 1966.
223. Simpson, E. R., and Estabrook, R. W. *Arch. Biochem. Biophys. 126*:977, 1968.
224. Skulachev, V. P. *The Relationship between Oxidation and Phosphorylation in the Respiratory Chain* (in Russian), Izd. AN SSSR, Moscow, 1962.
225. Skulachev, V. P. In: *Mitochondria. Biochemistry and Morphology* (in Russian), Nauka, Moscow, 1967, p. 119.
226. Skulachev, V. P. In: *Mechanisms of Respiration, Photosynthesis, and Nitrogen Fixation* (in Russian), Nauka, Moscow, 1967, p. 7.
227. Skulachev, V. P. *Usp. Sovr. Biol. 65*:152, 1968.
228. Skulachev, V. P. *The Accumulation of Energy in the Cell* (in Russian), Nauka, Moscow, 1969.
229. Skulachev, V. P. *Curr. Top. Bioenerg. 4*:127, 1971.

230. Skulachev, V. P. *The Transformation of Energy in Biological Membranes* (in Russian), Nauka, Moscow, 1972.
231. Slater, E. S. *Proceedings of the 5th International Biochemical Congress* (in Russian), vol. 5, Moscow, 1962, p. 343.
232. Slater, E. C., and Hülsmann, W. C. In: *Ciba Found. Symp. Regulation Cell Metabolism,* Boston, 1959, p. 58.
233. Smith, D. C., and Ewerett, G. M. (1943), cited by Prosser and Brown, 1967.
234. Smith, R. E. *Fed. Proc. 19*:146, 1960.
235. Smuckler, E. A., and Tata, J. R. *Nature 234*:33, 1971.
236. Sobel, B. E., Dempsey, P. J., and Cooper, T. *Proc. Soc. Exp. Biol. Med. 132*:6, 1969.
237. Sokoloff, L. In: *Regulatory Mechanisms for Protein Synthesis in Mammalian Cells,* Academic Press, New York, 1968, p. 345.
238. Sokoloff, L., Campbell, P. L., Francis, C. M., and Klee, C. B. *Biochim. Biophys. Acta 76*:329, 1963.
239. Sokoloff, L., Francis, C. M., and Campbell, P. L. *Proc. Nat. Acad. Sci. 52*:728, 1964.
240. Sokoloff, L., and Kaufman, S. *Science 129*:569, 1959.
241. Sokoloff, L., and Kaufman, S. *J. Biol. Chem. 236*:795, 1961.
242. Sokoloff, L., Kaufman, S., Campbell, P. L., Francis, C. M., and Gelboin, N. V. *J. Biol. Chem. 238*:1432, 1963.
243. Stein, A. M., Kaplan, N. O., and Clotti, M. M. *J. Biol. Chem. 234*:979, 1959.
244. Tabachnick, M. *J. Biol. Chem. 242*:1646, 1967.
245. Tapley, D. F., and Basso, N. *Biochim. Biophys. Acta 36*:486, 1959.
246. Tapley, D. F., and Cooper, C. *J. Biol. Chem. 222*:341, 1956.
247. Tarjan, E. M., and Kimata, S. I. *Endocrinology 78*:385, 1971.
248. Tata, J. R. In: *Action of Hormones on Molecular Process,* Wiley, New York, 1964, p. 58.
249. Tata, J. R. *Biochem. J. 97*:21P, 1965.
250. Tata, J. R. In: *Mechanisms of Hormone Actions* (1965), p. 173, cited by Bronk, J. R., 1966.
251. Tata, J. R. *Nature 213*:566, 1967.
252. Tata, J. R. *Acta Endocrinol. 124*:111, 1967.
253. Tata, J. R. In: *Regulatory Mechanisms for Protein Synthesis in Mammalian Cells,* Academic Press, New York, 1968, p. 299.
254. Tata, J. R. *Nature 219*:33, 1968.
255. Tata, J. R. *Biochem. J. 116*:617, 1970.
256. Tata, J. R., Ernster, L., Lindberg, O., Arrhenius, E., Pedersen, S., and Hedman, R. *Biochem. J. 86*:408, 1963.
257. Tata, J. R., and Widnell, C. C. *Biochem. J. 98*:604, 1966.
258. Tata, J. R., and Williams-Ashman, H. G. *Eur. J. Biochem. 2*;366, 1967.
259. Taxay, E. P. *Am. J. Med. Sci. 244*:191, 1962.
260. Turakulov, Ya. Kh. *The Biochemistry and Pathochemistry of the Thyroid Gland* (in Russian), Izd. AN Uzbek. SSR, Tashkent, 1963.
261. Turakulov, Ya. Kh. *Vestn. Akad. Med. Nauk SSSR 1969*(8):28.
262. Turakulov, Ya. Kh., Gagel'gans, A. I., Bekmukhametova, Z. U., and Tashmukhamedov, B. A. In: *Mitochondria. Enzymic Processes and Their Regulation* (in Russian), Nauka, Moscow, 1968, p. 79.
263. Turakulov, Ya. Kh., L'vovich, N. A., Gagel'gans, A. I., and Mirakhmedov, A. K. *Uzb. Biol. Zh. 1972*(1):3.
264. Turakulov, Ya. Kh., Mirakhmedov, A. K., L'vovich, N. A., and Khusainova, F. *Biokhimiya 35*:349, 1970.
265. Turakulov, Ya. Kh., Tashmukhamedov, B. A., and Gagel'gans, A. I. *Uzb. Biol. Zh. 1969*(4):6.

266. Turakulov, Ya. Kh., Tashmukhamedov, B. A., and Gagel'gans, A. I. In: *Mitochondria. Biochemical Functions in the System of Cell Organelles* (in Russian), Nauka, Moscow, 1969, p. 111.
267. Turakulov, Ya. Kh., Tashmukhamedov, B. A., Gagel'gans, A. I., and L'vovich, N. A. In: *Mitochondria. Structure and Function under Normal and Pathological Conditions* (in Russian), Nauka, Moscow, 1971, p. 177.
268. Turakulov, Ya. Kh., Tashmukhamedov, B. A., Gagel'gans, A. I., and Mamatkulov, Kh. M. In: *The Biophysics of Membranes* (in Russian), Moscow, 1969, p. 264.
269. Utsumi, K. *Acta Med. Okayama 18*:189, 1964.
270. Varonne, S., Consiglio, E., and Covelli, I. *Eur. J. Biochem. 13*:305, 1970.
271. Vasington, F. D., and Murphy, J. V. *J. Biol. Chem. 237*:2670, 1962.
272. Vasington, F. D. *J. Biol. Chem. 238*:1841, 1963.
273. Vinogradov, A. D., and Eftodienko, Yu. V. In: *Mitochondria, Biochemistry and Morphology* (in Russian), Nauka, Moscow, 1967, p. 5.
274. Vitale, J. J., Nakamura, M., and Hegsted, D. M. *J. Biol. Chem. 228*:573, 1957.
275. Volfin, P., Kaplay, S. S., and Sanadi, D. R. *J. Biol. Chem. 244*:5631, 1969.
276. Walter, P., Paetkau, V., and Lardy, H. A. *J. Biol. Chem. 241*:2523, 1966.
277. Warren, M. R. *J. Exp. Zool. 83*:127, 1940.
278. Weiss, W. P., Campbell, P. C., Deibler, G. E., and Sokoloff, L. *J. Pharm. Exp. Ther. 136*:366, 1962.
279. Whaley, R. A., Hart, T. M., and Klitgaard, H. M. *Am. J. Physiol. 196*:1258, 1959.
280. Wheeldok, L. W., and Lehninger, A. L. *Biochemistry 5*:3533, 1966.
281. Widnell, C. C., and Tata, J. R. *Biochem. J. 98*:621, 1966.
282. Williamson, J. R. *Biochem. J. 83*:377, 1962.
283. Wilson, D. F., Azzi, A. *Arch. Biochem. Biophys. 126*:724, 1968.
284. Wilt, F. H. *Biochem. J. 73*:13, 1959.
285. Wiswell, J. G., and Asper, S. P. *Bull. Johns Hopkins Hosp. 102*:115, 1958.
286. Wolf, G., and Rivlin, R. S. *Endocrinology 86*:1347, 1970.
287. Wolff, J. *J. Biol. Chem. 237*:230, 1962.
288. Wynn, J. *Arch. Biochem. Biophys. 126*:880, 1969.
289. Yang, S., and Criddle, R. S. *Biochem. Biophys. Res. Commun. 35*:429, 1969.
290. Yasaitis, A. A. In: *Abstracts of Proceedings of Symposia at the Second All-Union Biochemical Congress,* Fan, Tashkent, 1969, p. 233.
291. Yasaitis, A. A. *Separation and Reconstruction of Mitochondrial Systems Generating the Membrane Potential.* Author's abstract of doctoral dissertation, Moscow, 1972.

CONCLUSION

The new stage in the study of the thyroid gland which began only a little more than 30 years ago resulted from the introduction of two powerful methods of investigation—the use of the radioactive iodine isotope ^{131}I and of antithyroid compounds. These tools have lead within this comparatively short period to the elucidation of many of the unexplained problems of thyroid physiology and to the establishment of important facts in this field of endocrinology.

It must be accepted that the most important of these facts was the discovery made in 1953 simultaneously and independently by two groups of scientists—by Gross and Pitt-Rivers in England and by Roche and Michel in France—of a new iodinated thyronine in the thyroid gland and in the peripheral blood, namely, 3,5,3′-triiodothyronine, which not only had hormonal activity but was approximately five times more active than thyroxine itself. After this discovery, thyroxine could no longer be spoken of as the only hormone of the thyroid gland, as had hitherto been the case, but as one hormone of the thyroid gland.

The second important fact is the discovery and quantitative analysis of the free hormone fraction in the peripheral blood, in a state of equilibrium with the protein-bound thyroxine. The importance of this small fraction of circulating hormone is that it is the concentration of this fraction, precisely regulated through the combined participation of many factors, that determines the metabolic activity and physiological effect of thyroid function.

By the end of the 1950s all the chemical components of the thyroid gland, the principal stages in biosynthesis, the transport forms and peripheral distribution, and the pathways of intracellular conversion of the thyroid hormones had been studied reasonably fully. At that time the physiological effects of the thyroid hormones and their action on differentiation, respiration, and various aspects of the metabolism of individual organs and systems were being studied intensively. The problem of regulation of thyroid gland function was at the center of attention, the action of the thyroid-stimulating hormone of the anterior pituitary and of hypothalamic neurosecretion was being studied in detail, and the existence of a feedback mechanism between them had been established, although the chemical nature of the thyroid-stimulating hormone and the hypothalamic factors and the molecular mechanism for the control of thyroid activity were only just beginning to be worked out.

As regards the mechanism of action of the thyroid hormones, like that of other hormones, at the cellular and molecular levels there were no clear, soundly based concepts despite the profusion of facts, mainly to do with the action of thyroxine on enzyme activity, oxidative phosphorylation, and the mitochondria as a whole. This state of affairs can be explained by the level of our knowledge on the components of the cell, on their fine structure and metabolism, and on the mechanism of regulation of the biosynthesis of proteins and other macromolecules, as well as by the insufficiently refined methods available for the investigation of these structures and processes only 10 to 15 years ago.

The state of thyroid physiology and biochemistry as it was at the beginning of the 1960s was described in sufficient detail in my monograph, *The Biochemistry and Pathochemistry of the Thyroid Gland,* published in 1963.

In the last decade, research into the biochemistry of the thyroid hormones has continued to develop as intensively as ever. Attention has been concentrated on the structural organization and biosynthesis of thyroglobulin, the formation of hormonally active thyronines, and the connection between these processes and the degree of iodination of the thyroglobulin molecule. Our knowledge of the molecular mechanism of action of hypothalamic-releasing factor on the adenohypophysis and of the thyroid-stimulating hormone on the thyroid gland, on the place of the adenyl cyclase–cyclic-AMP system in the realization of the TSH effect, has widened considerably. Another and perhaps even more attractive aspect of the biochemistry of the thyroid hormones has been the investigation of the molecular mechanism of action of thyroxine and the attempt to find a link between the intracellular conversions in the structure of the hormone and its biological activity, on the one hand, and between its action on the fundamental processes of metabolism and its physiological effects, on the other hand.

Considerable progress has been made with this research, and some of the problems have been completely solved. The pathways of thyroglobulin biosynthesis have been studied in meticulous detail, but the mechanism of synthesis of thyroxine and triiodothyronine molecules still remains unexplained. The molecular interactions between the active centers of TSH and the regulatory site of the thyroid gland cell membrane and also the analogous reactions between thyrotropin-releasing factor and the specific cell of the adenohypophysis have still been incompletely elucidated.

The mechanism of action of the thyroid hormones must evidently be regarded from the standpoint of the existence of multiple points of application: A key position in the action of thyroxine on cell metabolism is occupied by the stimulation of cell respiration and of oxidative phosphorylation in the mitochondria and stimulation of the synthesis of specific proteins by activation of the genetic apparatus of the cell. This action perhaps takes place initially at the level of the mitochondria, and only later at the level of the cell nucleus. The discovery of the connection between these two centers, the cell targets for thyroid hormones, will be of the greatest importance. One of the most complex problems urgently in need of solution is how the hormonal effect is manifested in the form of the physiological function.

Some aspects of thyroid pathology are no less important. Advances in the study of the pathogenesis and treatment of the thyrotoxicoses, hypothyroidism, and thyroiditis have indisputably been made, and endemic goiter, a serious problem only 15 to 20 years ago, has now been eradicated as a mass disease in the USSR.

The manifestations of congenital thyroid disease, with a number of clearly defined forms reflecting defects in the biosynthesis, transport, and deiodination of the tyrosines, have still received comparatively little study. These inherited forms of thyroid pathology are of theoretical rather than practical interest, for because of the eradication of endemic foci of goiter, the genetic endocrine pathology of the thyroid gland, including cretinism, is hardly ever seen. However, from the point of view of current interest in the problem of inherited diseases, the elucidation of the molecular bases of congenital biochemical defects of hormone formation and of possible cretinism is of undoubted importance. However, no new substantial contributions have appeared in this field in the last decades.

Progress so far achieved in the fields of the biosynthesis, metabolism, and mechanism of action of the thyroid hormones has thus presented the research worker with new problems. Their successful solution will evidently mark progress toward a full and deep understanding of intracellular metabolic processes and the mechanisms regulating them and of the deiodination of the thyroid hormones.

MIX
Papier aus verantwortungsvollen Quellen
Paper from responsible sources
FSC® C105338
FSC
www.fsc.org

If you have any concerns about our products,
you can contact us on
ProductSafety@springernature.com

In case Publisher is established outside the EU,
the EU authorized representative is:
Springer Nature Customer Service Center GmbH
Europaplatz 3, 69115 Heidelberg, Germany

Printed by Libri Plureos GmbH
in Hamburg, Germany